Asthma and COPD Overlap: An Update

Editors

NICOLA A. HANANIA
LOUIS-PHILIPPE BOULET

IMMUNOLOGY AND ALLERGY CLINICS OF NORTH AMERICA

https://www.immunology.theclinics.com/

August 2022 • Volume 42 • Number 3

ELSEVIER

1600 John F. Kennedy Boulevard • Suite 1800 • Philadelphia, Pennsylvania, 19103-2899
http://www.theclinics.com

IMMUNOLOGY AND ALLERGY CLINICS OF NORTH AMERICA Volume 42, Number 3

August 2022 ISSN 0889-8561, ISBN-13: 978-0-323-98773-8

Editor: Taylor Hayes
Developmental Editor: Jessica Cañaberal

Immunology and Allergy Clinics of North America (ISSN 0889–8561) is published quarterly by Elsevier Inc., 360 Park Avenue South, New York, NY 10010-1710. Months of issue are February, May, August, and November. Periodicals postage paid at New York, NY and additional mailing offices. Subscription prices are $354.00 per year for US individuals, $844.00 per year for US institutions, $100.00 per year for US students and residents, $432.00 per year for Canadian individuals, $100.00 per year for Canadian students, $861.00 per year for Canadian institutions, $456.00 per year for international individuals, $861.00 per year for international institutions, $220.00 per year for international students. To receive student/resident rate, orders must be accompanied by name of affiliated institution, date of term, and the *signature* of program/residency coordinator on institution letterhead. Orders will be billed at individual rate until proof of status is received. Foreign air speed delivery is included in all *Clinics* subscription prices. All prices are subject to change without notice. **POSTMASTER**: Send address changes to *Immunology and Allergy Clinics of North America,* Elsevier Health Sciences Division, Subscription Customer Service, 3251 Riverport Lane, Maryland Heights, MO 63043. **Customer Service: 1-800-654-2452 (U.S. and Canada); 314-447-8871 (outside U.S. and Canada). Fax: 314-447-8029. E-mail: journalscustomerservice-usa@elsevier.com (for print support); journalsonlinesupport-usa@elsevier.com (for online support).**

Reprints. For copies of 100 or more, of articles in this publication, please contact the Commercial Reprints Department, Elsevier Inc., 360 Park Avenue South, New York, New York 10010-1710. Tel. 212-633-3874, Fax: 212-633-3820, E-mail: reprints@elsevier.com.

Immunology and Allergy Clinics of North America is covered in MEDLINE/PubMed (Index Medicus), Current Contents/Life Sciences, Science Citation Index, ISI/BIOMED, Chemical Abstracts, and EMBASE/Excerpta Medica.

Contributors

EDITORS

NICOLA A. HANANIA, MD, MS
Professor of Medicine, Section of Pulmonary, Critical Care Medicine, Baylor College of Medicine, Houston, Texas, USA

LOUIS-PHILIPPE BOULET, MD, FRCPC
Professor of Medicine, Québec Heart and Lung Institute, Université Laval, Québec, Canada

AUTHORS

MUHAMMAD ADRISH, MD, MBA
Associate Professor, Section of Pulmonary, Critical Care and Sleep Medicine, Department of Medicine, Baylor College of Medicine, Ben Taub Hospital, Houston, Texas, USA

MAHESH P. ANAND, MBBS
Department of Respiratory Medicine, JSS Medical College, JSSAHER, Mysore, Karnataka, India

JONATHAN A. BERNSTEIN, MD
Division of Immunology, Allergy and Rheumatology, Department of Internal Medicine, College of Medicine, University of Cincinnati, Cincinnati, Ohio, USA

LOUIS-PHILIPPE BOULET, MD, FRCPC
Professor of Medicine, Québec Heart and Lung Institute, Université Laval, Québec, Canada

CHRIS E. BRIGHTLING, PhD
Professor, Department of Respiratory Sciences, Leicester NIHR BRC, Institute for Lung Health, University of Leicester, Leicester, United Kingdom

MARIO CAZZOLA, MD
Unit of Respiratory Medicine, Department of Experimental Medicine, University of Rome "Tor Vergata", Rome, Italy

KIAN FAN CHUNG, MD, DSc, FRCP
Professor of Respiratory Medicine, National Heart and Lung Institute, Imperial College London and Royal Brompton and Harefield NHS Trust, London, United Kingdom

SARAH DIVER, PhD
Department of Respiratory Sciences, Leicester NIHR BRC, Institute for Lung Health, University of Leicester, Leicester, United Kingdom

ANNE L. FUHLBRIGGE, MD, MS
Associate Professor, Pulmonary Sciences and Critical Care Medicine, Department of Medicine, Senior Associate Dean for Clinical Affairs, University of Colorado School of Medicine, Aurora, Colorado, USA

PETER G. GIBSON, DMed, FRACP, FERS, F Thor Soc, FAPSR, FAHMS
Professor, Department of Respiratory and Sleep Medicine, John Hunter Hospital, Priority
Research Centre for Healthy Lungs, The University of Newcastle, Newcastle, New South
Wales, Australia

KRYSTELLE GODBOUT, MD, FRCPC
Quebec Heart and Lung Institute, Université Laval, Québec, Canada

NEIL J. GREENING, PhD
Department of Respiratory Sciences, Leicester NIHR BRC, Institute for Lung Health,
University of Leicester, Leicester, United Kingdom

NICOLA A. HANANIA, MD, MS
Professor of Medicine, Section of Pulmonary, Critical Care Medicine, Baylor College of
Medicine, Houston, Texas, USA

CRAIG P. HERSH, MD, MPH
Channing Division of Network Medicine, Harvard Medical School, Division of Pulmonary
and Critical Care Medicine, Brigham and Women's Hospital, Boston, Massachusetts, USA

FERNANDO HOLGUIN, MD, MPH
Division of Pulmonary Sciences and Critical Care Medicine, University of Colorado
Anschutz Medical Campus, Aurora, Colorado, USA

KEWU HUANG, MD
Professor of Medicine, Department of Pulmonary and Critical Care Medicine, Beijing
Chao-Yang Hospital, Capital Medical University, Beijing Institute of Respiratory Medicine,
Beijing, China

ANDI HUDLER, MD
Division of Pulmonary Sciences and Critical Care Medicine, University of Colorado
Anschutz Medical Campus, Aurora, Colorado, USA

CHARLES G. IRVIN, PhD
Professor of Medicine, Physiology and Biophysics, Pulmonary and Critical Care
Medicine, University of Vermont Larner College of Medicine, Burlington, Vermont, USA

DAVID A. KAMINSKY, MD
Professor of Medicine, Pulmonary and Critical Care Medicine, University of Vermont
Larner College of Medicine, Burlington, Vermont, USA

MIRANDA KIRBY, PhD
Department of Physics, Ryerson University, Institute for Biomedical Engineering, Science and
Technology (iBEST), St. Michael's Hospital, Unity Health Toronto, Toronto, Ontario, Canada

MARIA GABRIELLA MATERA, MD, PhD
Unit of Pharmacology, Department of Experimental Medicine, University of Campania
"Luigi Vanvitelli", Naples, Italy

MARC MIRAVITLLES, MD
Pneumology Department, Hospital Universitari Vall d'Hebron/Vall d'Hebron Research
Institute (VHIR), Vall d'Hebron Barcelona Hospital Campus, Barcelona, Spain

PAOLA ROGLIANI, MD
Unit of Respiratory Medicine, Department of Experimental Medicine, University of Rome
"Tor Vergata", Rome, Italy

AABIDA SAFERALI, PhD
Channing Division of Network Medicine, Brigham and Women's Hospital, Harvard Medical School, Boston, Massachusetts, USA

KASEY M. SHAO
Department of Molecular Biology, Princeton University, Princeton, NJ, USA

SUNITA SHARMA, MD, MPH
Division of Pulmonary Sciences and Critical Care Medicine, University of Colorado Anschutz Medical Campus, Aurora, Colorado, USA

SARAH SVENNINGSEN, PhD
Department of Medicine, Division of Respirology, McMaster University, Firestone Institute for Respiratory Health, Imaging Research Centre, St. Joseph's Healthcare Hamilton, Hamilton, Canada

NEIL C. THOMSON, MD, FRCP
Professor, Institute of Infection, Immunity & Inflammation, University of Glasgow, Glasgow, United Kingdom

Contents

Asthma and chronic obstructive pulmonary disease (COPD) are common diseases that often overlap. The term asthma-COPD overlap (ACO) has been used to define this entity but there remain several speculations on its exact definition, impact, pathophysiology, and clinical features. Patients with ACO have greater morbidity than those with asthma or COPD alone, but the information on the best therapeutic approach to this group of patients is still limited. Current treatment recommendations rely on expert opinions, roundtable discussions, and strategy documents. It is prudent to examine existing knowledge about ACO and determine the path for future research.

Much interest has been given to the asthma–chronic obstructive pulmonary disease (COPD) overlap (ACO) recently, but the condition is still ill defined. There is general agreement that a patient with long-standing asthma who develops fixed airflow obstruction after years of smoking has ACO, although defining asthma in the face of COPD can be challenging. Many features of asthma are found in patients with COPD without indicating an overlap, and no consensus exists on characteristics to include in the definition of ACO. Guidance has been issued to help clinicians and researchers make a diagnosis of ACO; these are reviewed here.

Asthma-chronic obstructive pulmonary disease (COPD) overlap (ACO) is a condition in which a person has clinical and biological features of both asthma and COPD. The pathophysiology behind the development of ACO is complex, with various inflammatory cells, cytokines, environmental factors, and architectural changes within the airways, all affecting a patient's clinical manifestation. A better understanding of the pathophysiologic mechanisms resulting in the development of ACO will help us to better identify potential drug targets and improve symptom burden and overall quality of life for patients living with ACO.

Asthma COPD Overlap has consistently reported to be associated with an increase burden of disease but the impact on lung function decline and mortality varies by study. The prevalence increases with age but the relationship with gender also varies with the study population. The variability in the prevalence and clinical characteristics of ACO is linked to differences in how chronic obstructive pulmonary disease (COPD) and asthma are defined, including diagnostic criteria (spirometry-based vs. clinical or symptom-based diagnoses vs. claims data), the population studied, the geographic region and environment and a consensus approach to the diagnosis of ACO is needed to allow meaningful and consistent epidemiologic information to be generated about this condition.

The diagnosis of asthma–chronic obstructive pulmonary disease (COPD) overlap (ACO) is considered when a patient presents features of both asthma and COPD, usually including a component of irreversible airway obstruction (IRAO). However, some patients with asthma, particularly smokers, may have various features typical of COPD in the absence of such component of IRAO. Features of early COPD can be found at a young age in such patients even with normal spirometry. More longitudinal studies should be conducted to determine steps needed to improve clinical outcomes of these patients including the early recognition of these changes and the application of preventative/therapeutic interventions.

Genome-wide association studies (GWAS) of asthma and chronic obstructive pulmonary disease (COPD) with ever-increasing sample sizes have found multiple genetic loci associated with either disease. However, there are few intersecting loci between asthma and COPD. GWAS specifically focused on asthma–COPD overlap (ACO) have been limited by smaller sample sizes and the lack of a consistent definition of ACO that has also hampered clinical and epidemiologic studies. Other genomic techniques, such as gene expression profiling, are feasible with smaller sample sizes. Genetic analyses of objective measures of airway reactivity and allergy/T2 biomarkers in COPD studies may be another strategy to overcome limitations in ACO definitions.

Asthma and chronic obstructive pulmonary disease (COPD) are both characterized by airway obstruction and share similar clinical manifestations. However, they differ in many respects related to underlying cause, mechanism of airway obstruction, pattern and progression of symptoms, and response to therapy. It remains unclear whether there is a unique physiologic phenotype that characterizes asthma-COPD overlap (ACO). This review describes the common and distinct physiologic tests that help define asthma and COPD and potentially how they may contribute to understanding the underlying physiology of ACO.

Asthma and chronic obstructive pulmonary disease (COPD) are 2 distinct diseases with different clinical presentations. Chronic inflammation and airway obstruction are key features of asthma and COPD. Increased morbidity and mortality rates seem to be an important characteristic associated with asthma-COPD overlap (ACO).Atopy is an important clinical characteristic of patients categorized as ACO. Herein, the authors review the recent advancements in basic research, clinical assessment, and defining characteristics of ACO and the role for allergy as well as highlight future potential for disease-specific therapeutics for this asthma subtype.

The purpose of this article is to review the imaging features in patients defined by researchers as having asthma-chronic obstructive pulmonary disease (COPD) overlap (ACO), highlight the existing imaging studies investigating patients with ACO when compared with those with asthma and COPD alone, and, finally, discuss some remaining gaps in the understanding of ACO that imaging may help resolve.

Exposure to cigarette smoke has a key role in the development, adverse health outcomes, and impaired response to some therapies among individuals with features of asthma and chronic obstructive pulmonary disease overlap (ACO). To aid the identification of clinical subtypes, the description of ever smokers with features of asthma and COPD should include data on smoking status, cumulative smoking history, and the phenotype of asthma and smoking-related chronic airway disease. Pathogenic mechanisms in smoking-related ACO involve poorly understood, complex interactions between smoking-induced and asthma-induced airway inflammation, corticosteroid insensitivity, and tissue remodeling. Evidence for the clinical effectiveness of interventions for adults with smoking-related ACO is limited. Management currently involves the identification and targeting of treatable traits such as current smoking, type 2 high eosinophilic inflammation, symptomatic airflow obstruction, and extrapulmonary comorbidities.

Although asthma and chronic obstructive pulmonary disease (COPD) are considered as 2 distinct airway disorders, asthma-COPD overlap (ACO) includes those with features of both asthma and COPD. ACO is distinguished by having more frequent exacerbations and being associated with higher medical costs. Several objective labels or biomarkers have been identified and recommended for diagnosing and guiding the management of ACO. This article reviews the recent advances in clinical assessment of and the utility of biomarkers in ACO, as well as highlights a treatable trait approach to identify and manage these chronic airway diseases.

Asthma and chronic obstructive pulmonary disease are considered unique diseases with distinct characteristics. Asthma–chronic obstructive pulmonary disease overlap is a disorder in which the clinical characteristics of asthma and chronic obstructive pulmonary disease coexist. Asthma–chronic obstructive pulmonary disease overlap is a heterogenous condition; patients can have varied clinical presentations. There are significant gender variations among different phenotypes overlap. Age of symptom onset is another important consideration. Severity of symptoms, spirometry findings, smoking history, and type of airway inflammation varies between the different phenotypes. Understanding disease pathophysiology and establishing phenotypic models will improve a precision approach.

The best therapeutic approach to patients with asthma-chronic obstructive pulmonary disease overlap (ACO) is unknown. Current treatment recommendations rely on expert opinions, roundtable discussions, and strategy documents, because patients with ACO have been excluded from most clinical studies in asthma and COPD. Because of the underlying asthma initial therapy, early use of inhaled corticosteroids along with a long-acting bronchodilator is recommended. If maintenance inhaler therapy is not effective, advanced therapies based on phenotyping and identification of treatable traits may be considered.

The term asthma-chronic obstructive pulmonary disease (COPD) overlap applies where there are features of asthma and COPD. Agents targeting eosinophilic inflammation have transformed asthma management and indicate promise across airways disease, whereas agents targeting neutrophilic inflammation have demonstrated limited efficacy. Successful treatment of airway dysbiosis, mucous hypersecretion, or airway remodeling may occur with better understanding of the impact of current agents on specific clinical end points or through novel approaches. Biomarkers indicating specific disease mechanisms are key to select appropriate populations for clinical trials and identify subgroups likely to benefit from targeted treatments.

If there is a need to consider the possible overlapping of features of asthma and chronic obstructive pulmonary disease (COPD) in the same patient as a clinical condition that deserves specific attention, an acceptable definition for it must be found. The identification of specific biomarkers using multi-omics platforms, may help in differentiating ACO from asthma and COPD and in choosing the right treatment. It is likely that an approach based on treatable traits and additional knowledge about the mechanisms underlying these treatable traits will be the solution to the problem.

IMMUNOLOGY AND ALLERGY CLINICS OF NORTH AMERICA

SERIES OF RELATED INTEREST

Medical Clinics
https://www.medical.theclinics.com/

THE CLINICS ARE AVAILABLE ONLINE!
Access your subscription at:
www.theclinics.com

Preface

Asthma–Chronic Obstructive Pulmonary Disease: An Update

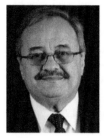 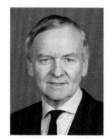

Nicola A. Hanania,
MD, MS

Louis-Philippe Boulet,
MD, FRCPC

Editors

Asthma and chronic obstructive pulmonary disease (COPD) are common airway diseases that often have overlapping clinical presentation, which may cause a major challenge for the health care providers. This overlap, although recognized for many years, has been called Asthma COPD Overlap (ACO). There is no consensus on the exact definition of ACO, although several epidemiologic studies suggest that its presence is associated with worse clinical outcomes than asthma or COPD. In the following series, our invited authors detail the various features associated with ACO, focusing on current knowledge and outlining future needs. The various articles discuss the definition, pathophysiology, and epidemiology of this entity. Other articles of this series deal with the development of early signs of COPD in asthmatic subjects, as well as the genetic determinants in addition to physiological changes and imaging features observed in patients with ACO. As most ACO patients have a significant history of smoking, the role of smoking in airway/lung changes is discussed. In other articles, the authors discuss the use of biomarkers and phenotyping of ACO subsets and provide an overview of pharmacologic and nonpharmacologic treatments of ACO. In addition, the

Immunol Allergy Clin N Am 42 (2022) xiii–xiv
https://doi.org/10.1016/j.iac.2022.04.010
0889-8561/22/© 2022 Published by Elsevier Inc.

potential new therapeutic targets and unmet needs to improve management of this condition are discussed.

Nicola A. Hanania, MD, MS
Section of Pulmonary and Critical Care Medicine
Baylor College of Medicine
1504 Taub Loop, Houston, TX 77030, USA

Louis-Philippe Boulet, MD, FRCPC
Centre de Pneumologie
Institut de Cardiologie et de Pneumologie de Québec
Université Laval
2725 Chemin Sainte-Foy
Québec, Canada G1V4G5

E-mail addresses:
hanania@bcm.edu (N.A. Hanania)
lpboulet@med.ulaval.ca (L.-P. Boulet)

When Asthma and Chronic Obstructive Pulmonary Disease Overlap; Current Knowledge and Unmet Needs

Louis-Philippe Boulet, MD, FRCPC[a], Nicola A. Hanania, MD, MS[b],*

KEYWORDS

- Asthma-COPD Overlap • Treatment • Obstructive airway disease • Phenotypes

KEY POINTS

- There is no consensus on the exact definition of asthma-chronic obstructive pulmonary disease (COPD) overlap (ACO).
- The molecular and pathophysiologic mechanisms of ACO result from the interaction of pathophysiological mechanisms typical seen in asthma and COPD.
- Epidemiologic studies suggest that the clinical impact of ACO is worse than that of asthma or COPD.
- Predisposing genetic risk factors have been observed both for asthma and COPD and they can co-occur in patients with ACO.
- Recent studies examined structural changes in ACO, using various imaging techniques such as computed tomography lung density measurement.
- ACO has multiple phenotypes that determine management strategies and outcomes.

Asthma and chronic obstructive pulmonary disease (COPD) are 2 common diseases that have been increasingly recognized as heterogeneous, but whose features overlap quite often.[1,2] The degree and type of overlap may vary, resulting in a variety of clinical phenotypes, probably related to different underlying pathophysiological mechanisms and risk factors.

DEFINING ASTHMA-CHRONIC OBSTRUCTIVE PULMONARY DISEASE OVERLAP

The association of asthma and COPD features in a single patient has been recognized for more than 60 years.[3] More recently the term asthma-COPD overlap (ACO) began to be used to reflect this association. However, there is no consensus about its exact

[a] Québec Heart and Lung Institute, Université Laval, Québec, Canada; [b] Section of Pulmonary, Critical Care Medicine, Baylor College of Medicine, 1504 Taub Loop, Houston, TX 77030, USA
* Corresponding author.
E-mail address: hanania@bcm.edu

Immunol Allergy Clin N Am 42 (2022) 499–505
https://doi.org/10.1016/j.iac.2022.05.001
0889-8561/22/© 2022 Elsevier Inc. All rights reserved.

definition, as it is unlikely to represent a single condition but reflects multiple pheno-types and endotypes.[4] The Global Initiative for Asthma (GINA) previously suggested that ACO can be considered if a patient has features of both asthma and COPD.[4] It states that: "'Asthma-COPD overlap' and 'asthma + COPD' are terms used to collec-tively describe patients who have persistent airflow limitation together with clinical fea-tures that are consistent with both asthma and COPD. This is not a definition of a single disease entity, but a descriptive term for clinical use that includes several different clin-ical phenotypes reflecting different underlying mechanisms."

Indeed, there has been a mounting controversy about the usefulness of naming obstructive airway diseases as asthma and COPD, and instead there has been a sug-gestion of simply defining these conditions in a given individual according to its spe-cific clinical characteristics or "treatable traits."[5,6] Although this may represent a "simplistic" way to the approach of these diseases, it is strongly believed that it is important for clinicians to be able distinguish between asthma, COPD, and overlap to enable a more precise approach to their respective treatment.[4]

MOLECULAR AND PATHOPHYSIOLOGICAL MECHANISMS OF ASTHMA-CHRONIC OBSTRUCTIVE PULMONARY DISEASE OVERLAP

The clinical and physiologic changes observed in ACO seem to result from the inter-action of pathophysiological mechanisms typically seen in asthma and COPD. ACO may be indeed particularly considered as a subset of airway diseases demonstrating overlapping characteristics of immune responses of patients with asthma and COPD. Therefore, understanding the pathophysiology of ACO requires a closer look at that of asthma and COPD. Airways or blood eosinophils are considered the key inflammatory cells in the pathophysiology of asthma, although they may also play an important role in the pathophysiology of 30% to 40% of patients with "classic" COPD.[7] In most pa-tients with COPD, airway inflammation is driven by non–type 2 mechanism and is char-acterized as neutrophilic. A cluster analysis of airway diseases based on cytokine profile demonstrated 3 specific clusters: (1) asthma predominant with a high type 2 cytokine profile and eosinophilia, (2) asthma and COPD predominant with mixed eosinophilia, and (3) neutrophilia.[8] In addition to the inflammatory features, some pa-tients with ACO may show evidence of airway and lung parenchyma structural changes similar to that seen in chronic asthma and COPD, but this remains to be confirmed in well-characterized subsets of ACO.[9] The pathophysiological conse-quences of ACO, particularly in smokers or ex-smokers, may therefore be related to the combined effect of parenchymal and airway changes resulting from inflammatory pathways and proteolytic cascade, in addition to airway changes/remodeling, both contributing to the development of a fixed component of airway narrowing.

EPIDEMIOLOGY OF ASTHMA-CHRONIC OBSTRUCTIVE PULMONARY DISEASE OVERLAP

Epidemiologic studies suggested that ACO is a common problem with a major impact on the patient and health care system, the fact that emphasizes the need for accurate recognition of this overlap to offer appropriate management.[10,11] There are, however, wide variations in its reported prevalence rates, from about 10% to more than 50% of patients with airway diseases, probably due to the various definitions used in such re-ports.[12,13] Furthermore, patients with ACO have greater burden of the disease, poorer outcomes and quality of life, and have increased health care use, compared with pa-tients with only asthma or COPD.[14,15] The risk factors of ACO include those associated to these 2 diseases, predominant ones being long-standing asthma, family history of asthma, atopy, and cigarette smoke exposure.[16]

EARLY FEATURES OF CHRONIC OBSTRUCTIVE PULMONARY DISEASE IN SMOKERS WITH ASTHMA

A fixed component of airway obstruction may arise in patients with early onset asthma, particularly if severe. However, in many instances, exposure to tobacco smoke or to other airway environmental pollutants may contribute to the development of such permanent airway obstructive component.[17,18]

Studies of early features of COPD in smokers with asthma not only allow us to understand the development of ACO but also open the door to possible preventative measures in this group, particularly in regard to smoking cessation. Indeed, even in young patients with asthma who smoke, we could observe physiologic alterations typically seen in early COPD.[19] We found, however, that smoking-associated ACO resulted in a more severe phenotype compared with patients with asthma with a similar degree of airway obstruction.[20] Thomson and colleagues reported that even if they had normal spirometry values, smokers with asthma had more respiratory symptoms, worse quality of life, increased frequency of exacerbations, reduced lung function, and more comorbidities than never-smokers with asthma or healthy never-smokers.[21] Comparisons between smokers and nonsmokers patients with asthma with a fixed airway obstruction can also help us understand the mechanisms associated with the development of COPD features in these subsets of patients with asthma.

GENETIC DETERMINANTS OF OBSTRUCTIVE AIRWAY DISEASES

Predisposing genetic risk factors have been observed both for asthma and COPD, and they can co-occur in patients with ACO.[8,22] Furthermore, genetic variations found in both diseases have been observed in a given individual.[8,23] Genome-wide association studies have provided valuable information on genetic variants in patients with the various airway obstructive diseases but more studies remain to be done to complete the whole picture in regard to the genetic makeup leading to COPD, asthma, and ACO.

LUNG PHYSIOLOGY IN ASTHMA-CHRONIC OBSTRUCTIVE PULMONARY DISEASE OVERLAP

Although the main physiologic characteristic of asthma is variable and reversible airflow limitation, whereas that for COPD is fixed or persistent airflow limitation, these are not mutually exclusive and may be found in both conditions.[24,25] Indeed, patients with ACO usually have a reduced FEV_1 but usually respond to bronchodilators and some may show airway hyperresponsiveness. The loss of lung function leading to persistent airway obstruction seems to result from the mixed processes involved, but more studies should explore these long-term changes in various subtypes of ACO.

IMAGING IN ASTHMA-CHRONIC OBSTRUCTIVE PULMONARY DISEASE OVERLAP

Recent studies looked at structural changes in ACO, using various imaging techniques such as computed tomography lung density measurement. It was shown that even when patients with ACO and those with COPD have a comparable smoking history and fixed airflow limitation, they have different physiologic and morphologic features of the airways.[26] We also showed that for patients with a history of asthma and persistent airway obstruction, bronchial structural changes were relatively similar in smoking and nonsmoking patients, although emphysematous changes were more predominant in smokers.[27] In that study, there was a correlation between airway neutrophilia and emphysematous features in smokers and between eosinophilia and both airway wall thickness and emphysematous changes in nonsmokers. More work remains to be done to improve assessment of structural changes over time in these patients using innovative imaging techniques.

THE ROLE OF ALLERGY AND ENVIRONMENTAL EXPOSURES IN ASTHMA AND CHRONIC OBSTRUCTIVE PULMONARY DISEASE OVERLAP

Allergen exposure in sensitized subjects can contribute to the development and clinical expression of asthma.[28] In ACO, allergy can play a similar role, although whether it is environmental, domestic, or occupational needs more exploration. Air pollution can also contribute to airways diseases and may affect the prevalence of ACO.[29]

THE ROLE OF SMOKING IN ASTHMA-CHRONIC OBSTRUCTIVE PULMONARY DISEASE OVERLAP

As mentioned previously, smoking is a major risk factor of ACO. Tobacco smoking is a risk factor for the development of COPD and may also contribute to the development and course of asthma in some individuals, even from secondary exposure.[30,31] Furthermore, smokers with asthma have more smoking-associated comorbidities that may influence the overall clinical features of ACO in addition to be associated with a worse clinical prognosis than in lifetime nonsmokers.[31,32]

CLINICAL ASSESSMENT AND UTILITY OF BIOMARKERS IN ASTHMA-CHRONIC OBSTRUCTIVE PULMONARY DISEASE OVERLAP

Clinical history and physical examination are essential to characterize obstructive airway diseases and exclude confounding or comorbid conditions. Variability of symptoms, exposure to risk factors, and other characteristics may suggest a predominant component of asthma or COPD.

Although we are limited in the number and types of biomarkers available to better characterize asthma and COPD, there is some progress in this field of research, fostered by the search for better markers to evaluate the potential efficacy of biologics. Currently, eosinophils have been considered a marker of better response to corticosteroids, both in asthma and COPD, and it should be so by extrapolation in ACO.[33,34] Blood and airway eosinophils, fractional exhaled nitric oxide, and serum immunoglobulin E are currently used for monitoring and predicting response to some biologics that may be useful in severe asthma. In this regard, using current biomarkers, agents such as omalizumab and mepolizumab have been shown to be useful in some subsets of patients with ACO.[35,36] The role of novel biomarkers, including metabolomics in the characterization of ACO, remain to be explored.[37,38]

PHENOTYPES OF ASTHMA-CHRONIC OBSTRUCTIVE PULMONARY DISEASE OVERLAP (INCLUDING AGE AND GENDER DIFFERENCES)

As we already mentioned, ACO encompasses a variety of phenotypes and endotypes. Many factors can influence these, including age, gender, race, and ethnicity.[39–43] However, we still need to know more about the various phenotypes of ACO, the mechanisms of development of chronic airflow limitation, their inflammatory features, clinical and physiologic characteristics, and outcomes. Further, additional research is needed to determine the optimal clinical assessment and management of overlap in addition to the consequences and outcomes of its various phenotypes.

Pharmacologic Management Strategies of Asthma-Chronic Obstructive Pulmonary Disease Overlap

Therapies for ACO share some similarities to those for asthma and COPD but the optimal strategies may vary from a patient to another. There have been, however, few studies looking at the best use of current drugs in ACO, as these patients are often be excluded from clinical trials. Current guidelines on asthma and COPD may, however, help us in this regard.[43] As suggested in the GINA report, when an asthmatic component is suspected in a patient with signs of COPD, an inhaled corticosteroid is essential to include in the treatment, whereas in "pure" COPD, long-acting bronchodilators should be the basis of treatment.[4]

Nonpharmacologic Treatments of Asthma-Chronic Obstructive Pulmonary Disease Overlap and Rehabilitation Programs

Smoking cessation, environmental control, weight loss in obese subjects, exercise, and rehabilitation programs can be useful in patients with ACO; this can be concluded mainly from indirect evidence; however, more studies are required to establish the benefits of these treatment in ACO.

Novel Targets for Therapy for Asthma-Chronic Obstructive Pulmonary Disease Overlap

Some biological agents used for severe asthma such as omalizumab and mepolizumab have been shown in some studies to be beneficial in patients with severe ACO with allergic or T2 inflammation.[35,36,44] Most of these agents may also contribute to reduce the use of oral corticosteroids in patients with severe disease. However, there is an unmet need to identify novel agents to treat patients with ACO with non-T2 inflammation.

SUMMARY

The present issue of *Immunology & Allergy Clinics* will provide an update on the aforementioned considerations about ACO. It will not only report current knowledge on ACO but also address the various controversies and care gaps related to this association and describe future needs.

REFERENCES

1. Boulet LP, Hanania NA. The many faces of asthma-chronic obstructive pulmonary disease overlap. Review. Curr Opin Pulm Med 2019;25:1–10.
2. Postma DS, Rabe KF. The Asthma-COPD Overlap Syndrome. N Engl J Med 2015; 373:1241–9.
3. American Thoracic Society. Standards for the diagnosis and care of patients with chronic obstructive pulmonary disease. Am J Respir Crit Care Med 1995;152: S77–121.
4. Global Initiative for Asthma (GINA). 2021. Available at: www.ginasthma.org.
5. Pavord ID, Beasley R, Agusti A, et al. After asthma: redefining airways diseases. Lancet 2018;391:350–400.
6. Agusti A, Bel E, Thomas M, et al. Treatable traits: toward precision medicine of chronic airway diseases. Eur Respir J 2016;47:410–9.
7. Singh D, Kolsum U, Brightling CE, et al. Eosinophilic inflammation in COPD: prevalence and clinical characteristics. Eur Respir J 2014;44:1697–700.

8. Ghebre MA, Bafadhel M, Desai D, et al. Biological clustering supports both "Dutch" and "British" hypotheses of asthma and chronic obstructive pulmonary disease. J Allergy Clin Immunol 2015;135:63–72.

9. Leung JM, Sin DD. Asthma-COPD overlap syndrome: pathogenesis, clinical feature, and therapeutic targets. BMJ 2017;358:j3772.

10. Inoue H, Nagase T, Morita S, et al. Prevalence and characteristics of asthma-COPD overlap syndrome identified by a stepwise approach. Int J Chron Obstruct Pulmon Dis 2017;12:1803–10.

11. Krishnan JA, Nibber A, Chisholm A, et al. Prevalence and characteristics of Asthma-Chronic Obstructive Pulmonary Disease Overlap in routine primary care practices. Ann Am Thorac Soc 2019;16:1143–50.

12. Ekerljung L, Mincheva R, Hagstad S, et al. Prevalence, clinical characteristics, and morbidity of the asthma-COPD overlap in a general population sample. J Asthma 2018;55:461–9.

13. Mendy A, Forno E, Niyonsenga T, et al. Prevalence and features of asthma-COPD overlap in the United States. Clin Respir J 2018;12:2369–77.

14. Kauppi P, Kupiainen H, Lindqvist A, et al. Overlap syndrome of asthma and COPD predicts low quality of life. J Asthma 2011;48:279–85.

15. Andersen H, Lampela P, Nevanlinna A, et al. High hospital burden in overlap syndrome of asthma and COPD. Clin Respir J 2013;7:342–6.

16. de Marco R, Pesce G, Marcon A, et al. The coexistence of asthma and chronic obstructive pulmonary disease (COPD): Prevalence and risk factors in young, middle-aged and elderly people from the general population. PLoS One 2013; 8:e62985.

17. ten Brinke A. Risk factors associated with irreversible airflow limitation in asthma. Curr Opin Allergy Clin Immunol 2008;8:63–9.

18. Golpe R, Perez de Llano L. Are the diagnostic criteria for asthma-COPD overlap syndrome appropriate in biomass smoke-induced chronic obstructive pulmonary disease? Arch Bronconeumol 2016;52:110.

19. Boulet LP, Lemière C, Archambault F, et al. Smoking and asthma: clinical and radiologic features, lung function, and airway inflammation. Chest 2006;129: 661–8.

20. Boulet LP, Boulay ME, Derival JL, et al. Asthma-COPD overlap phenotypes and smoking: Comparative features of asthma in smoking or non-smoking patients with an incomplete reversibility of airway obstruction. COPD 2018;15:130–8.

21. Thomson NC. Asthma and smoking-induced airway disease without spirometric COPD. Eur Respir J 2017;49:1602061.

22. Reséndiz-Hernández JM, et al. Genetic polymorphisms and their involvement in the regulation of the inflammatory response in asthma and COPD. Adv Clin Exp Med 2018;27:125–33.

23. Christenson SA, et al. Asthma-COPD overlap. Clinical relevance of genomic signatures of type 2 inflammation in chronic obstructive pulmonary disease. Am J Respir Crit Care Med 2015;191:758–66.

24. Gibson PG, Simpson JL. The overlap syndrome of asthma and COPD: What are its features and how important is it? Thorax 2009;64:728–35.

25. Hanania NA, Celli BR, Donohue JF, et al. Bronchodilator reversibility in COPD. Chest 2011;140:1055–63.

26. Karayama M, Inui N, Yasui H, et al. Suda T Physiological and morphological differences of airways between COPD and asthma-COPD overlap. Sci Rep 2019;9: 7818.

27. Boulet LP, Boulay ME, Coxson H, et al. Asthma with irreversible airway obstruction in smokers and non-smokers: links between airway inflammation and structural changes. Respiration 2020;1–11.

28. Tamaoki Jun, Izuhara Kenji. Asthma-chronic obstructive pulmonary disease overlap (ACO): an emerging entity in allergic respiratory diseases. Allergol Int 2018; 67:163–4.

29. To T, Zhu J, Larsen K, et al, Canadian Respiratory Research Network. Progression from asthma to chronic obstructive pulmonary disease. is air pollution a risk factor? Am J Respir Crit Care Med 2016;194:429–38.

30. Mannino DM, Buist AS. Global burden of COPD: risk factors, prevalence, and future trends. Lancet 2007;370(9589):765–73.

31. Polosa R, Thomson NC. Smoking and asthma: dangerous liaisons. Eur Respir J 2013;41:716–26.

32. Cerveri I, Cazzoletti L, Corsico A, et al. The impact of cigarette smoking on asthma: a population-based international cohort study. Int Arch Allergy Immunol 2012;158:175–83.

33. David B, Bafadhel M, Koenderman L, et al. Eosinophilic inflammation in COPD: from an inflammatory marker to a treatable trait. Thorax 2021;76:188–95.

34. Pavord ID, Sterk PJ, Hargreave FE, et al. Clinical applications of assessment of airway inflammation using induced sputum. Eur Respir J Suppl 2002;37:40s–3s.

35. Maltby S, Gibson PG, Powell H, et al. Omalizumab treatment response in a population with severe allergic asthma and overlapping COPD. CHEST 2017;151: 78–89.

36. Isoyama S, Ishikawa N, Hamai K, et al. Efficacy of mepolizumab in elderly patients with severe asthma and overlapping COPD in real-world settings: A retrospective observational study. Respir Investig 2021;59:478–86.

37. Izuhara K, Barnes PJ. Can We Define Asthma-COPD Overlap (ACO) by Biomarkers? J Allergy Clin Immunol Pract 2019;7:146–7.

38. Nilanjana Ghosh 1, Priyanka Choudhury 1, Elavarasan Subramani 1, Dipanjan Saha 2, Sayoni Sengupta 2, Mamata Joshi 3, Rintu Banerjee 4, Sushmita Roychowdhury 5, Parthasarathi Bhattacharyya 2, Koel Chaudhury 6 Metabolomic signatures of asthma-COPD overlap (ACO) are different from asthma and COPD. Metabolomics 2019;15:87.

39. King MJ, Hanania NA. Asthma in the elderly: current knowledge and future directions. Curr Opin Pulm Med 2010;16:55–9.

40. Han MK, Postma D, Mannino DM, et al. Gender and chronic obstructive pulmonary disease: why it matters. Am J Respir Crit Care Med 2007;176:1179–84.

41. Hanania NA, King MJ, Braman SS, et al. Asthma in the elderly: current understanding and future research needs—A report of a national Institute on Aging (NIA) workshop. J Allergy Clin Immunol 2011;128(Suppl. 3):S4–24.

42. Dunn RM, Lehman E, Chinchilli VM, et al. Impact of age and sex on response to asthma therapy. Am J Respir Crit Care Med 2015;192:551–8.

43. Reddel HK. Treatment of overlapping asthma-chronic obstructive pulmonary disease: can guidelines contribute in an evidence-free zone? J Allergy Clin Immunol 2015;136(3):546–52.

44. Bacharier LB, Mori A, Kita H. Advances in asthma, asthma-COPD overlap, and related biologics in 2018. J Allergy Clin Immunol 2019;144(4):906–19.

Defining Asthma–Chronic Obstructive Pulmonary Disease Overlap

Krystelle Godbout, MD, FRCPC[a],*,
Peter G. Gibson, DMed, FRACP, FERS, F Thor Soc, FAPSR, FAHMS[b,c]

KEYWORDS

- Asthma–COPD overlap • ACO • Asthma • COPD • Definition • Diagnosis

KEY POINTS

- Asthma–chronic obstructive pulmonary disease (COPD) overlap (ACO) is not usually considered a separate clinical entity but a concurrent occurrence of asthma and COPD in the same individual.
- No defining feature of asthma and COPD is pathognomonic, and their occurrence does not necessarily indicate overlap.
- There is no widely accepted definition of ACO.
- Most ACO definitions rely on the recognition of several features of asthma in an individual with persistent airflow obstruction and cigarette smoke exposure history.

INTRODUCTION

Asthma and chronic obstructive pulmonary disease (COPD) are the most common airways diseases, both affecting 5% to 15% of the population in developed countries.[1,2] With such high prevalence, the 2 conditions are bound to coexist in some individuals. The association of the 2 diseases has been recognized for decades but only recently received a proper designation: the asthma–COPD overlap (ACO). There is a growing interest in ACO among the medical community and although its components benefit from widely accepted definitions, the exact definition of ACO has yet to be agreed upon. Several attempts to define ACO have been made but have not been based

[a] Quebec Heart and Lung Institute - UL, Québec, Québec, Canada; [b] Department of Respiratory and Sleep Medicine, John Hunter Hospital, Newcastle, New South Wales, Australia; [c] Priority Research Centre for Healthy Lungs, The University of Newcastle, Newcastle, New South Wales, Australia
* Corresponding author. Institut universitaire de cardiologie et de pneumologie de Québec – Université Laval, 2725, chemin Sainte-Foy, Québec, Québec G1V 4G5, Canada.
E-mail address: krystelle.godbout@criucpq.ulaval.ca

Immunol Allergy Clin N Am 42 (2022) 507–519
https://doi.org/10.1016/j.iac.2022.04.007 immunology.theclinics.com
0889-8561/22/© 2022 Elsevier Inc. All rights reserved.

on evidence or proper validation. . Nevertheless, a proper definition of ACO is of paramount importance for clinicians and researchers.

IS ASTHMA–CHRONIC OBSTRUCTIVE PULMONARY DISEASE OVERLAP A SPECIFIC ENTITY?

Whether ACO is a distinct clinical entity or merely the combination of 2 common diseases has long been disputed. This parallels the longstanding debate around the origin of asthma and COPD whereby 2 theories prevail. The Dutch hypothesis put forward by Orie and Sluiter in 1961 hypothesizes that asthma and COPD are different clinical expressions of a common disease, modulated by environmental and genetic factors.[3] Following that theory, ACO could certainly be yet another expression of this original disease. On the other hand, the British hypothesis position asthma and COPD, and therefore ACO, as separate diseases with distinct causes.

The scientific community historically positioned asthma and COPD dichotomously but a recent understanding of the heterogeneity of the 2 diseases has shaken the established paradigm. Asthma and COPD are increasingly considered along a continuum of airway diseases in which patients position themselves according to their clinical and inflammatory characteristics.[4] Although the debate will likely be everlasting, ACO is now generally considered an important phenotype of airway diseases rather than a specific entity. Because of that conclusion, the disease formerly known as asthma–COPD overlap syndrome (ACOS), was renamed ACO in a 2017 ATS workshop.[5]

RELEVANCE OF DEFINING ASTHMA–CHRONIC OBSTRUCTIVE PULMONARY DISEASE OVERLAP

If ACO is merely the overlap of 2 frequent diseases, one could question the relevance of defining it specifically. Yet, for several reasons, it is of utmost importance to recognize ACO among the many patients presenting with airway diseases. First, with a prevalence of around 20% of airway diseases,[6] any recommendation specific to ACO would be relevant for a large number of individuals. ACO is also associated with a higher disease burden and worse prognosis than either asthma or COPD alone,[7] stressing a greater need for care and closer follow-up from physicians. Likewise, therapeutic choices differ in presence of ACO. And as making a diagnosis is not always straightforward, providing physicians with tools to recognize overlapping features of asthma and COPD would guide them toward more appropriate management strategies. Finally, and at least equally important are the implications for research. Patients with characteristics of both asthma and COPD have been systematically excluded from randomized-controlled trials.[8] Nevertheless, ACO became the subject of numerous studies in the past 2 decades, each applying a different, nonvalidated set of inclusion criteria. Without a consensus definition, the resulting outcomes are heterogeneous and external validity limited.

CURRENT DEFINITIONS AND DIAGNOSIS OF ASTHMA AND CHRONIC OBSTRUCTIVE PULMONARY DISEASE

To properly define ACO, the definition of its component conditions should be reviewed. Asthma and COPD have been recognized for centuries but the core elements of their respective definitions have evolved as the knowledge of their pathophysiology improved. Despite these scientific advances, asthma and COPD are still defined syndromically, by their recognizable symptoms and signs. Consequently, asthma and COPD populations are highly heterogeneous and likely composed of distinct entities sharing similar physiologic characteristics but different underlying mechanisms. Genome-wide association and transcriptomics studies have identified numerous distinct gene signatures among asthma and COPD populations, supporting this hypothesis.[9–11]

Asthma

According to the Global Initiative for Asthma (GINA), "asthma is a heterogeneous disease, usually characterized by chronic airway inflammation. It is defined by the history of respiratory symptoms such as wheeze, shortness of breath, chest tightness and cough that vary over time and in intensity, together with variable expiratory airflow limitation."[12] This definition recognizes the heterogeneity of the disease and the central role of chronic inflammation, usually of type 2 nature, in its development. Airway inflammation is, however, not required to establish a diagnosis of asthma that instead relies on airflow measurements. In an appropriate clinical setting, demonstrating airway obstruction together with an excessive variability in lung function provides a diagnosis of asthma.[12] It may, however, prove difficult to diagnose on a single spirometry or peak flow measurement as lung function frequently normalizes spontaneously in asthma. In these cases, testing for airway hyperresponsiveness (AHR) with provocation tests to direct (methacholine) or indirect (mannitol, exercise, hypertonic saline, or hyperventilation) stimuli may uncover the airflow hyperresponsiveness required for diagnosis.

Chronic Obstructive Pulmonary Disease

The Global Initiative for Chronic Obstructive Lung Disease (GOLD) defines COPD as "a common, preventable, and treatable disease that is characterized by persistent respiratory symptoms and airflow limitation that is due to airway and/or alveolar abnormalities usually caused by significant exposure to noxious particles or gases and influenced by host factors including abnormal lung development."[13] This definition reinforces the key elements required for its development that is exposure to noxious particles, most commonly cigarette smoke, and individual susceptibility. It also acknowledges that COPD pathophysiology is not restricted to the airways and that parenchymal destruction (emphysema) may contribute to respiratory symptoms and airflow limitation. Unlike asthma, airway obstruction in COPD is persistent and considered less variable. It can easily be diagnosed on spirometry in the presence of a postbronchodilator FEV_1/FVC less than 0.70,[13] although controversy exists on the use of lower limit of normal (LLN) as the defining threshold instead.[14] Using a fixed FEV_1/FVC ratio has been linked to overdiagnosis in healthy older adults[15] and underdiagnosis in the young adult population.[16]

Other important COPD characteristics did not make their way in the core definition. Chronic inflammation, for instance, is central to the development of the disease, underlying the many structural changes that lead to the clinical disease. Once part of the GOLD definition, it was subsequently removed in favor of more central characteristics.[13] Also omitted was mucociliary dysfunction, another important feature that manifests clinically as the chronic bronchitis phenotype.

THE COMPLEXITY OF DEFINING ASTHMA–CHRONIC OBSTRUCTIVE PULMONARY DISEASE OVERLAP

As stated above, our knowledge of asthma and COPD pathophysiology and clinical expression allowed the scientific community to achieve widely accepted definitions and diagnostic criteria for both diseases. In that case, one could then question whether ACO should simply be identified in an individual who simultaneously meets the definition and diagnostic criteria for asthma and COPD. However, the reality is that no defining feature of asthma and COPD is pathognomonic and there is a considerable overlap in the characteristics of the 2 conditions. Relying solely on these nonspecific features, therefore, increases the risk of diagnostic inaccuracies.

Two situations arise in which a diagnosis of ACO should be raised: the smoker with asthma who develops chronic airway obstruction and patients with COPD with features of asthma. Whether a patient with longstanding asthma and no history of smoking or exposure to noxious particles but with irreversible airway obstruction should be labeled as ACO has been debated. Research has shown that fundamental differences exist in the clinico-physiological characteristics and inflammatory patterns of smoker and nonsmoker patients with asthma and irreversible airflow obstruction, establishing that they are, in fact, different clinical entities.[17–21] Therefore, to reduce the heterogeneity of ACO, it is common practice to exclude nonsmoking asthmatics with persistent obstruction from its definition.[22]

A Smoker with Asthma and Persistent Airflow Obstruction

The most intuitive situation in which ACO develops is after years of smoking in an individual with a diagnosis of asthma at an earlier age. As asthma interacts with smoking to increase the risk of developing COPD by more than 10-fold,[23] it is not surprising to find a high prevalence of chronic airway obstruction in patients with asthma and a history of smoking.[24] And the increased emphysema index found on computed tomography of these patients supports that the irreversible obstruction of this population is, indeed, an added COPD component.[20]

As long as the diagnosis of asthma has been properly established before the emergence of the fixed airflow limitation, identifying ACO in this population is simple. It relies on the demonstration of a persistent postbronchodilator airway obstruction together with a significant smoking history, usually more than 10 pack-years. Radiological emphysematous changes can support the diagnosis although they are not essential.

A Patient with Chronic Obstructive Pulmonary Disease with Features of Asthma

Identifying ACO in an individual without a prior history of asthma has proven more challenging as the defining characteristics of asthma are also more prevalent in COPD (**Table 1**). As asthmatic features are not exclusive to asthma, which ones accurately identify an asthma component in a patient with COPD? Compared with COPD, ACO is associated with a higher disease burden, worse prognosis, and different treatment responses and selecting characteristics with the ability to predict these different ACO characteristics could address the issue. **Table 1** summarizes our current state of knowledge on the topic.

Bronchodilator reversibility (BDR) is the hallmark of asthma but is also commonly seen in the COPD population[30] whereby it does not predict a different course or treatment response, hence its poor value to identify ACO. To increase its specificity, rising

Table 1
Value of features of asthma to identify ACO in a COPD population

Features	Prevalence	Risk Prediction	Treatment Response
Atopy	Up to 20%[25] Less frequent than in asthma[25,26]	More respiratory symptoms and higher risk of exacerbation[27]	Better improvement in FEV_1 with ICS but weak evidence[28]
BDR 200 mL and 12%	Up to 50% but highly variable[29] Similar to asthma[30]	No value[31]	No value[29]
400 mL	5% or less[29]	Does not predict severe exacerbations[32]	Unknown
AHR	25%–70% and related to baseline FEV_1[33,34]	Higher rate of disease progression and increased mortality[34]	ICS improve PC_{20}[35] but little is known about the ability to predict ICS response
Eosinophilia	20%–40% airway eosinophilia Similar to asthma[26,36,37]	Higher risk of exacerbation but some inconsistencies[38–41]	Strong evidence that it predicts response to ICS and OCS[42,43]
FeNO	More than a third with a FeNO $\geq$25 ppb[44]	Variable associations between FeNO and exacerbations[45]	Weak evidence that it identifies responders to ICS[28,46]

Abbreviations: AHR, airway hyperresponsiveness; BDR, bronchodilator reversibility; FeNO, fraction of exhaled nitric oxide; FEV_1, forced expiratory volume in the first second the reversibility threshold to 400 mL has been advocated but the usefulness of such a proposal remains unknown. And while AHR, the other physiologic feature of asthma predicts a poorer prognosis in COPD that could certainly fit ACO,[34] little is known about its therapeutic implication. The most promising tools to identify asthma in a COPD population are inflammatory biomarkers. A large body of evidence already supports the use of blood eosinophils to predict inhaled corticosteroids (ICS) response in COPD.[42] FeNO and sputum eosinophils have shown similar benefits[28,43,46] but further research is required to refine their role.

PROPOSED DEFINITIONS FOR ASTHMA–CHRONIC OBSTRUCTIVE PULMONARY DISEASE OVERLAP
Definition Suggested by Published Studies

ACO has already been the subject of numerous publications. But given the lack of a universally accepted definition, investigators had to decide on their own criteria for its identification. This led to a wide range of definitions across studies, although they usually involved either self-reporting, physician diagnosis, or clinico-physiological features of both asthma and COPD. **Table 2** illustrates the array of definitions found in ACO studies. Results of these investigations are highly dependent on the selected definition, hampering external validity.[55]

Table 2
Sample of ACO definitions used in studies

Study	Definition
Marsh et al,[47] 2008	Postbronchodilator $FEV_1/FVC < 0.7$ BDR >12% and 200 mL or PEF variability >20% over 1 wk or physician diagnosis of asthma with current symptoms or inhaler use
Hardin et al,[48] 2011	≥10 pack-years and $FEV_1/FVC < 0.7$ and $FEV_1 < 80\%$ predicted Self-reported doctor diagnosis of asthma before age 40
Andersen et al,[49] 2013	ICD code related to COPD (chronic bronchitis, emphysema, COPD) ICD code related to asthma (asthma, status asthmaticus)
De Marco et al,[25] 2013	Self-reported doctor diagnosis of COPD Self-reported doctor diagnosis of asthma
Lim et al,[50] 2014	Age ≥40 and ≥ 10 pack-years and postbronchodilator $FEV_1/FVC < 0.7$ BDR >12% and 200 mL or $PC_{20} < 16$ mg/mL
Menezes et al,[51] 2014	$FEV_1/FVC < 0.7$ Wheeze in the past 12 mo and BDR >12% and 200 mL
Lange et al,[52] 2016	Postbronchodilator $FEV_1/FVC < 0.7$ Self-reported current diagnosis of asthma
CHAIN study, 2016[53]	≥10 pack-years and postbronchodilator $FEV_1/FVC < 0.7$ 1 major or 2 minor criteria Major criteria: previous diagnosis of asthma, BDR >15%, and 400 mL Minor criteria: IgE >100 IU, history of atopy, 2 BDR >12% and 200 mL, blood eosinophils >5%
POPE study, 2017[54]	≥10 pack-years and postbronchodilator $FEV_1/FVC < 0.7$ Asthma diagnosis before 40 year old or BDR >12% and 200 mL in the past year + history of atopy and/or allergy
NOVELTY study, 2020[26]	Physician diagnosis of COPD Physician diagnosis of asthma

Abbreviations: BDR, bronchodilator response; COPD, chronic obstructive pulmonary disease; ICD, International classification of disease; PC_{20}, provocation concentration causing a decrease in FEV_1 of 20%; PEF, peak expiratory flow.

Table 3
ACO definitions arising from guidelines

	Feature	Spanish Experts 2012[56]	CPPS 2013[57]	GINA/GOLD[12,58]	International Experts 2016[8]	Belgian Experts 2017[59]	GesPOC/GEMA 2017[60]
COPD CRITERIA	Feature	COPD + 2 major or 1 major and 2 minor	COPD + 2 major or 1 major and 2 minor	Features of both asthma and COPD	COPD + 1 major and 1 minor	COPD + 2 major and 1 minor	COPD + 1 clinical and 1 physiological asthma or 1 alternative
	Post-bronchodilator obstruction	Not specified	FEV$_1$/FVC < LLN	FEV$_1$/FVC < 0.7	FEV$_1$/FVC < 0.7 or LLN	Not specified	FEV$_1$/FVC < 0.7
	Age			No specific criteria aside from persistent obstruction. Diagnosis is based on simultaneous features of both asthma and COPD	≥40 years		≥35 years
	Exposure	≥10 pack-yr smoking	≥10 pack-yr smoking		≥10 pack-yr smoking or equivalent		≥10 pack-yr smoking
ASTHMA CRITERIA	Symptoms					Variable MINOR	Variable or upper airway disease CLINICAL
	History of asthma	Before age 40 MAJOR	MAJOR		Before age 40 MAJOR	Before age 40 or age in favor of asthma MINOR	Family history or personal in childhood CLINICAL
	Atopy	Personal history MINOR	Personal history MINOR		Documented MINOR	Personal of family history or specific IgE MINOR	
	BDR	≥12% and 200 ml on ≥2 occasions MINOR	≥12% and 200 ml MINOR		≥12% and 200 ml on ≥2 visits MINOR	≥12% and 200 ml MAJOR	≥12% and 200 ml PHYSIOLOGICAL
	Very high BDR	≥400 ml and 15% MAJOR	≥400 ml and 15% MAJOR		≥400 ml MAJOR	Variability ≥400ml over time MAJOR	≥400 ml and 15% ALTERNATIVE
	AHR		MAJOR				
	Blood eosinophils				≥300 cell/µL MINOR	MINOR	≥300 cell/µL ALTERNATIVE
	Sputum eosinophils	≥3% MAJOR	≥3% MAJOR				
	High total IgE	MINOR	MINOR				
	FeNO		≥45-50ppb MAJOR			MINOR	≥50ppb PHYSIOLOGICAL

Abbreviations: AHR, airway hyperresponsiveness; BDR, bronchodilator reversibility; FeNO, fraction of exhaled nitric oxide; LLN, lower limit of normal.

Definition Suggested by Practice Guidelines

Despite the lack of high-quality evidence to support recommendations, some expert groups and respiratory societies attempted to provide clinicians with guidance on defining and diagnosing ACO. These are reviewed in **Table 3**. The Spanish have been the most proactive in their effort to define ACO. Based on the results of a modified Delphi method, they were first to issue specific diagnostic criteria for ACO in 2012.[56,57] They further refined their definition in 2017 with a joined consensus guidelines from the COPD and asthma societies.[59,60]

GINA and GOLD have, in turn, attempted to define ACO in 2015. Faced with a lack of evidence, they were unable to reach an agreement on clear diagnostic criteria. They instead provided a syndromic approach in which classical features of asthma and COPD are compared and ACO is considered when a proportionate number of each are identified in a patient with persistent airflow obstruction.[58] The result, being imprecise, is difficult to implement in clinical practice. After this joint effort, GOLD decided to stop referring to ACO in its annual COPD report, handling asthma and COPD as 2 separate diseases.[13] An updated article is, however, still available in GINA asthma reports.[12]

More pragmatic guidance was subsequently given by an international expert panel[8] after an extensive review of the existing scientific literature. They agreed on a consensus definition involving major and minor criteria that, although unvalidated, meant to act as an operational definition for clinicians and investigators to increase our knowledge of the disease.

FUTURE STRATEGIES

Much effort has been made to adequately define ACO and distinguish it from other airway diseases. However, the population selected using ACO definitions ended up being as heterogeneous as asthma and COPD, making ACO another "umbrella" term.[26] In this era of precision medicine, using diagnostic labels, however well-defined they may be, is insufficient to guide clinical decisions. Phenotyping has been developed for that purpose and allows further distill diseases into more uniform clusters. It is now widely accepted and implemented as the preferred method to individualize the treatment of airway diseases.

Another approach to airway disease management has been introduced in recent years. It moves away from diagnostic labels to concentrate on characteristics that can be identified and targeted for treatment, the "treatable traits."[61] This label-free approach is promising for patients with overlapping features but is still in its infancy. There is currently a lack of consensus on which features should be designated as treatable traits, reflecting the paucity of high-quality evidence to support the concept. A treatable trait should be clinically relevant, measurable, have a treatable nature, and lead to a clinically meaningful outcome once treated with a favorable risk-benefit ratio. The concept is slowly being substantiated,[62,63] but its promising nature has already earned it a place in the GOLD recommendations.[13]

SUMMARY

Asthma and COPD benefit from well-accepted definitions that include typical clinical and physiologic features. However, significant overlap exists in the defining features of both conditions leading to considerable heterogeneity in their populations. Much interest has been given to these overlapping features in recent years, leading to the creation of the ACO designation. ACO is, however, still ill-defined as the criteria required for its diagnosis are being debated. This lack of consensus limits to research and diagnosis in clinical practice. Then again, current diagnostic labels of airway diseases, including ACO, hamper individualized medicine and new taxonomies are being developed to address this issue. Whether ACO in its actual separate form will last remains to be seen.

CLINICS CARE POINTS

- A patient with longstanding asthma who develops a fixed airway obstruction after more than 10 pack-years of cigarette smoking can be diagnosed with ACO.
- A bronchodilator response of 200 mL and 12% occurs frequently in COPD and does not, by itself, indicate the presence of asthma. Increasing the threshold to 400 mL is more specific but its usefulness to diagnose ACO is still unvalidated.
- A high blood or sputum eosinophils count is associated with worse clinical outcomes and better response corticosteroids in COPD, making it a favored feature to define asthma in a patient with COPD.

DISCLOSURE

Dr K. Godbout reports grants and personal fees from AstraZeneca, personal fees from Covis, personal fees from GSK, personal fees from Merck, grants and personal fees from Novartis, grants and personal fees from Sanofi, personal fees from TEVA, personal fees from Valeo, outside the submitted work; Dr P.G. Gibson reports grants and personal fees from GlaxoSmithKline, and personal fees from AstraZeneca, Novartis, and Sanofi.

REFERENCES

1. To T, Stanojevic S, Moores G, et al. Global asthma prevalence in adults: findings from the cross-sectional world health survey. BMC Public Health 2012;12:204 [published correction appears in BMC Public Health. 2021;21(1):1809].
2. Raherison C, Girodet PO. Epidemiology of COPD. Eur Respir Rev 2009;18(114): 213–21.
3. Orie NG, Sluiter HJ. Bronchitis. Chrles C Thomas; 1961.
4. Leung JM, Sin DD. Asthma-COPD overlap syndrome: pathogenesis, clinical features, and therapeutic targets. BMJ 2017;358:j3772.
5. Woodruff PG, van den Berge M, Boucher RC, et al. American Thoracic Society/ National Heart, Lung, and Blood Institute Asthma-Chronic Obstructive Pulmonary Disease Overlap Workshop Report. Am J Respir Crit Care Med 2017;196(3): 375–81.
6. Gibson PG, McDonald VM. Asthma-COPD overlap 2015: now we are six. Thorax 2015;70(7):683–91.
7. Barrecheguren M, Esquinas C, Miravitlles M. The asthma-COPD overlap syndrome: a new entity? COPD Res Pract 2015;1(8):1–6.
8. Sin DD, Miravitlles M, Mannino DM, et al. What is asthma-COPD overlap syndrome? Towards a consensus definition from a round table discussion. Eur Respir J 2016;48(3):664–73.
9. Kim KW, Ober C. Lessons Learned From GWAS of Asthma. Allergy Asthma Immunol Res 2019;11(2):170–87.

10. Kuo CS, Pavlidis S, Loza M, et al. A Transcriptome-driven Analysis of Epithelial Brushings and Bronchial Biopsies to Define Asthma Phenotypes in U-BIOPRED. Am J Respir Crit Care Med 2017;195(4):443–55.
11. Silverman EK. Genetics of COPD. Annu Rev Physiol 2020;82:413–31.
12. Global Initiative for Asthma (GINA). Global strategy for asthma management and prevention. 2021. Available at: www.ginasthma.org. Accessed December 4, 2021.
13. Global Initiative for Chronic Obstructive Lung Disease (GOLD). Global strategy for the diagnosis, management, and prevention of chronic obstructive pulmonary disease. 2022 Report. 2022. Available at: http://www.goldcopd.org/. Accessed December 4, 2022.
14. van Dijk WD, Gupta N, Tan WC, et al. Clinical relevance of diagnosing COPD by fixed ratio or lower limit of normal: a systematic review. COPD 2014;11(1):113–20.
15. Hardie JA, Buist AS, Vollmer WM, et al. Risk of over-diagnosis of COPD in asymptomatic elderly never-smokers. Eur Respir J 2002;20(5):1117–22.
16. Cerveri I, Corsico AG, Accordini S, et al. Underestimation of airflow obstruction among young adults using FEV1/FVC <70% as a fixed cut-off: a longitudinal evaluation of clinical and functional outcomes. Thorax 2008;63(12):1040–5.
17. Tommola M, Ilmarinen P, Tuomisto LE, et al. Differences between asthma-COPD overlap syndrome and adult-onset asthma. Eur Respir J 2017;49(5):1602383.
18. Cosío BG, Pérez de Llano L, Lopez Viña A, et al. Th-2 signature in chronic airway diseases: towards the extinction of asthma-COPD overlap syndrome? Eur Respir J 2017;49(5):1602397.
19. Kitaguchi Y, Yasuo M, Hanaoka M. Comparison of pulmonary function in patients with COPD, asthma-COPD overlap syndrome, and asthma with airflow limitation. Int J Chron Obstruct Pulmon Dis 2016;11:991–7.
20. Xie M, Wang W, Dou S, et al. Quantitative computed tomography measurements of emphysema for diagnosing asthma-chronic obstructive pulmonary disease overlap syndrome. Int J Chron Obstruct Pulmon Dis 2016;11:953–61.
21. Boulet LP, Boulay MÈ, Dérival JL, et al. Asthma-COPD Overlap Phenotypes and Smoking :Comparative features of asthma in smoking or non-smoking patients with an incomplete reversibility of airway obstruction. COPD 2018;15(2):130–8.
22. Miravitlles M. Diagnosis of asthma-COPD overlap: the five commandments. Eur Respir J 2017;49(5):1700506.
23. Silva GE, Sherrill DL, Guerra S, et al. Asthma as a risk factor for COPD in a longitudinal study. Chest 2004;126(1):59–65.
24. Aanerud M, Carsin AE, Sunyer J, et al. Interaction between asthma and smoking increases the risk of adult airway obstruction. Eur Respir J 2015;45(3):635–43.
25. de Marco R, Pesce G, Marcon A, et al. The coexistence of asthma and chronic obstructive pulmonary disease (COPD): prevalence and risk factors in young, middle-aged and elderly people from the general population. PLoS One 2013; 8(5):e62985.
26. Reddel HK, Vestbo J, Agustí A, et al. Heterogeneity within and between physician-diagnosed asthma and/or COPD: NOVELTY cohort. Eur Respir J 2021;58(3):2003927.
27. Jamieson DB, Matsui EC, Belli A, et al. Effects of allergic phenotype on respiratory symptoms and exacerbations in patients with chronic obstructive pulmonary disease. Am J Respir Crit Care Med 2013;188(2):187–92.
28. Akamatsu K, Matsunaga K, Sugiura H, et al. Improvement of Airflow Limitation by Fluticasone Propionate/Salmeterol in Chronic Obstructive Pulmonary Disease: What is the Specific Marker? Front Pharmacol 2011;2:36.

29. Calverley PM, Albert P, Walker PP. Bronchodilator reversibility in chronic obstructive pulmonary disease: use and limitations. Lancet Respir Med 2013;1(7): 564–73.

30. Janson C, Malinovschi A, Amaral AFS, et al. Bronchodilator reversibility in asthma and COPD: findings from three large population studies. Eur Respir J 2019;54(3): 1900561.

31. Albert P, Agusti A, Edwards L, et al. Bronchodilator responsiveness as a phenotypic characteristic of established chronic obstructive pulmonary disease. Thorax 2012;67(8):701–8.

32. Kim J, Kim WJ, Lee CH, et al. Which bronchodilator reversibility criteria can predict severe acute exacerbation in chronic obstructive pulmonary disease patients? Respir Res 2017;18(1):107.

33. Tashkin DP, Altose MD, Bleecker ER, et al. The lung health study: airway responsiveness to inhaled methacholine in smokers with mild to moderate airflow limitation. The Lung Health Study Research Group. Am Rev Respir Dis 1992;145(2 Pt 1):301–10.

34. Tkacova R, Dai DLY, Vonk JM, et al. Airway hyperresponsiveness in chronic obstructive pulmonary disease: A marker of asthma-chronic obstructive pulmonary disease overlap syndrome? J Allergy Clin Immunol 2016;138(6):1571–9.

35. Lapperre TS, Snoeck-Stroband JB, Gosman MM, et al. Effect of fluticasone with and without salmeterol on pulmonary outcomes in chronic obstructive pulmonary disease: a randomized trial. Ann Intern Med 2009;151(8):517–27.

36. Saha S, Brightling CE. Eosinophilic airway inflammation in COPD. Int J Chron Obstruct Pulmon Dis 2006;1(1):39–47.

37. Bafadhel M, Pavord ID, Russell REK. Eosinophils in COPD: just another biomarker? Lancet Respir Med 2017;5(9):747–59 [published correction appears in Lancet Respir Med. 2017 Aug;5(8):e28].

38. Vedel-Krogh S, Nielsen SF, Lange P, et al. Blood Eosinophils and Exacerbations in Chronic Obstructive Pulmonary Disease. The Copenhagen General Population Study. Am J Respir Crit Care Med 2016;193(9):965–74.

39. Wedzicha JA. Eosinophils as Biomarkers of Chronic Obstructive Pulmonary Disease Exacerbation Risk. Maybe Just for Some? Am J Respir Crit Care Med 2016; 193(9):937–8.

40. Zanini A, Cherubino F, Zampogna E, et al. Bronchial hyperresponsiveness, airway inflammation, and reversibility in patients with chronic obstructive pulmonary disease. Int J Chron Obstruct Pulmon Dis 2015;10:1155–61.

41. Singh D, Wedzicha JA, Siddiqui S, et al. Blood eosinophils as a biomarker of future COPD exacerbation risk: pooled data from 11 clinical trials. Respir Res 2020;21(1):240.

42. Brusselle G, Pavord ID, Landis S, et al. Blood eosinophil levels as a biomarker in COPD. Respir Med 2018;138:21–31.

43. Singh D. Blood Eosinophil Counts in Chronic Obstructive Pulmonary Disease: A Biomarker of Inhaled Corticosteroid Effects. Tuberc Respir Dis (Seoul) 2020; 83(3):185–94.

44. Tamada T, Sugiura H, Takahashi T, et al. Biomarker-based detection of asthma-COPD overlap syndrome in COPD populations. Int J Chron Obstruct Pulmon Dis 2015;10:2169–76.

45. Mostafavi-Pour-Manshadi SM, Naderi N, Barrecheguren M, et al. Investigating Fractional Exhaled Nitric Oxide in Chronic Obstructive Pulmonary Disease (COPD) and Asthma-COPD Overlap (ACO): A Scoping Review [published correction appears in COPD. 2019 Apr;16(2):x]. COPD 2018;15(4):377–91.

46. Yamaji Y, Oishi K, Hamada K, et al. Detection of type2 biomarkers for response in COPD. J Breath Res 2020;14(2):026007.
47. Marsh SE, Travers J, Weatherall M, et al. Proportional classifications of COPD phenotypes. Thorax 2008;63(9):761–7 [published correction appears in Thorax. 2014;69(7):672] [published correction appears in Thorax. 2015;70(9):905].
48. Hardin M, Silverman EK, Barr RG, et al. The clinical features of the overlap between COPD and asthma. Respir Res 2011;12(1):127.
49. Andersén H, Lampela P, Nevanlinna A, et al. High hospital burden in overlap syndrome of asthma and COPD. Clin Respir J 2013;7(4):342–6.
50. Lim HS, Choi SM, Lee J, et al. Responsiveness to inhaled corticosteroid treatment in patients with asthma-chronic obstructive pulmonary disease overlap syndrome. Ann Allergy Asthma Immunol 2014;113(6):652–7.
51. Menezes AMB, Montes de Oca M, Pérez-Padilla R, et al. Increased risk of exacerbation and hospitalization in subjects with an overlap phenotype: COPD-asthma. Chest 2014;145(2):297–304.
52. Lange P, Çolak Y, Ingebrigtsen TS, et al. Long-term prognosis of asthma, chronic obstructive pulmonary disease, and asthma-chronic obstructive pulmonary disease overlap in the Copenhagen City Heart study: a prospective population-based analysis. Lancet Respir Med 2016;4(6):454–62.
53. Cosio BG, Soriano JB, López-Campos JL, et al. Defining the Asthma-COPD Overlap Syndrome in a COPD Cohort. Chest 2016;149(1):45–52.
54. Koblizek V, Milenkovic B, Barczyk A, et al. Phenotypes of COPD patients with a smoking history in Central and Eastern Europe: the POPE Study. Eur Respir J 2017;49(5):1601446.
55. Barrecheguren M, Pinto L, Mostafavi-Pour-Manshadi SM, et al. Identification and definition of asthma-COPD overlap: The CanCOLD study. Respirology 2020; 25(8):836–49.
56. Soler-Cataluña JJ, Cosío B, Izquierdo JL, et al. Consensus document on the overlap phenotype COPD-asthma in COPD. Arch Bronconeumol 2012;48(9):331–7.
57. Koblizek V, Chlumsky J, Zindr V, et al. Chronic Obstructive Pulmonary Disease: official diagnosis and treatment guidelines of the Czech Pneumological and Phthisiological Society; a novel phenotypic approach to COPD with patient-oriented care. Biomed Pap Med Fac Univ Palacky Olomouc Czech Repub 2013;157(2):189–201.
58. Global Initiative for Asthma (GINA) and Global Initiative for Chronic Obstructive Lung Disease (GOLD). Asthma, COPD and Asthma-COPD Overlap Syndrome (ACOS). 2015. Available at: http://www.goldcopd.org/. Accessed December 4, 2022.
59. Cataldo D, Corhay JL, Derom E, et al. A Belgian survey on the diagnosis of asthma-COPD overlap syndrome. Int J Chron Obstruct Pulmon Dis 2017;12: 601–13.
60. Plaza V, Álvarez F, Calle M, et al. Consensus on the Asthma-COPD Overlap Syndrome (ACOS) Between the Spanish COPD Guidelines (GesEPOC) and the Spanish Guidelines on the Management of Asthma (GEMA). Consenso sobre el solapamiento de asma y EPOC (ACO) entre la Guía española de la EPOC (GesEPOC) y la Guía Española para el Manejo del Asma (GEMA). Arch Bronconeumol 2017;53(8):443–9.

61. Agusti A, Bel E, Thomas M, et al. Treatable traits: toward precision medicine of chronic airway diseases. Eur Respir J 2016;47(2):410–9.
62. McDonald VM, Clark VL, Cordova-Rivera L, et al. Targeting treatable traits in severe asthma: a randomised controlled trial. Eur Respir J 2020;55(3):1901509.
63. Ulrik CS, Vijverberg S, Hanania NA, et al. Precision medicine and treatable traits in chronic airway diseases - where do we stand? Curr Opin Pulm Med 2020; 26(1):33–9.

Pathophysiology of Asthma-Chronic Obstructive Pulmonary Disease Overlap

Andi Hudler, MD, Fernando Holguin, MD, MPH*,
Sunita Sharma, MD, MPH

KEYWORDS

- Asthma-COPD overlap • Pathophysiology • Asthma • COPD

KEY POINTS

- Patients with asthma-chronic obstructive pulmonary disease (COPD) overlap (ACO) exhibit overlapping clinical characteristics of both asthma and COPD but the underlying pathophysiology for this subset of patients with airway disease has not been entirely explained.
- The development of ACO involves the innate and adaptive immune responses with contributions from various inflammatory cells, cytokines, chemokines, and architectural distortion/remodeling of the airways.
- Further investigations into the biological mechanisms behind the development of ACO is warranted to better elucidate the natural history of the disease course by defining the underlying pathophysiology of this clinically relevant syndrome.

INTRODUCTION

Asthma and chronic obstructive pulmonary disease (COPD) comprise 2 of the most common chronic respiratory diseases encountered globally. In 2019, it was estimated that there were approximately 262 million people worldwide living with asthma,[1] whereas the global prevalence of COPD was estimated at 13.1% and caused 3.23 million deaths.[2,3] Estimates of asthma-COPD overlap (ACO) can very due to differences in definitions of the disease, but worldwide prevalence is somewhere between 2% and 4% of the general population.[4,5]

Asthma is a heterogenous disease characterized by chronic airway inflammation. It is associated with airway hyperresponsiveness and variable airflow limitation and is defined by the history of typical respiratory symptoms that vary over time and can be worsened by exposure to specific triggers.[6] In contrast, COPD is characterized

Division of Pulmonary Sciences and Critical Care Medicine, University of Colorado Anschutz Medical Campus, 12700 East 19th Avenue, 9C03, Aurora, CO 80045, USA
* Corresponding author.
E-mail address: Fernando.Holguin@cuanschutz.edu

Immunol Allergy Clin N Am 42 (2022) 521–532
https://doi.org/10.1016/j.iac.2022.04.008
0889-8561/22/© 2022 Elsevier Inc. All rights reserved.

by fixed airflow limitation that is often progressive and associated with chronic, pathologic inflammatory responses to various noxious stimuli, such as tobacco smoke exposure.[7,8]

Although asthma and COPD are considered distinct disease entities, there is increasing recognition that they are heterogeneous conditions with often overlapping features. For example, there is a subset of patients with COPD who exhibit markers of inflammation associated with type 2 immune responses that are classically exhibited by patients with asthma.[9] ACO is a condition in which a person has clinical and biological features of both asthma and COPD.[6] ACO is associated with high morbidity including increased respiratory symptoms, disease exacerbations, and hospitalizations as compared with those with asthma or COPD alone.[4] Although epidemiologic studies suggest that ACO effects approximately 2.0% of the global population,[10] definitions of the syndrome are highly variable across studies complicating the assessment of the true global health burden. ACO defines a subgroup of patients with asthma who have persistent airflow limitation or patients with COPD who may also exhibit variable airflow limitation with or without evidence of type 2–mediated inflammation. A better understanding of the pathophysiological mechanisms that underlie this clinical syndrome is essential to better understand the natural history and optimal treatment modalities for this patient population.

OVERVIEW OF THE PATHOPHYSIOLOGY OF ASTHMA

The pathophysiology of asthma is extremely complex, with multiple cell types and inflammatory pathways contributing to each patient's disease process. There is considerable disease heterogeneity in asthma, with patients displaying varying levels of inflammation related to type 1 and type 2 immune responses. Type 1 inflammation is predominantly regulated by subpopulations of CD4+ T cells referred to as T helper 1 cells that stimulate phagocyte activity through the secretion of interleukin-2 (IL-2), interferon-gamma, and lymphotoxin-alpha.[11] Alternatively, type 2 inflammation is usually characterized by eosinophilia and high antibody titers through the effects of IL-4, IL-5, and IL-13.[11] It is regulated by a subpopulation of CD4+ T cells known as T helper 2 cells and also involves concerted effects through eosinophils, mast cells, basophils, group 2 innate lymphoid cells, and immunoglobulin E (IgE)-producing B cells.[12] These inflammatory indices are observed in patients with type 2 (T2) asthma, whereas patients with non-type 2 asthma do not exhibit increased levels of these inflammatory markers. This constellation of inflammatory signaling results in pathologic changes in the airways, including subepithelial fibrosis, smooth muscle hypertrophy/hyperplasia, increased volume of submucosal glands, and goblet cell hyperplasia.[12]

OVERVIEW OF THE PATHOPHYSIOLOGY OF CHRONIC OBSTRUCTIVE PULMONARY DISEASE

Similar to asthma, the pathophysiology of COPD is complicated with many routes of inflammation contributing to the pathologic changes observed on a cellular level. For most cases, the pathogenesis of COPD is thought to be due to an abnormal inflammatory response to the inhalation of noxious stimuli such as tobacco smoke or biomass fuel. Prior studies have shown that the airways of patients with COPD exhibit increased levels of inflammatory cell infiltration, predominantly driven by macrophages (CD68+) and CD8+ lymphocytes.[13,14]

Patients with COPD also exhibit increased neutrophils in sputum and bronchoalveolar lavage (BAL) samples.[15] Although the exact role of neutrophils in the pathogenesis of COPD is not entirely clear, it is thought that alveolar destruction may be due in part to secretion of serum proteinases by neutrophils, as prior studies have shown a relationship between circulating neutrophil count and disease severity.[16] As the disease process progresses, patients with COPD also exhibit an increased level of B lymphocytes and bronchial-associated lymphoid tissue, which suggests a role of the adaptive immune response in the pathogenesis of the permanent airway damage seen in patients with COPD.[8,17]

The abnormal concentration of inflammatory cells found in patients with COPD results in abnormal levels of cytokines and chemokines within the airways of patients with COPD. Increased levels of IL-8, IL-6, tumor necrosis factor-alpha (TNF-α), monocyte chemotactic protein, metalloproteinases, transforming growth factor-beta (TGF-β), and epidermal growth factor have all been shown to be present in patients with COPD.[18] These extracellular signaling proteins can then go on to enhance inflammation and damage through a variety of processes, including chemotaxis of inflammatory cells, proliferation of fibroblasts, and increased levels of mucin production within the airways.[18] In addition, prior studies have demonstrated increased levels of reactive oxygen species within the airways of patients with COPD, which result in tissue damage and carbonyl stress that causes a variety of pathologic processes, including mitochondrial dysfunction and increased proinflammatory signaling.[19] The constellation of pathologic inflammatory processes seen in COPD results in increased levels of fibrosis, alveolar wall destruction, loss of lung elastic recoil, and mucous hypersecretion.[8]

PATHOPHYSIOLOGY OF ASTHMA-CHRONIC OBSTRUCTIVE PULMONARY DISEASE OVERLAP

Although much is known about the pathophysiology of asthma and COPD as distinct disease entities, ACO is a disease process for which the underlying pathophysiology is not entirely clear. The Global Initiative for Asthma and Global Initiative for Chronic Obstructive Lung Disease describe ACO as a disease process characterized by persistent airflow limitation with multiple features of asthma and COPD present, including symptom patterns, lung function, age of onset, and time course of illness.[20] Although it is evident that patients with ACO exhibit overlapping clinical characteristics of both asthma and COPD, the underlying pathophysiology for this subset of patients with airway disease has not been entirely elucidated at this point in time. In addition, there are likely multiple phenotypes present within the broad category of patients with ACO, as patients with ACO may have varying clinical manifestations depending on the underlying pathophysiologic mechanisms present. This article focuses on the cellular and molecular mechanisms that may underlie the development of ACO with the understanding that further investigation is required to better understand the undoubtedly complex mechanisms at play in the development of this disease process.

DISCUSSION
Eosinophilic Versus Noneosinophilic Disease

In patients with overlapping features of asthma and COPD, it is difficult to determine which disease process determines a patient's clinical course. Some patients with asthma go on to develop irreversible, permanent airflow limitation associated with permanent structural airway remodeling changes. This process is often associated with a decrease in bronchodilator responsiveness and an increase in symptoms.[9] Conversely, there can be patients with established COPD who have concomitant features that resemble asthma with features of increased T2-mediated inflammation and clinical evidence of airway hyperresponsiveness, atopy, and significant reversibility of airflow limitation with administration of bronchodilators.[9]

Patients with asthma and COPD exist along a phenotypic continuum with marked heterogeneity due to clinical, symptom, and pathophysiologic variability among subjects; this is also likely true for patients with ACO, but further investigation is warranted to determine how eosinophilic versus neutrophilic/macrophage predominant inflammation early versus late in the disease process relates to the development of ACO as well as the phenotypic heterogeneity seen in clinical manifestations of the disease.

Role of Environmental Triggers

Environmental triggers including tobacco smoke, air pollution, and environmental allergens play a large role in the development of COPD and asthma and are likely significant contributors to the development of ACO.

Tobacco smoke

In patients with asthma, exposure to tobacco smoke has been shown to increase neutrophilic inflammation and create a mixed neutrophilic/eosinophilic picture in lieu of the eosinophil predominance typically seen.[21,22] This effect has also been shown to occur in mouse models of asthma in which attenuated eosinophilic responses to known allergic triggers were seen in subjects that were exposed to tobacco smoke.[23] Although the pathophysiological mechanisms that explain increased disease severity in subjects with ACO are unclear, the development of ACO may be due in part to the shift toward more neutrophil-predominant inflammatory mechanisms. In addition, this transition to a more neutrophil-predominant infiltration of the airways has been shown to result in airway remodeling, which can lead to fixed airflow limitation that characterizes ACO.[4,24]

Exposure to tobacco smoke has also been shown to increase the concentration of CD8+ T cells within the airway epithelium of patients with asthma in a similar fashion to that seen in patients with COPD.[25,26] This increase in CD8+ T cells results in abnormal inflammatory indices, which can result in chronic inflammation, airway remodeling, and persistent airflow limitation characteristic of ACO. For further discussion on this topic, please see the full paper on smoking and ACO by Thomson within this series.

Air pollution

Air pollutants are contaminants that enter the atmosphere at concentrations high enough to result in detrimental effects, including negative effects on human health.[27] Prior studies have evaluated the link between increased levels of air pollution with the development of asthma[28] and COPD.[29] Air pollution contributes to worsening lung disease through a complex cascade of inflammation, oxidative stress, and immunomodulatory effects.[30] In addition, prior studies have shown that patients with asthma may have enhanced susceptibility to air pollution, as they have increased permeability of airway epithelium, which may place them at increased risk for continued inflammation and damage from inhaled irritants in air pollution.[31] Thus, this chronic inflammation may play a role in continued damage to the airways of patients with asthma, resulting in irreversible airflow limitation characteristic of ACO.

Indoor air pollutants also influence the development of airways disease. Biomass fuel exposure, including the burning of wood, garbage, charcoal, and crops, is a known risk factor for the development of COPD. Additional studies have shown that exposure to biomass fuels used for cooking is associated with increased rates of asthma in children.[32] Exposure to biomass fuel has also been shown to be a risk factor for the development of ACO in low- and middle-income countries and may represent an overlooked risk factor for the development of the disease in these populations.[5] Long-term ozone exposure has been associated with a more rapid decline in forced expiratory volume in 1 second (FEV1), whereas nitrogen dioxide, fine particulate matter, and black carbon have been linked to having greater percentage of emphysema.[33] Further investigation is warranted to better elucidate the mechanisms behind how air pollution may contribute to the development of ACO, as this represents a potentially modifiable risk factor for development of the disease. This is a topic of great interest in the field, particularly in the setting of the current global climate crisis resulting in continually increasing concentrations of various air pollutants around the world.

Environmental allergens

There is an association between exposure to certain allergens with increased risk for development of asthma. Prior studies have shown that pediatric patients with increased exposure to specific molds, dust mites, cockroaches, and mice exhibit increased rates of asthma and worse asthma control.[34] Recurrent exposure to known allergens may contribute to the development of ACO in patients with asthma due to chronic inflammation within the airways resulting in permanent remodeling and subsequent fixed airflow limitation. Alternatively, patients with COPD may become sensitized to allergens following repeated exposure, and this may cause an imbalance in the adaptive immune response, with subsequent development of hypersensitivity and airway hyperreactivity, consistent with ACO.

Role of Inflammatory Cells

The inflammatory response in both asthma and COPD involves a concerted effort between innate and adaptive immunity. Unfortunately, the body of literature looking at inflammatory endotypes observed in patients with asthma or COPD has traditionally excluded patients with features of ACO. Although inferences can be made by looking at inflammatory profiles noted in patients with asthma or COPD, dedicated research investigating the inflammatory endotypes seen in patients with ACO is required to better classify the underlying pathophysiology in this patient population.

Macrophages

Macrophages are key players in the coordination of the chronic inflammatory state that results in airway remodeling and irreversible damage in the airways of patients with COPD. As previously discussed, patients with COPD have been shown to have increased levels of macrophage infiltration in the airways and lung parenchyma as well as increased concentrations in sputum and BAL samples. It is likely that proinflammatory macrophages predominate in COPD and contribute to the defective airway remodeling seen in this disease process.[35,36] Macrophages isolated from patients with COPD have also been shown to release increased levels of inflammatory mediators, including TNF-alpha, IL-1β, and IL-6.[37,38]

The role of macrophages in the pathophysiology of asthma is less clear, as they may have proinflammatory or antiinflammatory effects depending on their surrounding environment and activation state.[37] However, it can be hypothesized that patients with asthma with increased levels of macrophages present in airway epithelium may be at increased risk for developing irreversible airflow limitation resulting from an imbalance of proinflammatory and antiinflammatory macrophage activation similar to what is observed in patients with COPD.

Lymphocytes

Lymphocytes likely play a key role in the pathophysiology of the development of ACO, as they mediate the inflammatory states seen in both asthma and COPD. In asthma, the T2 endotype of inflammation is driven by the coordination of CD4+ T2 lymphocytes that release IL-5 to drive eosinophilic inflammation and IL-4 and IL-13 that result in increased IgE production.[12,37] Conversely, patients with COPD have an increased concentration of CD8+ lymphocytes with increased T-cell infiltration correlating with higher levels of alveolar damage and more severe airflow limitation.[15,37] Prior studies have shown that patients with asthma who have a smoking history display a distinct pattern of airway pathology including high concentrations of CD8+ T cells.[25] This transition from predominantly CD4+ to CD8+ T-cell infiltration can result in alveolar destruction and the irreversible airflow limitation characteristic of patients with ACO.

In addition, patients with asthma and COPD have been shown to have increased levels of Th17 lymphocytes, which have been shown to be instrumental in the orchestration of airway hyperresponsiveness and tissue destruction seen in asthma and COPD, respectively.[39] This common pathway of inflammation may be key in understanding the role of lymphocytes in the pathogenesis of ACO, but dedicated research into the topic is required to better elucidate the effects of this subpopulation of lymphocytes in this particular disease process.

Eosinophils

Eosinophils were previously thought of as differentiated cytotoxic effector cells but have since been shown to have a more robust role in the orchestration of function of other immune cells.[40] Eosinophilic inflammation is characteristic of the T2 inflammation seen in patients with asthma. Increased levels of sputum eosinophils have been shown to correlate with increased frequency of airway mucous plugs and lower FEV1 in patients with asthma, which is one proposed mechanism of chronic airflow limitation in this population.[41] Some patients with COPD exhibit increased numbers of eosinophils within the airways, which may place them at increased risk for airway hyperresponsiveness consistent with ACO[4]; this is further supported by studies that have shown that (1) there is more beneficial therapeutic outcome to corticosteroids and bronchodilators in patients with COPD who have elevated eosinophils in comparison to patients with COPD without eosinophilia[37] and (2) reducing peripheral eosinophils with mepolizumab, an anti-IL-5 monoclonal antibody, is associated with a lower annual rate of moderate or severe exacerbations than placebo among patients with COPD and an eosinophilic phenotype.[42]

Neutrophils

Some patients with asthma display a neutrophil-predominant inflammatory phenotype within the airways, and the inflammation seen in COPD is classically characterized as being neutrophilic.[43] Neutrophils secrete serine proteases, which may contribute to alveolar destruction, and have also been shown to be linked with mucous hypersecretion via stimulation of submucosal glands and goblet cells.[37,44] At this time, there are not any studies looking at the role of neutrophils resulting in irreversible airflow limitation in patients with asthma with a neutrophil-predominant inflammatory endotype, but this mechanism could certainly contribute to the development of ACO.

Role of Cytokines and Chemokines

Patients with COPD and asthma have been shown to have abnormal levels of cytokines that orchestrate the chronic inflammatory states seen in each disease process by recruiting, activating, or promoting the survival of various inflammatory cells and pathways within airway epithelium.[37,45] Patients with asthma often exhibit increased markers of Th2-mediated inflammation with elevated levels of IL-4, IL-5, IL-9, and IL-13 as well as proinflammatory cytokines including TNF-α and IL-1β that help to intensify the inflammatory response.[37] Patients with COPD have been shown to have increased levels of IL-6, IL-β, TNF-α, and IL-8 in sputum.[46]

Th17 cells release IL-17A and IL-22, both of which have been found to be elevated in patients with asthma and COPD and are believed to play a role in increasing neutrophilic inflammation in the airways.[39] Airway epithelial cells in patients with asthma and COPD have also been found to release increased levels of thymic stromal lymphopoietin (TSLP), an upstream cytokine that has been shown to selectively attract Th2 cells in asthma and orchestrate the function of innate lymphoid cells in COPD.[47,48] These shared inflammatory pathways may play a role in the underlying pathophysiology of ACO by causing neutrophilic airway infiltration, resulting in remodeling and permanent airflow limitation in patients with asthma. Increased levels of TSLP in patients with COPD can cause increased recruitment of Th2 cells, resulting in upregulation of allergy-mediated inflammation and bronchial hyperreactivity characteristic of ACO.[47]

Chemokines have been shown to increase inflammation in the airways of patients with asthma and COPD through their role in attracting inflammatory cells from the circulation into the lungs by activation of G-protein–coupled receptors.[37] This recruitment of inflammatory cells into the airways likely contributes to ongoing damage and may be in an important mechanism by which patients develop ACO.

The body of scientific literature looking at cytokine and chemokine balance in patients with ACO is sparse at this time, as patients with features of ACO have traditionally been excluded from studies looking at the inflammatory profiles present in patients with COPD or asthma. Dedicated work looking at this subject may be of benefit to better classify the inflammatory endotypes seen in patients with ACO.

Role of Genetics and the Microbiome

Asthma and COPD are complex diseases with contributions from both genetics and environmental exposures. Substantial previous work has demonstrated a genetic predisposition to asthma[49,50] and COPD.[51,52] Investigating the role of genetic variation to the development of ACO is a growing field, but genetic studies in well-characterized cohorts of ACO remain limited. With the advent of more widely available genome-wide association techniques, the literature on this topic is expanding. One recent study looking at more than 8000 patients with ACO found 8 novel signals for ACO that suggest a shared genetic influence that may predispose individuals to the development of the disease.[53] Further research is warranted to look at the interplay between each of these genetic predispositions and their role in the development of ACO as well as their influence on the phenotypic heterogeneity of the disease process.

The human microbiome affects the development of airways disease. Prior studies have looked at the effects of the microbiome on development of asthma and chronic wheeze in children and have found that colonization with certain organisms, including *Streptococcus pneumoniae*, *Haemophilus Influenzae*, or *Moraxella catarrhalis*, increases the risk of developing asthma.[54,55] One study looking at the microbiome of patients with exacerbations of asthma or COPD revealed biological clusters with distinct inflammatory mediator and microbiome profiles despite having similar clinical presentations.[56] Additional investigation is required to better elucidate how the lung microbiome affects the development of ACO, as this may reveal novel treatment or prevention strategies for patients.

Architectural Destruction and Airway Remodeling

Prior studies looking at patients with COPD and asthma have shown elevated levels of cytokines that not only result in the differentiation and promotion of inflammatory cells but also act to promote and activate various structural cells that result in airway remodeling.[45] Biopsies from patients with asthma have been shown to demonstrate increased collagen type III deposition, larger mucous glands and airway smooth

Table 1
Pathophysiologic features of asthma, chronic obstructive pulmonary disease, and asthma-chronic obstructive pulmonary disease overlap

	Asthma	COPD	ACO
Macrophage infiltration within the airways	-	+	+
CD8+ T lymphocyte predominance	-	++	+/−
CD4+ T lymphocyte predominance	++	-	+/−
Eosinophilic inflammation predominates	+	-	+/−
Neutrophilic inflammation predominates	+	++	+/−
Elevated IL-5, IL-4, IL-13	+	-	+
Elevated IL-6, IL-8	-	+	+

Legend: "+", typically present in the disease process; "-", not typically observed in the disease process; "+/−", can be present or absent in the disease process.

Table represents the phenotypic traits classically recognized in each disease process with the knowledge that there are cases that will not fit into the classic pattern typically observed.

muscle (ASM) areas, augmented ASM size, and increased myosin light chain expression in patients with severe asthma, which has then been correlated with lower FEV1 values.[57,58] Two mechanisms of particular importance may be mucous hypersecretion and airway fibrosis, as these are shared between patients with asthma and COPD at differing degrees of severity.

The effect of tobacco smoke also influences airway remodeling and progression from the reversible bronchoconstriction seen in asthma to the fixed airway limitation characteristic of ACO. Prior studies looking at mouse models of allergen-induced asthma have shown exposure to tobacco smoke along with a pathogenic allergen resulted in increased collagen deposition in comparison to subjects only exposed to the allergen itself.[23] In addition, when looking at epithelial changes in patients with asthma who smoke versus those who do not smoke, it was shown that patients with asthma who smoke had increased numbers of goblet cells and mucous-positive epithelium, increased epithelial thickness, and an increased proliferation rate of basal epithelium.[24]

SUMMARY

Although there are many potential mechanisms at play in the development of ACO, we have not yet identified the exact pathways of inflammation and airway remodeling that result in the clinical phenotypes we see in patients with ACO (**Table 1**). Further investigations with a dedicated focus on this subgroup of patients is warranted to better elucidate the natural history of their disease course by defining the underlying pathophysiology of this clinically relevant syndrome. A better understanding of the pathophysiologic mechanisms that result in increased disease severity in patients with ACO will help us to better identify potential drug targets and improve symptom burden and overall quality of life for patients living with ACO.

CLINICS CARE POINTS

- The development of ACO involves the innate and adaptive immune responses with contributions from environmental and genetic influences.

- Further research into the pathophysiology of ACO is warranted to help better elucidate the mechanisms underlying this disease to provide treatments to improve the lives of patients living with this condition.
- There is likely considerable phenotypic heterogeneity within the disease process, but additional research focused on the evaluation of this is needed to better classify the inflammatory and clinical characteristics of patients with ACO.
- When evaluating for ACO, it may be helpful to characterize the inflammatory profile present within the airways, but further research is warranted to better classify the inflammatory phenotypes seen in patients with ACO.
- The interaction between airway inflammation and environmental triggers, such as tobacco smoke and air pollution, can play a pivotal role in the development of ACO, so a thorough history is key when making the diagnosis.
- Exposure to tobacco smoke may be of particular importance in regard to the architectural destruction and airway remodeling in patients with ACO, so emphasis on smoking cessation remains of utmost importance.

DISCLOSURE

Dr F. Holguin is a member of the ASPEN trial adjudication committee, INSMED.

REFERENCES

1. World Health Organization. Asthma. Available at: https://www.who.int/news-room/fact-sheets/detail/asthma. Accessed November 20, 2021.
2. Blanco I, Diego I, Bueno P, et al. Geographic distribution of COPD prevalence in the world displayed by geographic information system maps. Eur Respir J 2019; 54(1). https://doi.org/10.1183/13993003.00610-2019.
3. World Health Organization. Chronic obstructive pulmonary disease (COPD). Available at: https://www.who.int/news-room/fact-sheets/detail/chronic-obstructive-pulmonary-disease-(copd). Accessed November 20, 2021.
4. Sharma S, Khurana S, Federman AD, et al. Asthma-chronic obstructive pulmonary disease overlap. Immunol Allergy Clin North Am 2020;40(4):565–73.
5. Morgan BW, Grigsby MR, Siddharthan T, et al. Epidemiology and risk factors of asthma-chronic obstructive pulmonary disease overlap in low- and middle-income countries. J Allergy Clin Immunol 2019;143(4):1598–606.
6. Global Strategy for Asthma Management and Prevention. Global strategy for asthma management and preventsion (2021 update). 2021. Available at: https://ginasthma.org/wp-content/uploads/2021/05/GINA-Main-Report-2021-V2-WMS.pdf. Accessed Novermber 20, 2021.
7. Celli BR, MacNee W, Force AET. Standards for the diagnosis and treatment of patients with COPD: a summary of the ATS/ERS position paper. Eur Respir J 2004; 23(6):932–46.
8. Broaddus VC, Mason RJ, Ernst JD, Murray, et al. Nadel's textbook of respiratory medicine. 6th edition. Elsevier Saunders; 2016.
9. Desai M, Oppenheimer J, Tashkin DP. Asthma-chronic obstructive pulmonary disease overlap syndrome: What we know and what we need to find out. Ann Allergy Asthma Immunol 2017;118(3):241–5.
10. Hosseini M, Almasi-Hashiani A, Sepidarkish M, et al. Global prevalence of asthma-COPD overlap (ACO) in the general population: a systematic review and meta-analysis. Respir Res 2019;20(1):229.

11. Spellberg B, Edwards JE Jr. Type 1/Type 2 immunity in infectious diseases. Clin Infect Dis 2001;32(1):76–102.
12. Fahy JV. Type 2 inflammation in asthma–present in most, absent in many. Nat Rev Immunol 2015;15(1):57–65.
13. Saetta M, Di Stefano A, Maestrelli P, et al. Activated T-lymphocytes and macrophages in bronchial mucosa of subjects with chronic bronchitis. Am Rev Respir Dis 1993;147(2):301–6.
14. O'Shaughnessy TC, Ansari TW, Barnes NC, et al. Inflammation in bronchial biopsies of subjects with chronic bronchitis: inverse relationship of CD8+ T lymphocytes with FEV1. Am J Respir Crit Care Med 1997;155(3):852–7.
15. Di Stefano A, Caramori G, Ricciardolo FL, et al. Cellular and molecular mechanisms in chronic obstructive pulmonary disease: an overview. Clin Exp Allergy 2004;34(8):1156–67.
16. Di Stefano A, Capelli A, Lusuardi M, et al. Severity of airflow limitation is associated with severity of airway inflammation in smokers. Am J Respir Crit Care Med 1998;158(4):1277–85.
17. Hogg JC, Chu F, Utokaparch S, et al. The nature of small-airway obstruction in chronic obstructive pulmonary disease. N Engl J Med 2004;350(26):2645–53.
18. Chung KF. Cytokines in chronic obstructive pulmonary disease. Eur Respir J Suppl 2001;34:50s–9s.
19. Kirkham PA, Barnes PJ. Oxidative stress in COPD. Chest 2013;144(1):266–73.
20. Global Initiative for Asthma, and Global Initiative for Chronic Obstructive Lung Disease. Diagnosis and Initial treatment of asthma, COPD and asthma-COPD overlap. Available at: ginasthma.org, 2017. Accessed December 2, 2021.
21. Boulet LP, Lemiere C, Archambault F, et al. Smoking and asthma: clinical and radiologic features, lung function, and airway inflammation. Chest 2006;129(3):661–8.
22. Morissette M, Godbout K, Cote A, et al. Asthma COPD overlap: insights into cellular and molecular mechanisms. Mol Aspects Med 2021;11:101021.
23. Botelho FM, Llop-Guevara A, Trimble NJ, et al. Cigarette smoke differentially affects eosinophilia and remodeling in a model of house dust mite asthma. Am J Respir Cell Mol Biol 2011;45(4):753–60.
24. Broekema M, ten Hacken NH, Volbeda F, et al. Airway epithelial changes in smokers but not in ex-smokers with asthma. Am J Respir Crit Care Med 2009;180(12):1170–8.
25. Ravensberg AJ, Slats AM, van Wetering S, et al. CD8(+) T cells characterize early smoking-related airway pathology in patients with asthma. Respir Med 2013;107(7):959–66.
26. Saetta M, Baraldo S, Corbino L, et al. CD8+ve cells in the lungs of smokers with chronic obstructive pulmonary disease. Am J Respir Crit Care Med 1999;160(2):711–7.
27. Almetwally AA, Bin-Jumah M, Allam AA. Ambient air pollution and its influence on human health and welfare: an overview. Environ Sci Pollut Res Int 2020;27(20):24815–30.
28. Hehua Z, Qing C, Shanyan G, et al. The impact of prenatal exposure to air pollution on childhood wheezing and asthma: a systematic review. Environ Res 2017;159:519–30.
29. Arbex MA, de Souza Conceicao GM, Cendon SP, et al. Urban air pollution and chronic obstructive pulmonary disease-related emergency department visits. J Epidemiol Community Health 2009;63(10):777–83.

30. Mocelin HT, Fischer GB, Bush A. Adverse early-life environmental exposures and their repercussions on adult respiratory health. J Pediatr (Rio J) 2022;98(Suppl 1): S86–95.
31. Holgate ST. Pathogenesis of asthma. Clin Exp Allergy 2008;38(6):872–97.
32. Wong GW, Brunekreef B, Ellwood P, et al. Cooking fuels and prevalence of asthma: a global analysis of phase three of the international study of asthma and allergies in childhood (ISAAC). Lancet Respir Med 2013;1(5):386–94.
33. Wang M, Aaron CP, Madrigano J, et al. Association between long-term exposure to ambient air pollution and change in quantitatively assessed emphysema and lung function. JAMA 2019;322(6):546–56.
34. Seth D, Saini S, Poowuttikul P. Pediatric inner-city asthma. Immunol Allergy Clin North Am 2021;41(4):599–611.
35. Chana KK, Fenwick PS, Nicholson AG, et al. Identification of a distinct glucocorticosteroid-insensitive pulmonary macrophage phenotype in patients with chronic obstructive pulmonary disease. J Allergy Clin Immunol 2014; 133(1):207–16.e1-11.
36. Vlahos R, Bozinovski S. Role of alveolar macrophages in chronic obstructive pulmonary disease. Front Immunol 2014;5:435.
37. Barnes PJ. Cellular and molecular mechanisms of asthma and COPD. Clin Sci (Lond) 2017;131(13):1541–58.
38. Culpitt SV, Rogers DF, Shah P, et al. Impaired inhibition by dexamethasone of cytokine release by alveolar macrophages from patients with chronic obstructive pulmonary disease. Am J Respir Crit Care Med 2003;167(1):24–31.
39. Halwani R, Al-Muhsen S, Hamid Q. T helper 17 cells in airway diseases: from laboratory bench to bedside. Chest 2013;143(2):494–501.
40. Rosenberg HF, Dyer KD, Foster PS. Eosinophils: changing perspectives in health and disease. Nat Rev Immunol 2013;13(1):9–22.
41. Dunican EM, Elicker BM, Gierada DS, et al. Mucus plugs in patients with asthma linked to eosinophilia and airflow obstruction. J Clin Invest 2018;128(3): 997–1009.
42. Pavord ID, Chanez P, Criner GJ, et al. Mepolizumab for eosinophilic chronic obstructive pulmonary disease. N Engl J Med 2017;377(17):1613–29.
43. Trejo Bittar HE, Yousem SA, Wenzel SE. Pathobiology of severe asthma. Annu Rev Pathol 2015;10:511–45.
44. Fahy JV, Dickey BF. Airway mucus function and dysfunction. N Engl J Med 2010; 363(23):2233–47.
45. Barnes PJ. The cytokine network in asthma and chronic obstructive pulmonary disease. J Clin Invest 2008;118(11):3546–56.
46. Chung KF. Inflammatory mediators in chronic obstructive pulmonary disease. Curr Drug Targets Inflamm Allergy 2005;4(6):619–25.
47. Ying S, O'Connor B, Ratoff J, et al. Expression and cellular provenance of thymic stromal lymphopoietin and chemokines in patients with severe asthma and chronic obstructive pulmonary disease. J Immunol 2008;181(4):2790–8.
48. Mitchell PD, O'Byrne PM. Biologics and the lung: TSLP and other epithelial cell-derived cytokines in asthma. Pharmacol Ther 2017;169:104–12.
49. Demenais F, Margaritte-Jeannin P, Barnes KC, et al. Multiancestry association study identifies new asthma risk loci that colocalize with immune-cell enhancer marks. Nat Genet 2018;50(1):42–53.
50. Moffatt MF, Gut IG, Demenais F, et al. A large-scale, consortium-based genome-wide association study of asthma. N Engl J Med 2010;363(13):1211–21.

51. Sakornsakolpat P, Prokopenko D, Lamontagne M, et al. Genetic landscape of chronic obstructive pulmonary disease identifies heterogeneous cell-type and phenotype associations. Nat Genet 2019;51(3):494–505.

52. Zhao X, Qiao D, Yang C, et al. Whole genome sequence analysis of pulmonary function and COPD in 19,996 multi-ethnic participants. Nat Commun 2020; 11(1):5182.

53. John C, Guyatt AL, Shrine N, et al. Genetic associations and architecture of asthma-COPD overlap. Chest 2022. https://doi.org/10.1016/j.chest.2021.12.674.

54. Bisgaard H, Hermansen MN, Buchvald F, et al. Childhood asthma after bacterial colonization of the airway in neonates. N Engl J Med 2007;357(15):1487–95.

55. Teo SM, Tang HHF, Mok D, et al. Airway microbiota dynamics uncover a critical window for interplay of pathogenic bacteria and allergy in childhood respiratory disease. Cell Host Microbe 2018;24(3):341–52.e5.

56. Ghebre MA, Pang PH, Diver S, et al. Biological exacerbation clusters demonstrate asthma and chronic obstructive pulmonary disease overlap with distinct mediator and microbiome profiles. J Allergy Clin Immunol 2018;141(6): 2027–36.e12.

57. Benayoun L, Druilhe A, Dombret MC, et al. Airway structural alterations selectively associated with severe asthma. Am J Respir Crit Care Med 2003;167(10): 1360–8.

58. Pepe C, Foley S, Shannon J, et al. Differences in airway remodeling between subjects with severe and moderate asthma. J Allergy Clin Immunol 2005;116(3): 544–9.

Epidemiology of Asthma-Chronic Obstructive Pulmonary Disease Overlap

Anne L. Fuhlbrigge, MD, MS

KEYWORDS

- Asthma COPD overlap • Epidemiology • Prevalence • Risk factors

KEY POINTS

- The prevalence of ACO increases with age but the relationship with gender varies with the study population.
- The variability in the prevalence and clinical characteristics of ACO is linked to differences in how chronic obstructive pulmonary disease (COPD) and asthma are defined, including diagnostic criteria (spirometry-based vs. clinical or symptom-based diagnoses vs. claims data), the population studied, the geographic region and environment
- A consensus approach to the diagnosis of ACO is needed to allow meaningful and consistent epidemiologic information to be generated for this condition.

INTRODUCTION

As Godbout and Gibson outline in this issue of the Journal, our understanding, and the definition of Asthma-chronic obstructive pulmonary disease (COPD) Overlap (ACO) continues to evolve. Because of a lack of consensus on the definition of ACO, epidemiologic studies have used disparate definitions; including the use of claims data using ICD-9/10 codes, self-reported physician/health professional diagnosis, combinations of pulmonary function, laboratory testing and symptom descriptions and algorithms that combine these into sets of major/minor clinical criteria. This variation limits our ability to accurately capture the prevalence of ACO. Highlighting the importance of different definitions, Turner and colleagues used a claims-based definition and identified 10,250 patients meeting the criteria for both asthma and COPD. The authors then reviewed records for a random sample of the patients identified with the claims-based definition of ACO to validate the claims-based diagnosis. They confirmed a diagnosis of ACO in only 50.1% of the patients on medical record review.[1]

Pulmonary Sciences and Critical Care Medicine, Department of Medicine, University of Colorado School of Medicine, Fitzsimons Building | 13001 East 17th Place, Aurora, CO 80045, USA
E-mail address: Anne.Fuhlbrigge@cuanschutz.edu

Immunol Allergy Clin N Am 42 (2022) 533–547
https://doi.org/10.1016/j.iac.2022.03.001
0889-8561/22/© 2022 Elsevier Inc. All rights reserved.
immunology.theclinics.com

Adding to the variation, the prevalence of ACO varies widely according to the study design and the population studied (general vs specialty clinic population with known respiratory disease (asthma, COPD)). Further, it has long been recognized that some patients with asthma develop fixed airflow obstruction (FAO); airflow obstruction that does not fully reverse.[2] The prevalence of FAO in severe or difficult-to-treat asthma has been reported to be as high as 55% to 60%.[3] In the Childhood Asthma Management Program (CAMP) population, a longitudinal cohort of children followed until young adulthood, 11% of the cohort met the Global Initiative for Chronic Obstructive Lung Disease spirometry criteria for COPD.[4] Similarly, Tan and colleagues[5] examined data from the CanCOLD study and observed that the prevalence of FAO (FEV$_1$/FVC < lower limits of normal) in never-smokers was 6.4%, constituting 27% of all "COPD" subjects. The common independent predictors of COPD in never-smokers and ever-smokers were older age, self-reported asthma, and lower education. In never-smokers, a history of asthma, hospitalization in childhood for respiratory illness, and age greater than 70 yrs. was identified as risk factors for "COPD." Shirtcliffe and colleagues[6] found that among a random population sample, aged 25 to 75 years, a diagnosis of childhood asthma was associated with an increased risk for developing "COPD" that equated to a 22-year increase in age or a 62-pack year smoking exposure. Bui and colleagues[7] investigated the role of childhood lung function in adult COPD phenotypes in a cohort of 7-year-old Tasmanian children (n = 8583) who were resurveyed at age 45 years. Asthma–COPD overlap syndrome (ACOS) was defined as the coexistence of both current asthma and COPD (spirometrically defined by (postbronchodilator FEV1/FVC less than the lower limit of normal)). Being in the lowest quartile for lung function at age 7 had an impact on the development of spirometrically defined COPD and therefore "ACO" by middle age. Finally, Perret and colleagues[8] demonstrated an interaction between the effects of smoking, asthma, and atopy on FEV$_1$/FVC, indicating that the deleterious effect of smoking on lung function is more pronounced in patients with asthma and atopy.

IS ASTHMA WITH FIXED AIRFLOW OBSTRUCTION ASTHMA-CHRONIC OBSTRUCTIVE PULMONARY DISEASE OVERLAP?

The presence of FAO complicates the differentiation of asthma from COPD, as COPD is also defined by the presence of "irreversible airflow obstruction." The ATS/ERS defines COPD as a disease state characterized by airflow limitation that is not fully reversible and associated with a chronic inflammatory response of the lungs to noxious particles or gases.[9] Cigarette smoking is the most common risk factor,[10] but other exposures are increasingly being recognized (eg, biomass fuels and α_1-antitrypsin deficiency). Therefore, a critical feature for the diagnosis of COPD, and therefore ACO, is a history of significant exposure to noxious particles or gases. Yet, despite the clear link/requirement between such exposures and the development/diagnosis of COPD, a significant proportion of the population-based studies rely on self-report of COPD and/or claims data that do not clearly outline whether such exposures were included as part of the diagnosis of COPD. Similarly, other studies use postbronchodilator irreversible airflow obstruction as a sole diagnostic criterion for COPD and do not outline whether environmental exposures (either cigarette smoke or biomass fuel) are a key component. Adding further uncertainty, the absence of a smoking history does not eliminate the possibility of developing COPD, and a quarter of patients with asthma are current cigarette smokers.[11] Further, at least one quarter of people with COPD are nonsmokers[5] with epidemiologic studies demonstrating the impact of air pollution and environmental (passive) tobacco smoke on lung function and risk of developing COPD.[12–16] It has been proposed that asthma with FAO, is a distinct subpopulation and should not be included in estimates of the prevalence of ACO.[17]

PREVALENCE OF ASTHMA-CHRONIC OBSTRUCTIVE PULMONARY DISEASE OVERLAP

Meta-analyses have summarized the growing body of literature on the epidemiology of ACO. Alshabanat and colleagues[18] pooled data on the prevalence of ACO. They observed a pooled prevalence of ACO among patients with COPD was 27% (95% CI: 0.16–0.38, $P < .0001$) and 28% (95% CI: 0.09–0.47, $P = .0032$) in the population and hospital-based studies, respectively. Of note, only 13 studies used post-BD values for COPD diagnosis. While most studies included in the above systematic review were matched or adjusted for potential confounders, including smoking status, it is not stated how many of the studies included exposures to noxious gases in the diagnosis of COPD. Hosseini and colleagues[19] performed a systematic review that adhered to the PRISMA (Preferred Reporting Items for Systematic Reviews and Meta-Analyses) checklist.[20] The authors reanalyzed the data to examine the presence of ACO in the population studied as a whole and stratified by underlying asthma and COPD. The ACO prevalence reported in the various studies showed considerable variability in patients with asthma (ranging from 3.2% to 51.4%) and COPD (ranging from 13.0% to 55.7%) and when the results were pooled, the prevalence of ACO was 26.5% (95% CI: 19.5%–33.6%) in patients with asthma and 29.6% (95% CI: 19.3%–39.9%) in patients with COPD (**Table 1**). Most of the studies originated from either North America or Europe, but studies from Latin America, China, Korea, and six low- and middle-income countries were included but no studies from Africa, the Middle East, and Eastern Europe were not included.

THE PREVALENCE OF ASTHMA-CHRONIC OBSTRUCTIVE PULMONARY DISEASE OVERLAP ACROSS DIFFERENT CRITERIA IN THE SAME POPULATION

Several analyses have looked at how the prevalence of ACO varies across different criteria in the same population. Barczyk and colleagues[21] conducted a prospective study on a population of patients with asthma and COPD recruited from outpatient pulmonary clinics in university teaching hospitals and pulmonary specialist offices. They applied 5 different published definitions of ACO; GINA/GOLD[22]; Spanish

Table 1
Summary of meta-analysis results

Outcomes	Pooled Estimates	
	# Studies	Prevalence (95% CI)
ACO	27	2.0% (1.4–2.6)
ACO in patients with asthma	19	26.5% (19.5–33.6)
ACO in patients with COPD	22	29.6% (19.3–39.9)

Abbreviations: ACO, Asthma COPD overlap; CI, confidence interval; COPD, chronic obstructive pulmonary disease.

Data from Hosseini M, Almasi-Hashiani A, Sepidarkish M, Maroufizadeh S. Global prevalence of asthma-COPD overlap (ACO) in the general population: a systematic review and meta-analysis. Respir Res. 2019 Oct 23;20(1):229.

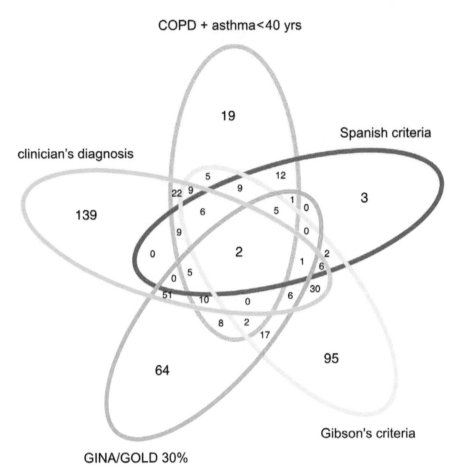

COPD + asthma<40 yrs

Spanish criteria

clinician's diagnosis

Gibson's criteria

GINA/GOLD 30%

Fig. 1. Venn diagram of the prevalence of ACO (absolute numbers) as defined by different diagnostic criteria; GINA/GOLD in blue; Spanish criteria in red; COPD + asthma less than 40 years in orange; Gibson's criteria in yellow; and clinician's diagnosis in green. (*From* Barczyk A, Maskey-Warzęchowska M, Górska K, et al. Asthma-COPD Overlap-A Discordance Between Patient Populations Defined by Different Diagnostic Criteria. *J Allergy Clin Immunol Pract.* 2019;7(7):2326-2336.e5.)

criteria[23]; COPD + asthma and less than 40 years; Gibson's criteria[24]; and clinician's diagnosis. The ACO prevalence ranged between 3.8% (Spanish criteria) and 18.4% (clinician's diagnosis) based on the definition used. A Venn diagram of the prevalence of ACO as defined by different diagnostic criteria is shown in **Fig. 1**. Incorporating all 5 definitions resulted in 31 ACO subpopulations. A total of 573 (33.4%) patients met the criteria from at least one ACO definition, but the level of agreement between different ACO definitions was poor, with only 2 patients (0.12%) meeting all the ACO definitions.

Jo and colleagues[25] examined patients that were part of the Seoul National University Airway Registry between April 2013 and November 2016. The registry is a prospective, observational, multicenter cohort study that enrolled patients, 40 years or older with chronic airway disease, including COPD. COPD was defined by a smoking history of 10 pack-years or more and persistent airflow limitation (postbronchodilator forced expiratory volume in 1 second [FEV1]/forced vital capacity [FVC] ratio <0.7). The authors compared the prevalence of ACO using 4 published definitions. Among 301 patients with COPD, 31.3%, 11.9%, 48.3%, and 46.15% were diagnosed with ACO according to the modified Spanish,[26] ATS Roundtable criteria,[27] PLATINO,[28] and GINA/GOLD criteria,[22] respectively.

The Canadian Cohort Obstructive Lung Disease CanCOLD) study is a prospective, multicenter study that recruited patients with COPD (spirometric GOLD categories 1–4).[29] From a total of 1561 CanCOLD participants, Barrecheguren and colleagues[30] randomly recruited 522 individuals with COPD (53.1% GOLD 1% and 46.9% GOLD 2–4) to describe the prevalence of ACO using various definitions. The most used features of ACO in the literature were selected and tested alone and in combination: (1) reversibility pre–postbronchodilator (>12% and >200 mL of increment in the postbronchodilator FEV1); (2) large reversibility pre–postbronchodilator (>15% and >400 mL of increment in the FEV1); (3) atopy (as reported in a self-reported questionnaire when asked about the presence of respiratory allergies or hay fever); (4) physician diagnosis of asthma (as reported in a self-reported questionnaire); (5) reversibility pre–postbronchodilator and atopy; (6) atopy and a physician diagnosis of asthma; and (7) reversibility pre–postbronchodilator, atopy and physician diagnosis of asthma. Of the 522 individuals with COPD, 264 fulfilled at least one of the 7 definitions of ACO, with the prevalence of ACO varying from 3.8% (definition 7) to 31% (definition 4). Importantly, regardless of the definition, individuals with ACO had worse outcomes (lung function and higher percentage of fast decliners, symptoms and exacerbations, health-related quality of life, and comorbidities) than the remaining patients with COPD.

Inoue and colleagues[31] used data from a multicenter, cross-sectional, observational study of patients with COPD treated by pulmonary specialists in Japan. Patients were eligible for analysis if they fulfilled the following criteria: FEV1/FVC ratio less than 0.7 in past medical records, age ≥40 years at the time of COPD diagnosis, and availability of past (≥1 year) medical records detailing COPD, including spirometry results. Importantly, patients needed to be current or ex-smoker with a history of greater than 10 pack-years of exposure. Patients with ACO syndrome were identified using a stepwise approach as stated in the GINA/GOLD report.[22] Patients who had both 3 or more features favoring asthma plus 3 or more features favoring COPD, were selected as candidates for ACO. Patients were then further classified by the degree of bronchodilator response (≥12% and ≥200 mL FEV1 vs ≥12% and ≥400 mL FEV1 variability). Of the 1008 patients, 167 (16.6%) were identified as having syndromic features of ACO (both 3 or more features favoring asthma and 3 or more features favoring COPD), with 135 (13.4%) patients fulfilling the additional bronchodilation criteria; 93 (9.2%) patients had ≥12% and ≥200 mL FEV1 variability and 42 (4.2%) patients had ≥12% and ≥400 mL FEV1 variability. Of the total population, 595 patients (59.0%; 95% CI 56.0%–62.1%) met either syndromic or spirometric reversibility criteria (≥12%/≥200 mL FEV1 variability). Patients identified as having ACO syndrome were of significantly younger age, had a shorter duration of COPD, lower number of pack-years, better lung function, milder dyspnea symptoms, and higher peripheral blood eosinophil values compared with patients with COPD alone. The rate of exacerbations in the previous year was not significantly different between the ACO and COPD groups.

Variation in the prevalence of ACO, across various definitions, within the same population, underscores the inability to accurately capture the prevalence of ACO. This highlights the importance of clearly outlining the definition used and whether exposure to noxious particles or gases was included. Therefore, Supplementary Tables S1–S4 included in this review, outline the prevalence of ACO across different populations and indicate whether tobacco use/biomass exposure was formally assessed and included in the definition of COPD and therefore ACO. Many but not all studies included in Tables S1–S4 overlap with the meta-analyses published by Hosseini and Alshabanat discussed earlier.[18,19] In addition, several studies have reported results based on sub-populations (asthma vs COPD vs mixed obstructive disease) baseline populations) and are included in more than one table. Table S2 outlines the prevalence of ACO in general populations, while Tables S3 and S4 present the prevalence of ACO among populations with underlying mixed obstructive airway disease, asthma, and COPD, respectively.

ASTHMA-CHRONIC OBSTRUCTIVE PULMONARY DISEASE OVERLAP IN PERSONS WITH KNOWN OBSTRUCTIVE DISEASE (ASTHMA OR CHRONIC OBSTRUCTIVE PULMONARY DISEASE OVERLAP)

Among populations with known obstructive airway disease, the prevalence of ACO is higher compared with general populations but varies depending on the population being studied (mixed obstructive disease, asthma vs COPD alone), the definition of ACO being used, and how that information is being gathered (eg, self-report, medical records, or prospective/retrospective review).[32] Table S2 outlines the prevalence estimates among studies looking at patients with any airway obstruction (defined by either patient report or diagnosis in the medical record of asthma or COPD or through spirometry), outlining prevalence estimates ranging from 14.5% to 55.5%.

ASTHMA-CHRONIC OBSTRUCTIVE PULMONARY DISEASE OVERLAP IN PERSONS WITH KNOWN ASTHMA

Prevalence of ACO has also been reported in patients with asthma. Milanese and colleagues[33] performed a survey on patients with asthma aged $\geq$65 years and found a prevalence of ACO of 29% using the GINA-GOLD ACO definition. 43% of patients with ACO were smokers or former smokers and interestingly 84% reported chronic bronchitis and 35% demonstrated impaired DLCO. Kiljander and colleagues[34] investigated patients in the primary care setting with a smoking history of at least 10 pack-years and found that 27.4% of these patients demonstrated irreversible airflow limitation and were diagnosed with ACO. This prevalence increased up to 37.8% in a population of 256 patients with asthma from a tertiary referral hospital. Table S3 outlines prevalence estimates in persons with underlying asthma which range from 15.3% to 31%. In the meta-analysis performed by Hosseini and colleagues[19] pooled estimates gave an ACO prevalence of 26.5% (95% CI 19.5%–33.6%) among patients with asthma, but with substantial heterogeneity between studies.

ASTHMA-CHRONIC OBSTRUCTIVE PULMONARY DISEASE OVERLAP IN PERSONS WITH KNOWN CHRONIC OBSTRUCTIVE PULMONARY DISEASE OVERLAP

Jo and colleagues[25] found a prevalence of ACO according to various well-known definitions of between 3% and 24.7% among 1067 patients with COPD from the KOCOSS cohort. As highlighted previously, Barrecheguren and colleagues[30] reported a prevalence of ACO among patients with COPD ranging from 3.8% to 50.6% according to 7 different ACO criteria. with pooled estimates from a meta-analysis suggesting a prevalence of just more than 25%.[18] Table S4 outlines studies that reported on ACO prevalence among patients with COPD specifically, with prevalence estimates ranging from 3.8% to 50.6%.

ASTHMA-CHRONIC OBSTRUCTIVE PULMONARY DISEASE OVERLAP IN GENERAL POPULATION

The prevalence of ACO in pooled estimates from the meta-analysis suggests a prevalence of ACO in general population of 2.0%.[19] In Table S1, values ranging from 0.61% to 11.1% in the general population are outlined. Yet the prevalence of ACO has been shown to increase with age[35] and the high estimate of 11.1% comes from the study by Sorino and colleagues,[36] which enrolled subjects aged 65 to 100 years (mean 73.7) in a multicenter project involving 24 pulmonary or geriatric institutions distributed throughout Italy. As expected the values in the general population are lower compared with estimates in patients with obstructive airway disease, asthma, or COPD as outlined in Tables S2–S4. General populations tend to avoid the bias of predefined inclusion and exclusion criteria, yet frequently rely on databases that only have access to a physician diagnosis or diagnostic codes and lack detailed characterization of pulmonary function or other diagnostic tests. Alternatively, cohort studies may not be representative of the general population because patients are usually enrolled in referral (or tertiary) hospitals.

Interestingly, Kendzerska and colleagues[37] published on the temporal trend of ACO prevalence, suggesting that ACO prevalence is increasing over time. This is consistent with the increasing prevalence that has been reported in multiple studies over the same time period in both asthma and COPD.[38] Related, Cosio and colleagues, looked at the stability of ACO classification over time. They observed that among 831 patients with COPD, 125 (15%) fulfilled the criteria for ACO, and 98.4% of them sustained these criteria after 1 year.[26]

REGIONAL VARIATION IN ASTHMA-CHRONIC OBSTRUCTIVE PULMONARY DISEASE OVERLAP PREVALENCE

As highlighted earlier, the prevalence of ACO can vary according to geographic region. However, many of these reports also vary with regard to baseline population, study design, and definition for ACO. A few reports have documented variability in the prevalence of ACO by country and region within a single country using a similar definition for ACO.[39] Morgan and colleagues combined data from 4 studies that included 6 low and middle-income countries (Peru, Argentina, Chile, Uruguay, Bangladesh and Uganda). The prevalence of ACO was 3.8% overall but varied from 0% in rural Peru to 7.8% in Bangladesh. Risk factors for ACO included, low education, and biomass exposure when compared with the asthma-only, nonobstructed nonasthma, and general population groups. Koleade and colleagues[40] used data from the 2012 Aboriginal Peoples Survey (APS) and evaluated the prevalence of ACO in the aboriginal people in Canada. ACO was defined by self-reported diagnosis by a health profession of asthma and chronic bronchitis/emphysema/COPD. The overall prevalence of ACO in the aboriginal population was 2.7% with prevalence varying from 1.01% to 5.68% by region within Canada.

ASTHMA-CHRONIC OBSTRUCTIVE PULMONARY DISEASE OVERLAP AND DEMOGRAPHIC VARIABLES

The prevalence of ACO increases with age.[35] In general populations, patients with ACO are older than those with asthma alone and younger or similar in age to COPD cohorts, based on the age range for the COPD cohort.[35] Kumbhare and colleagues[41] analyzed the 2012 Behavioral Risk Factor Surveillance System (BRFSS) to examine the relative distribution of asthma, COPD, and ACO within the United States. Overall, the prevalence of ACO was lower than the prevalence of either asthma or COPD alone. However, the relative distribution of each diagnosis changed with age. For persons between the ages of 35 to 45 yers, the relative prevalence of asthma is greater than the prevalence of either COPD or ACO. However, between the ages of 45 and 85 years, the prevalence of COPD and ACO increases while the prevalence of asthma decreases. After age 85, the absolute prevalence of all 3 conditions declines but the relative prevalence of COPD remains higher than that of either asthma or ACO.[41] Similarly the prevalence of ACO in an Italian general population sample varied by age, De Marco and colleagues[42] reported estimates of 1.6%, 2.1%, and 4.5%, for person's age 20 to 44 yrs versus 45 to 64 years versus 65 to 84 years, respectively. Henriksen demonstrated that in a Norwegian population the prevalence varied by age; 5% less than 40 yrs, 12% 40 to 60 yrs., 22% greater than 60 yrs.[43] Alshabanat observed that in comparison to subject with only COPD, ACO subjects were significantly younger, along with having higher BMI, health care utilization/health care costs, and lower HRQoL.[18]

Other demographic factors play a role in the prevalence of ACO. The relationship with gender varies with the study population. In populations whereby biomass exposure is one of the causes of COPD, there is a large population of female patients, while in populations whereby tobacco use if the main exposure there may be a male predominance. Yet, reviews have concluded there is no significant association between ACO and gender.[18,35]

ACO seems to be more prevalent among persons of non-white race, lower income, and those with a lower education level relative to persons diagnosed with asthma or COPD.[41,44] The literature is mixed on the impact of obesity on the prevalence of ACO; some reports suggest a greater prevalence of ACO among obese and morbidly obese subjects,[41] while others have suggested higher body mass index has a protective effect.[39] Alshabanat concluded that in comparison to subject with only COPD, ACO subjects had significantly higher BMI[18] and Leung and Sin highlighted a consistent finding of higher body mass index in ACO compared with asthma or COPD in their review.[17]

VARIATION IN ASTHMA-CHRONIC OBSTRUCTIVE PULMONARY DISEASE OVERLAP PREVALENCE WITH EXPOSURE

As expected, the prevalence of ACO varies with smoking status. Patients with ACO report rates of current or former cigarette smoking that are intermediate between rates reported for patients with COPD alone and persons with asthma. However, there are reports that observe no difference in smoking history between COPD and ACO subjects.[28] Among patients with asthma who smoke, the degree of smoking is a significant predictor of ACO.[34] Finally, differences in the predominant exposure associated with COPD may influence the prevalence of COPD and therefore ACO. Whether cigarette smoking versus biomass fuels are the predominant exposure varies by region and may contribute to some of the variation seen in the reported prevalence of ACO by country. Morgan and colleagues[39] observed that ACO may be as prevalent and more severe in LMICs than has been reported in high-income settings and that exposure to biomass fuel smoke may be an overlooked risk factor. Inclusion of smoking or other "noxious particle or gases" in defining COPD is an important criterion that impacts estimates of ACO in the literature. Others have highlighted the risk of ACO with specific exposures. Haghighi and colleagues[45] published on ACO in the World Trade Center Health Registry enrollees. Probable ACO was defined as self-reported post-9/11 physician-diagnosed asthma and either emphysema, chronic bronchitis, or COPD. Of 36,864 Wave 4 participants, 29,911 were eligible for this analysis, and 1495 (5.0%) had self-reported post-9/11 probable ACO. After adjusting for demographics and smoking status, they found 38% increased odds of having ACO in enrollees with exposure to the dust cloud, and up to 3.39 times the odds in those with greater than 3 injuries sustained on 9/11. Among rescue/recovery workers, ever working on the pile, on the pile on 9/11 or 9/12/01, or working on the World Trade Center (WTC) site for greater than 7 days showed increased odds ratios of having ACO.

ASTHMA-CHRONIC OBSTRUCTIVE PULMONARY DISEASE OVERLAP AND COMORBIDITY

Reviews have observed the burden of comorbid medical conditions is higher in ACO than in asthma and is possibly higher than in COPD.[17] A population survey in the US found that 90% of respondents with ACO had at least 1 comorbidity compared with 84% in COPD and 71% in asthma.[41] Kumbhare and colleagues[41] reported that patients with ACO had a higher prevalence of comorbidities compared with asthma or patients with COPD alone and this relationship persisted despite controlling for age, sex, race, marital status, income, employment, body mass index, and smoking status. Some authors have suggested the increase morbidity associated with ACO is secondary to health impairment of the comorbid conditions,[46] yet this is not a universal finding. Peltola and colleagues,[47] observed the negative effect of having 3 or more comorbidities on survival was significant in both ACO and COPD subpopulations and they didn't see differences in the profiles of comorbidity patterns in the underlying cause of deaths or in the pulmonary function between ACO and COPD groups. The variation in demographic predictors of ACO likely relates to differences in the populations being studied, varying definitions of asthma, COPD, and ACO as well as obstructive disease severity, comorbid influences, and uncontrolled differences in environmental exposures.

ASTHMA-CHRONIC OBSTRUCTIVE PULMONARY DISEASE OVERLAP AND LUNG FUNCTION DECLINE

Data on the rate of lung function decline in ACO are limited and mixed. Park and colleagues showed that patients with ACO experience a slower rate of annual decline in prebronchodilator FEV_1 compared with patients with COPD (-13.9 mL/y vs -29.3 mL/y), over a median follow-up duration of 5.8 years. The difference was persistent after adjustment for confounders affecting lung function decline. In contrast, De Marco and colleagues demonstrated more rapid disease progression, as measured by lung function compared with either COPD or asthma alone.[42,48] and Lange and colleagues observed that ACO had an accelerated rate of decline but only in individuals with late-onset asthma (onset > 40 years of age). ACO based on late-onset asthma had the worst prognosis with an FEV1 decline of 49.6 mL/y compared with 39.5 mL/y in COPD, and 27.3 mL/y in patients with ACO with early-onset asthma.[49] Others have shown that FEV1 decline in ACO was similar to that in asthma but better than in COPD,[48] or that no difference existed between ACO, asthma, and COPD groups.[50]

MORBIDITY AND MORTALITY

ACO has been consistently reported to be associated with an increased burden of disease. De Marco and colleagues[42,48] demonstrated more frequent exacerbations and poorer quality of life c/w either COPD or asthma alone. with the frequency of exacerbations up to 5-fold higher with 4-fold risk of hospitalization in some studies.[28] In the COPDGene cohort, patients with ACO were more likely to be frequent exacerbators (defined as 2 or more exacerbations in the year before study enrollment) and almost twice as likely to have a history of severe exacerbation (hospital presentation in the year before study enrollment).[51]

Other have highlighted that individuals with ACO have increased disease severity,[28] poorer quality of life,[52] and have higher health care costs when compared with patients with asthma or COPD alone.[18,53] Kauppi reported that HRQoL was the poorer in an ACO population as assessed by the AQ20.[54] Among the ACO group, the mean AQ20 summary score was 8.8 at the 1-year follow-up, which was significantly higher (patients reporting more symptoms) than in the asthma-only (6.8, $P \leq .001$) or the COPD-only group (7.4, $P \leq .05$).[55] The proportion of disability pensioners and patients with ≥ 10 days of sickness absence during the past year was higher in the ACO group than in the other 2 groups. Similarly, in their meta-analysis, Alshabanat and colleagues,[18] observed that in comparison to subject with only COPD, ACO subjects had significantly lower HRQoL. Patients with ACO have been reported to incur twice the health-related costs of asthma and patients with COPD,[56,57] mainly through outpatient visits and drugs.[56,58] Izquierdo-Alonso and colleagues[59]. found that the use of the fixed-dose combination of LABA and ICS was significantly higher in ACO than in the pure COPD phenotype ($P < .05$).

Data on the association between ACO and mortality compared with either asthma or COPD are also mixed. Diaz-Guzman and colleagues[60] evaluated data from the National Health and Nutrition Examination Survey III (NHANES-III) cohort. In survival models adjusting for all factors except baseline lung function, coexisting COPD and asthma had the highest risk for mortality, followed by COPD only, and asthma only (HR (hazard ratio: 1.83, 1.44, 1.16, respectively). These effects were attenuated but the trend remained after controlling for baseline lung function: coexisting asthma and COPD. In contrast, other studies did not confirm an increased risk of mortality in ACO compared with asthma or COPD.[50] Other studies report decreased mortality in ACO compared with COPD,[61] but no difference in mortality compared with asthma.[36] This mixed picture with regard to mortality has also been highlighted in the review by Leung and Sin.[17] Variable follow-up times and differences in case definition and may account for these discordant results.

SUMMARY

The ability to accurately define and characterize ACO remains elusive. This variability in the prevalence and clinical characteristics of ACO is linked to differences in COPD and asthma diagnostic criteria, disease ascertainment methods (spirometry-based vs clinical or symptom-based diagnoses and claims data), and the population studied including age, gender, and environmental exposures (tobacco, biomass fuels vs environmental exposures). The prevalence of ACO increases with age but can vary according to geographic region and the relationship with gender varies with the study population. The burden of comorbid medical conditions is higher in ACO and ACO has been consistently reported to be associated with an increase burden of disease. However, the impact of ACO on lung function decline and mortality is mixed. As our knowledge of the clinical phenotypes and underlying mechanisms within asthma, COPD, and Asthma-COPD Overlap improve, the epidemiology will continue to evolve. Given the continued lack of consensus definition for ACO a "diagnostic label–free" (ie, COPD vs asthma vs ACO) approach has been recommended [62] and others propose focusing on the unique phenotypes that have therapeutic and/or prognostic implications.[63,64] Regardless, a consensus approach to the diagnosis of ACO is essential for generating meaningful and consistent worldwide epidemiologic information about this condition.

CLINICS CARE POINTS

- The variability in the prevalence and clinical characteristics of ACO is linked to differences in how chronic obstructive pulmonary disease (COPD) and asthma are defined.

- Including persons that meet criteria for COPD, (exposure to smoking or other noxious particles or gases) is critical for accurate diagnosis.

- Asthma with fixed airflow obstruction (FAO) is a distinct entity and should not be included in estimates of ACO.

DISCLOSURE

The authors have nothing to disclose.

SUPPLEMENTARY DATA

Supplementary data related to this article can be found online at https://doi.org/10.1016/j.iac.2022.03.001.

REFERENCES

1. Turner RM, DePietro M, Ding B. Overlap of asthma and chronic obstructive pulmonary disease in patients in the united states: analysis of prevalence, features, and subtypes. JMIR Public Health Surveill 2018;4(3):e60.
2. Ulrik CS. Outcome of asthma: longitudinal changes in lung function. Eur Respir J 1999;13(4):904–18.
3. Lee JH, Haselkorn T, Borish L, et al. Risk factors associated with persistent airflow limitation in severe or difficult-to-treat asthma: insights from the TENOR study. Chest 2007;132(6):1882–9.
4. McGeachie MJ, Yates KP, Zhou X, et al. Patterns of growth and decline in lung function in persistent childhood asthma. N Engl J Med 2016;374(19):1842–52.
5. Tan WC, Sin DD, Bourbeau J, et al. Characteristics of COPD in never-smokers and ever-smokers in the general population: results from the CanCOLD study. Thorax 2015;70(9):822–9.
6. Shirtcliffe P, Marsh S, Travers J, et al. Childhood asthma and GOLD-defined chronic obstructive pulmonary disease. Intern Med J 2012;42(1):83–8.
7. Bui DS, Burgess JA, Lowe AJ, et al. Childhood Lung Function Predicts Adult Chronic Obstructive Pulmonary Disease and Asthma-Chronic Obstructive Pulmonary Disease Overlap Syndrome. Am J Respir Crit Care Med 2017;196(1):39–46.
8. Perret JL, Dharmage SC, Matheson MC, et al. The interplay between the effects of lifetime asthma, smoking, and atopy on fixed airflow obstruction in middle age. Am J Respir Crit Care Med 2013;187(1):42–8.
9. Celli BR, MacNee W, ATS/ERS Task Force. Standards for the diagnosis and treatment of patients with COPD: a summary of the ATS/ERS position paper. Eur Respir J 2004;23(6):932–46.

10. Rostron BL, Chang CM, Pechacek TF. Estimation of cigarette smoking-attributable morbidity in the United States. JAMA Intern Med 2014;174(12):1922–8.

11. Thomson NC, Chaudhuri R, Livingston E. Asthma and cigarette smoking. Eur Respir J 2004;24(5):822–33.

12. To T, Shu J, Larsen K, et al. Progression from asthma to chronic obstructive pulmonary disease. is air pollution a risk factor? Am J Respir Crit Care Med 2016; 194(4):429–38.

13. Park J, Kim Hyung-Jun, Lee Chan-Hoon, et al. Impact of long-term exposure to ambient air pollution on the incidence of chronic obstructive pulmonary disease: a systematic review and meta-analysis. Environ Res 2021;194:110703.

14. Eisner MD, Balmes J, Katz PP, et al. Lifetime environmental tobacco smoke exposure and the risk of chronic obstructive pulmonary disease. Environ Health 2005; 4(1):7.

15. Walter R, Gottlieb DJ, O'Connor GT. Environmental and genetic risk factors and gene-environment interactions in the pathogenesis of chronic obstructive lung disease. Environ Health Perspect 2000;108(Suppl 4):733–42.

16. Liu Y, Pleasants RA, Croft JB, et al. Smoking duration, respiratory symptoms, and COPD in adults aged >/=45 years with a smoking history. Int J Chron Obstruct Pulmon Dis 2015;10:1409–16.

17. Leung JM, Sin DD. Asthma-COPD overlap syndrome: pathogenesis, clinical features, and therapeutic targets. BMJ 2017;358:j3772.

18. Alshabanat A, Zafari Z, Albanyan O, et al. Asthma and COPD Overlap Syndrome (ACOS): A Systematic Review and Meta Analysis. PLoS One 2015;10(9): e0136065.

19. Hosseini M, Amir Almasi-Hashiani, Sepidarkish M, et al. Global prevalence of asthma-COPD overlap (ACO) in the general population: a systematic review and meta-analysis. Respir Res 2019;20(1):229.

20. Moher D, Liberati A, Tetzlaff J, et al. Preferred reporting items for systematic reviews and meta-analyses: the PRISMA statement. Ann Intern Med 2009;151(4): 264–9. W64.

21. Barczyk A, Maskey-Warzechowska M, Gorska K, et al. Asthma-COPD Overlap-A Discordance Between Patient Populations Defined by Different Diagnostic Criteria. J Allergy Clin Immunol Pract 2019;7(7):2326–2336 e5.

22. Global Initiative for Chronic Obstructive Lung Disease: The GOLD Report. Diagnosis of diseases of chronic airflow limitation: asthma, COPD, and asthma-COPD overlap syndrome (ACOS). Available at: https://goldcopd.org/2022-gold-reports-2/. Accessed December 29, 2021.

23. Soler-Cataluna JJ, Cosio B, Izquierdo JL, et al. Consensus document on the overlap phenotype COPD-asthma in COPD. Arch Bronconeumol 2012;48(9): 331–7.

24. Gibson PG, Simpson JL. The overlap syndrome of asthma and COPD: what are its features and how important is it? Thorax 2009;64(8):728–35.

25. Jo YS, Lee J, Kim DK, et al. Different prevalence and clinical characteristics of asthma-chronic obstructive pulmonary disease overlap syndrome according to accepted criteria. Ann Allergy Asthma Immunol 2017;118(6):696–703 e1.

26. Cosio BG, Soriano JB, Lopez-Campos JL, et al. Defining the Asthma-COPD Overlap Syndrome in a COPD Cohort. Chest 2016;149(1):45–52.

27. Sin DD, Miravitlles M, Mannino DM, et al. What is asthma-COPD overlap syndrome? Towards a consensus definition from a round table discussion. Eur Respir J 2016;48(3):664–73.

28. Menezes AMB, Montes de OM, Perez-Padilla R, et al. Increased risk of exacerbation and hospitalization in subjects with an overlap phenotype: COPD-asthma. Chest 2014;145(2):297–304.

29. Bourbeau J, Tan WC, Benedetti A, et al. Canadian Cohort Obstructive Lung Disease (CanCOLD): Fulfilling the need for longitudinal observational studies in COPD. COPD 2014;11(2):125–32.

30. Barrecheguren M, Pinto L, Mostafavi-Pour-Manshadi Seyed-Mohammad-Yousof, et al. Identification and definition of asthma-COPD overlap: The CanCOLD study. Respirology 2020;25(8):836–49.

31. Inoue H, Nagase T, Morita S, et al. Prevalence and characteristics of asthma-COPD overlap syndrome identified by a stepwise approach. Int J Chron Obstruct Pulmon Dis 2017;12:1803–10.

32. Ding B, Enstone A. Asthma and chronic obstructive pulmonary disease overlap syndrome (ACOS): structured literature review and physician insights. Expert Rev Respir Med 2016;10(3):363–71.

33. Milanese M, Di Marco F, Corsico AG, et al. Asthma control in elderly asthmatics. An Italian observational study. Respir Med 2014;108(8):1091–9.

34. Kiljander T, Helin T, Venho K, et al. Prevalence of asthma-COPD overlap syndrome among primary care asthmatics with a smoking history: a cross-sectional study. NPJ Prim Care Respir Med 2015;25:15047.

35. Uchida A, Sakaue K, Inoue H. Epidemiology of asthma-chronic obstructive pulmonary disease overlap (ACO). Allergol Int 2018;67(2):165–71.

36. Sorino C, Pedone C, Scichilone N. Fifteen-year mortality of patients with asthma-COPD overlap syndrome. Eur J Intern Med 2016;34:72–7.

37. Kendzerska T, Sadatsafavi M, Aaron SD, et al. Concurrent physician-diagnosed asthma and chronic obstructive pulmonary disease: A population study of prevalence, incidence and mortality. PLoS One 2017;12(3):e0173830.

38. GBD 2016 Disease and Injury Incidence and Prevalence Collaborators. Prevalence, Global, regional, and national incidence, prevalence, and years lived with disability for 328 diseases and injuries for 195 countries, 1990-2016: a systematic analysis for the Global Burden of Disease Study 2016. Lancet 2017; 390(10100):1211–59.

39. Morgan BW, Grigsby MR, Siddharthan T, et al. Epidemiology and risk factors of asthma-chronic obstructive pulmonary disease overlap in low- and middle-income countries. J Allergy Clin Immunol 2019;143(4):1598–606.

40. Koleade A, Farrell J, Mugford G, et al. Prevalence and Risk Factors of ACO (Asthma-COPD Overlap) in Aboriginal People. J Environ Public Health 2018;21: 4657420.

41. Kumbhare S, Pleasants R, Ohar JA, et al. Characteristics and Prevalence of Asthma/Chronic Obstructive Pulmonary Disease Overlap in the United States. Ann Am Thorac Soc 2016;13(6):803–10.

42. de Marco R, Pesce G, Marcon A, et al. The coexistence of asthma and chronic obstructive pulmonary disease (COPD): prevalence and risk factors in young, middle-aged and elderly people from the general population. PLoS One 2013; 8(5):e62985.

43. Henriksen AH, Langhammer A, Steinshamn S, et al. The Prevalence and Symptom Profile of Asthma-COPD Overlap: The HUNT Study. COPD 2018; 15(1):27–35.

44. Chung J, Kong K, Lee JH, et al. Characteristics and self-rated health of overlap syndrome. Int J Chron Obstruct Pulmon Dis 2014;9:795–804.

45. Haghighi A, Cone JE, Li J, et al. Asthma-COPD overlap in World Trade Center Health Registry enrollees, 2015-2016. J Asthma 2021;58(11):1415–23.

46. Akmatov MK, Ermakova T, Holstiege J, et al. Comorbidity profile of patients with concurrent diagnoses of asthma and COPD in Germany. Sci Rep 2020;10(1): 17945.

47. Peltola L, Patsi H, Harju T. COPD Comorbidities Predict High Mortality - Asthma-COPD-Overlap Has Better Prognosis. COPD 2020;17(4):366–72.

48. de Marco R, Marcon A, Rossi A, et al. Asthma, COPD and overlap syndrome: a longitudinal study in young European adults. Eur Respir J 2015;46(3):671–9.

49. Lange P, Colak Y, Ingebrigtsen TS, et al. Long-term prognosis of asthma, chronic obstructive pulmonary disease, and asthma-chronic obstructive pulmonary disease overlap in the Copenhagen City Heart study: a prospective population-based analysis. Lancet Respir Med 2016;4(6):454–62.

50. Fu Juna-Juan, Gibson PG, Simpson JL, et al. Longitudinal changes in clinical outcomes in older patients with asthma, COPD and asthma-COPD overlap syndrome. Respiration 2014;87(1):63–74.

51. Hardin M, Silverman EK, Barr RG, et al. The clinical features of the overlap between COPD and asthma. Respir Res 2011;12:127.

52. Miravitlles M, Soriano JB, Ancochea J, et al. Characterisation of the overlap COPD-asthma phenotype. Focus on physical activity and health status. Respir Med 2013;107(7):1053–60.

53. Kim M, Tillis W, {ate; Preeti, et al. Association between asthma/chronic obstructive pulmonary disease overlap syndrome and healthcare utilization among the US adult population. Curr Med Res Opin 2019;35(7):1191–6.

54. Alemayehu B, Aubert RE, Feifer RA, et al. Comparative analysis of two quality-of-life instruments for patients with chronic obstructive pulmonary disease. Value Health 2002;5(5):437–42.

55. Kauppi P, Kupianinen H, Lindqvist A, et al. Overlap syndrome of asthma and COPD predicts low quality of life. J Asthma 2011;48(3):279–85.

56. Rhee C, Yoon HK, Yoo KH, et al. Medical utilization and cost in patients with overlap syndrome of chronic obstructive pulmonary disease and asthma. COPD 2014;11(2):163–70.

57. Gerhardsson de Verdier M, Andersson M, Kern DM, et al. Asthma and chronic obstructive pulmonary disease overlap syndrome: doubled costs compared with patients with asthma alone. Value Health 2015;18(6):759–66.

58. Sadatsafavi M, Tavakoli H, Kendzerska T, et al. History of asthma in patients with chronic obstructive pulmonary disease. a comparative study of economic burden. Ann Am Thorac Soc 2016;13(2):188–96.

59. Izquierdo-Alonso JL, Rodriguez-Gonzalezmoro JM, de Lucas-Ramos P, et al. Prevalence and characteristics of three clinical phenotypes of chronic obstructive pulmonary disease (COPD). Respir Med 2013;107(5):724–31.

60. Diaz-Guzman E, Khosravi M, Mannino D. Asthma, chronic obstructive pulmonary disease, and mortality in the U.S. population. COPD 2011;8(6):400–7.

61. Bai J-W, Mao B, Yang W-L, et al. Asthma-COPD overlap syndrome showed more exacerbations however lower mortality than COPD. QJM 2017;110(7): 431–6.
62. Agusti A, Bel E, Thomas M, et al. Treatable traits: toward precision medicine of chronic airway diseases. Eur Respir J 2016;47:410–9.
63. Turner AM, Tamasi L, Schleich F, et al. Clinically relevant subgroups in COPD and asthma. Eur Respir Rev 2015;24(136):283–98.
64. Barnes PJ. Therapeutic approaches to asthma–chronic obstructive pulmonary disease overlap syndromes. J Allergy Clin Immunol 2015;136:531–45.

Early Features of Chronic Obstructive Pulmonary Disease in Patients with Asthma

Is there ACO before ACO?

Louis-Philippe Boulet, MD, FRCPC

KEYWORDS

- Asthma • COPD • ACO • Asthma–COPD overlap • Obstructive airway diseases
- Irreversible airway obstruction (IRAO)

KEY POINTS

- An irreversible component of airway obstruction (IRAO) can be found in patients with asthma, particularly in smokers, who have worse clinical outcomes than nonsmokers.
- Features of early COPD can be encountered at a young age in some smokers with asthma, even before showing the classic criteria of ACO such as IRAO, possibly representing a "pre-ACO" stage.
- Long-term clinical outcomes and optimal management of such "pre-ACO" are still unknown.
- Early recognition of COPD features in smokers with asthma may emphasize the need for preventative and therapeutic measures.
- More research is needed on this population.

INTRODUCTION

About 15% to 20% of the general population has either asthma, chronic obstructive pulmonary disease (COPD), or both.[1–4] However, asthma and COPD are not single

Potential conflicts of interest: The author consider to have no conflicts of interest in regard to this publication but would like to report the following: *Research grants for participation in clinical studies:* Amgen, AstraZeneca, Biohaven, GlaxoSmithKline, Merck, Novartis, Sanofi-Regeneron *Consulting and advisory boards:* Astra Zeneca, Novartis, GlaxoSmithKline, Merck, Sanofi-Regeneron *Nonprofit grants for the production of educational materials:* AstraZeneca, Covis, GlaxoSmithKline, Merck, Novartis *Lecture fees:* AstraZeneca, Covis, Cipla, GlaxoSmithKline, Novartis, Merck, Sanofi.
Institut Universitaire de Cardiologie et de Pneumologie de Québec, Université Laval, 2725, Chemin Sainte-Foy, Québec, Québec G1V 4G5, Canada
E-mail address: lpboulet@med.ulaval.ca

Immunol Allergy Clin N Am 42 (2022) 549–558
https://doi.org/10.1016/j.iac.2022.03.002
0889-8561/22/© 2022 Elsevier Inc. All rights reserved.

Abbreviations	
IRAO	Irrreversible component of airway obstruction
COPD	Chronic Obstructive Pulmonary Disease
ACO	Asthma-COPD Overlap
FEV1	Forced expiratory volume in 1 second
FVC	Forced vital capacity
GINA	Global Initiative for Asthma
GOLD	Global Initiative for Chronic Obstructive Lung Disease
INF	Interferon
IL	Interleukin
CT	Chest Tomodensitometry
ICS	Inhaled Corticosteroid
LABA	Long Acting Beta2-Agonist
FAO	Fixed Airway Obstruction

entities and an increasing number of phenotypes and endotypes have been described for these airway diseases.[3–7]

Although it has been recognized for a long time that features of asthma and COPD may be observed in the same patient, there has been a renewed interest in this condition called "the Asthma-COPD Overlap (ACO)," or "asthma with associated COPD," and its various phenotypes.[7–10] The possible relationship between asthma and COPD was first discussed in the 1960s and led to the "Dutch Hypothesis" suggesting common pathways between the 2 diseases.[11] Then in 1995, the American Thoracic Society (ATS) formally recognized the possible overlap between those 2 entities although no formal recommendations were made about its diagnosis or management.[12]

More recently, it became obvious that ACO was associated with in an increased mortality and morbidity.[8,10,13,14] Furthermore, because patients with ACO have traditionally been excluded from clinical trials, little is known about its optimal management. Recent attempts to better define its pathophysiology, outcomes, and treatment needs to face the problem of an absent consensus on its definition and the presence of multiple phenotypes involved.

DEFINITIONS OF ASTHMA AND CHRONIC OBSTRUCTIVE PULMONARY DISEASE –WHAT ABOUT ASTHMA–CHRONIC OBSTRUCTIVE PULMONARY DISEASE OVERLAP?
Asthma

The Global Initiative for Asthma (GINA) defines asthma as "*A heterogeneous disease, usually characterized by chronic airway inflammation. It is defined by the history of respiratory symptoms such as wheeze, shortness of breath, chest tightness and cough that vary over time and in intensity, together with variable expiratory airflow limitation.*"[3,15] Its features include variable airway obstruction, chronic airway inflammation, and airway hyperresponsiveness (AHR), in addition to recurrent or intermittent episodes of the above respiratory symptoms. Although expiratory flows, as a mean of assessing airway obstruction, can normalize after treatment in most controlled asthmatic patients, a certain proportion of those have persistent airway obstruction, also described as a component of irreversible airway obstruction (IRAO), with a ratio of forced expiratory volume in 1 second (FEV_1) over forced vital capacity (FVC), and also often FEV_1, remaining under the lower limit of normality despite optimal treatment, even in never smokers. However, these features seemed somewhat different from those of classic COPD, regarding associated clinical features and airway inflammation.[16–18] Compared with patients with asthma with completely reversible airway obstruction, those showing IRAO tend to be older, males, with a longer duration of disease, and have increased asthma-related morbidity and risk of death from airway disease.[16,18,19]

Chronic Obstructive Pulmonary Disease

The Global Initiative for Chronic Lung Disease (GOLD) defines COPD as "a common, preventable and treatable disease that is characterized by persistent respiratory symptoms and airflow limitation that is due to airway and/or alveolar abnormalities usually caused by significant exposure to noxious particles or gases."[20]Cigarrete smoke-induced COPD includes the phenotypes of "chronic bronchitis," with cough and sputum production daily for at least 3 months and for at least 2 consecutive years, and pulmonary emphysema, characterized by the destruction of the lung, loss of elastic recoil and distention of peripheral airspaces as revealed on imaging tests, notably lung density on chest CT scans.[21] These 2 last phenotypes of COPD, often amalgamated in a given patient and not distinguished in recent reports/guidelines, are usually associated with fixed airway obstruction (FAO), although, particularly at their early stages, spirometry can be within normal limits.

The "classical" diagnosis of COPD requires the demonstration of IRAO in a patient with typical symptoms, exposure to a risk factor (eg, smoking), often associated with a family history of COPD. COPD is often a mixture of phenotypes, which sometimes show asthma-like features such as marked bronchodilator response, AHR, and/or airway eosinophilia.[22–24] COPD with AHR has been associated with an accelerated decline in lung function.[24,25] Furthermore, an eosinophilic bronchitis may be seen in COPD in about 10% to 20% of patients.[26,27] Finally, blood and sputum eosinophilia predict short-term clinical benefit from high-dose inhaled corticosteroid (ICS) treatment in patients with stable moderate-to-severe COPD.[28]

The features of COPD can take years to develop in a smoker, and the term "pre-COPD" has been proposed for smokers or ex-smokers with normal spirometry at risk of developing COPD but also for smokers with long-standing asthma.[29,30]

Asthma–Chronic Obstructive Pulmonary Disease Overlap

In 2015, the GINA and GOLD reports suggested a set of characteristics defining such overlap and a strategy for its evaluation and treatment.[3,4] ACO was *"characterized by persistent airflow limitation with several features usually associated with asthma and several features usually associated with COPD."* This definition can, however, be interpreted in many ways and may include a large variety of features, showing the heterogeneity of this condition and its various phenotypes.

Many "consensus reports," therefore, suggested various criteria to define ACO, initially called ACOS, the S being dropped as it did not seem to fill the criteria to be named a syndrome.[3,31,32] Among criteria considered essential to define ACO were the presence of IRAO despite optimal treatment in patients older than 40 years old with a history of smoking in addition to a previous diagnosis of asthma, although definitions varied significantly from a report to another.[9,31–36] A common criterion provided for a diagnosis of ACO was the presence of a persistent component of airflow limitation—defined as postbronchodilator FEV_1/FVC ratio (either < 0.7 or inferior to the lower limit of normality)—usually associated with a significant bronchodilator response.

Gibson and colleagues[9] suggested defining the Overlap as "Asthma and COPD—that is, symptoms of increased variability of airflow and incompletely reversible airflow obstruction." Later these authors suggested that "ACO could be diagnosed when a patient has the defining characteristic of COPD, namely incompletely reversible airflow limitation as well as features of asthma," in keeping with the GINA report.[3,37]

COULD THERE BE ASTHMA–CHRONIC OBSTRUCTIVE PULMONARY DISEASE OVERLAP WITHOUT IRREVERSIBLE COMPONENT OF AIRWAY OBSTRUCTION?

Some patients with asthma may show features similar to COPD, or early COPD, in the absence of a FAO.[30,38,39] These may not be considered as having "typical" ACO or "asthma + COPD," although they may share characteristics of both diseases. The debate about the definition of ACO, its specific features, and its optimal management continues. Guidelines suggest some specific criteria to define overlap but overall, they recommend evaluating if there are sufficient features of both asthma and COPD to make such a diagnosis.[37] Nevertheless, while establishing this in specialized centers is relatively easy, it often constitutes a challenge in primary care, whereby access to tools such as lung function tests, imaging, and inflammatory biomarkers are not always available.

Even young smoking or nonsmoking patients with asthma may show features of early COPD including IRAO, but as we demonstrated, this phenotype does not seem as severe in nonsmoking compared with smoking patients with IRAO or COPD.[16,40] Regarding smoking, when started at a young age, it may induce its effects on airways/lung as young as in the 20s or 30s, altering morphologic and inflammatory processes in patients with asthma.[16,18,40,41] It also has the potential to modulate asthma treatment responses and lead to worse clinical outcomes, in addition to promoting faster decline in lung function.[19,42] In this regard, we reported that, compared with nonsmokers with asthma, smokers had more respiratory symptoms despite a possible reduction of perception of bronchoconstriction, a higher functional residual capacity and more severe airway obstruction, particularly at mid-expiratory flow rates, in addition to lower lung diffusion capacity-even if most of these parameters remained in the normal range.[18,40]

SHOULD WE ONLY CARE ABOUT "TREATABLE TREATS"?

In its recent iterations, the GOLD report no longer refers to asthma–COPD overlap (ACO), but instead emphasizes that asthma and COPD are different disorders, which may share common traits and clinical features such as eosinophilia or some degree of reversibility.[20] This goes along a proposal to stop using "umbrella" terms such as asthma, COPD or ACO and simply define which "treatable treats" are present in a given patients, as these last help determine the treatment needs and requirements regarding its management.[43,44] However, clinicians often use these general terms and therefore it is important to differentiate between them. Indeed, for example, if a patient is considered to have asthma, it is imperative to prescribe an ICS even if the inflammatory biomarker profile does not necessarily show significant eosinophilia. On the other hand, if a patient has a "classic form" of COPD, long-acting bronchodilators are the mainstay of treatment and monotherapy with ICS is not recommended in the absence of eosinophilia and may increase the risk of adverse effects such as pneumonia.[15,20]

Miravitlles adequately pointed out that *"Eliminating the concept of ACO may create confusion among clinicians and scientists, because the scientific community will then use different terms or expressions to name what we now call ACO."*[45] One way to describe a patient does not exclude the possibility to use another, considering that both can help guide clinicians in the overall management of these conditions while treatable traits should be considered for therapeutic choices when needed. This approach may suggest that we should "phenotype" all patients with airway obstructive diseases, although for example, for mild to moderate asthma, up to now, phenotyping is not considered necessary.[15]

ETIOLOGY OF OBSTRUCTIVE AIRWAY DISEASES

Many patients with both asthma and COPD features are long-time smokers, suggesting that the mechanisms linked to the effects of tobacco smoke on the airways and the lung have been superimposed on asthma pathophysiological mechanisms. Although it may vary significantly from a country to another, about 25% of patients with asthma patients smoke.[46,47] The "smoking asthma patient" phenotype is probably the most common and unequivocal form of ACO. Studies in smokers with asthma provide useful clues on the pathophysiology of this condition and its optimal management.[47] However, in contrast to COPD, the natural history of lung function in smokers with asthma, particularly the factors influencing the risk of development and degree of IRAO, remain to be further explored.

The reader is invited to consult the article by Thomson in this series, on the effects of smoking on asthma. In summary, smoking is generally associated with a more neutrophilic type of asthma, a reduced response to corticosteroids, and accelerated loss of lung function.[16,47,48] Smoking influences asthma in many ways. Not only it induced more neutrophilic airway inflammation, making asthma more difficult to control, but it may also impair the perception of bronchoconstriction and worsen asthma-related morbidity.[40,41,47] Compared with nonsmokers with asthma, the bronchial mucosa in smokers with asthma show squamous cell metaplasia, increased expression of subepithelial neutrophil elastase, IFN-γ, and intraepithelial IL-8.[41,47,48]

As for patients with asthma or COPD, the mechanisms responsible for the development of IRAO in nonsmokers with asthma remains to be further explored. This IRAO could be observed in poorly controlled asthma but when on optimal therapy, it may be due to asthma itself, particularly if severe, probably related to airway structural changes.[49–52]

ASTHMA–CHRONIC OBSTRUCTIVE PULMONARY DISEASE OVERLAP IN YOUNG PATIENTS WITH ASTHMA AND IN THE ELDERLY

We previously showed that induced-sputum neutrophil and bronchial cell counts were higher and high-resolution CT showed more common airway and parenchymal abnormalities in smokers with asthma with IRAO compared with nonsmokers.[18,51] In asthma with IRAO, we found a correlation between airway neutrophilia and emphysematous features in smokers and between eosinophilia and both airway wall thickness and emphysematous changes in nonsmokers. It is, therefore, possible that the type of airway inflammation could influence airways/parenchymal changes in asthma.

In patients with asthma who never smoked, features such as IRAO or lung emphysematous changes may also result from past respiratory infections or be associated with congenital diseases (eg, congenital emphysema, Mikiti–Wilson syndrome, and so forth) which may impair lung function and modulate the treatment choices for this condition.[53]

Following many years of smoking, smokers with asthma often show the predominance of COPD features over those related to asthma, because of the effects of cigarette smoke on airways and lung parenchyma.[54] Furthermore, an interaction between the effects of smoking, asthma, and atopy on airway obstruction have been described, suggesting that the deleterious effect of smoking on lung function is more pronounced in patients with allergic asthma compared with those nonallergic patients.[55] In elderly never-smokers with asthma, an IRAO can follow a long-term decline in lung function compared with normal individuals, possibly more marked in those who had initially small airways/lung, as shown in COPD.[42]

In addition to some viral infections, pollutants, occupational sensitizers/irritants, biomass burning, and other types of aggressions to the airways may also induce COPD-like features in patients with or without asthma.[56] To and colleagues[57] suggested that individuals exposed to higher levels of air pollution had nearly 3-fold greater odds of developing ACO. However, a significant proportion of individuals considered to have COPD had no significant environmental exposure and/or never smoked, as reported in the CanCOLD group studies, showing a prevalence of COPD was 6.4% in never smokers, constituting 27% of all patients with COPD.[58] The factors involved in the development of COPD in never-smokers included older age and previous asthma.

SO, IS THERE ACO BEFORE ACO?

The answer to this question obviously depends on the criteria used to define ACO, but it is evident that some patients, even at an early age, particularly if they smoked, even less than 10 packs. Years may present with features "classically" belonging to both asthma and to COPD. Should we then call these patients early ACO or "pre-ACO" or "asthma with early signs of COPD"? We may further discuss the usefulness for the clinician of making such characterization but revealing these findings to these patients can help them to stop smoking and have a more regular follow-up, as we observed during our studies on young smokers with asthma who have COPD features.

Long-term ICS could reduce the loss of lung function among smoking asthmatic patients although compared with nonsmokers with asthma, it was less effective for the prevention of severe exacerbations.[59-61] A reduced "sensitivity" to ICS has, indeed, been shown in smokers with asthma.[47,54,59] This may be related to the type of exacerbations and/or the type of airway inflammation associated. Furthermore, these "pre-ACO" patients may possibly benefit from the early introduction of daily long-acting bronchodilator associated with an ICS. Smokers with asthma have better clinical outcomes with medium/high dose ICS-LABA compared with ICS alone.[60,61] This remains, however, to be confirmed in the "pre-ACO" population.

THE NEED FOR FURTHER RESEARCH

We need to gather more information on the early stages of ACO, particularly in smokers. We also need to know if long-term cannabis smoking or vaping can lead to this type of problem in patients with asthma as there is a lack of data on this. Furthermore, current treatment of ACO is based mostly on recommendations for asthma and the role of the different treatment strategies for ACO and its various stages or phenotypes remain to be examined. Using a strategy to focus therapy on treatable traits may be an alternative but there may be other features to consider in our general management of these patients. The role of vaccinations or exercise/rehabilitation in these patients should also be further investigated.[62] Some data suggest that biologics may be beneficial in some patients with ACO, but here again, we need to know more about this, particularly in patients with "pre-ACO."[63]

SUMMARY

In summary, asthma, COPD and ACO include a wide variety of phenotypes, with either asthma or a COPD predominance. Using the terms "ACO" or "asthma + COPD" is still debated, but it remains important to assess its different features in a given patient and examine early features of COPD in patients with asthma, particularly in young smokers, even before the development of an IRAO component.

CLINICS CARE POINTS

- When suspecting an airway obstructive disease in a given patient, always perform spirometry (pre and postbronchodilator) in addition to document smoking and allergic history.

- A diagnosis of asthma–COPD Overlap may be considered in a patient with both features of asthma and COPD, particularly if significant smoking history

- In a smoking asthmatic patient, even with only a few years of smoking, we should look at potential early signs of COPD superimposed to asthma, to emphasize smoking cessation and adequately assess treatment needs.

- In patients suspected of Pre-ACO, as for asthma and COPD, search for "treatable traits" can provide relevant information for the adjustment of treatment, and the treatment of these patients, as for all patients with features of asthma, should include an inhaled corticosteroid.

REFERENCES

1. To T, Stanojevic S, Moores G, et al. Global asthma prevalence in adults: findings from the cross-sectional world health survey. BMC public health 2012; 12:204.
2. Adeloye D, Chua S, Lee C, et al. Global and regional estimates of COPD prevalence: systematic review and meta-analysis. J Glob Health 2015;5: 020415.
3. GINA. Global strategy for asthma management and prevention. 2015. Available at: http://www.ginasthma.org. Accessed February 10, 2022.
4. GOLD. Global strategy for the diagnosis, management, and prevention of COPD. 2015. Available at: http://www.goldcopd.org/. Accessed February 10, 2022.
5. Wenzel SE. Complex phenotypes in asthma: current definitions. Pulm Pharmacol Ther 2013;26:710–5.
6. Agache I, Akdis C, Jutel M, et al. Untangling asthma phenotypes and endotypes. Allergy 2012;67:835–46.
7. Postma DS, van den Berge M. The different faces of the asthma-COPD overlap syndrome. Eur Respir J 2015;46:587–90.
8. Boulet LP, Hanania NA. The many faces of asthma-chronic obstructive pulmonary disease overlap. Review. Curr Opin Pulm Med 2019;25:1–10.
9. Gibson PG, Simpson JL. The overlap syndrome of asthma and COPD: what are its features and how important is it? Thorax 2009;64:728–35.
10. Konstantellou E, Papaioannou AI, Loukides S, et al. Persistent airflow obstruction in patients with asthma: Characteristics of a distinct clinical phenotype. Respir Med 2015;109:1404–9.
11. Orie N, Sluiter HJ, De Vries K, et al. The host factor in bronchitis. In: Orie N, Sluiter HJ, editors. Bronchitis. Assen: Royal Van Gorcum; 1961. p. 43–9.
12. No author. Standards for the diagnosis and care of patients with chronic obstructive pulmonary diseases. Am J Respir Crit Care Med 1995;152:S77–121.
13. Leung JM, Sin DD. Asthma-COPD Overlap syndrome: pathogenesis, clinical features, and therapeutic targets. BMJ 2017;358:j3772.
14. Postma DS, Rabe KF. The Asthma-COPD Overlap Syndrome. N Engl J Med 2015; 373:1241–9.

15. Reddel HK, Bacharier LB, Bateman ED, et al. Global initiative for asthma (GINA) strategy 2021 - executive summary and rationale for key changes. Am J Respir Crit Care Med 2021. https://doi.org/10.1164/rccm.202109-2205PP.

16. Boulet LP, Turcotte H, Hudon C, et al. Clinical, physiological, and radiological features of asthma with incomplete reversibility of airflow obstruction compared with those of COPD. Can Respir J 1998;5:270–7.

17. Fabbri LM, Romagnoli M, Corbetta L, et al. Differences in airway inflammation in patients with fixed airflow obstruction due to asthma or chronic obstructive pulmonary disease. Am J Respir Crit Care Med 2003;167:418–24.

18. Boulet LP, Lemiere C, Archambault F, et al. Smoking and asthma: clinical and radiologic features, lung function, and airway inflammation. Chest 2006;129: 661–8.

19. Lange P. Persistent airway obstruction in asthma. Am J Respir Crit Care Med 2013;187:1–2.

20. Global strategy for the diagnosis, management, and prevention of chronic obstructive pulmonary disease. 2021. Available at: http://www.goldcopd.org. Accessed 18th December 2021.

21. Rabe KF, Watz H. Chronic obstructive pulmonary disease. Lancet 2017;389: 1931–40.

22. Calverley PM, Burge PS, Spencer S, et al. Bronchodilator reversibility testing in chronic obstructive pulmonary disease. Thorax 2003;58:659–64.

23. Tashkin DP, Celli B, Decramer M, et al. Bronchodilator responsiveness in patients with COPD. Eur Resp J 2008;31:742–50.

24. Tashkin DP, Altose MD, Bleecker ER, et al. The lung health study: airway responsiveness to inhaled methacholine in smokers with mild to moderate airflow limitation. Am Rev Respir Dis 1992;145(2 II SUPPL):301–10.

25. van den Berge M, Vonk JM, Gosman M, et al. Clinical and inflammatory determinants of bronchial hyperresponsiveness in COPD. Eur Resp J 2012;40:1098–105.

26. Saha S, Brightling CE. Eosinophilic airway inflammation in COPD. Int J COPD 2006;1:39–47.

27. Saetta M, Di Stefano A, Maestrelli P, et al. Eosinophilia in chronic bronchitis during exacerbations. Am J Respir Crit Care Med 1994;150(6 Pt 1):1646–52.

28. Kitaguchi Y, Komatsu Y, Fujimoto K, et al. Sputum eosinophilia can predict responsiveness to inhaled corticosteroid treatment in patients with overlap syndrome of COPD and asthma. Int J COPD 2012;7:283–9.

29. Han MK, Agusti A, Celli BR, et al. From GOLD 0 to Pre-COPD. Am J Respir Crit Care Med 2021;203:414–23.

30. Thomson NC. Asthma with a smoking history and pre–chronic obstructive pulmonary disease. Am J Respir Crit Care Med 2021;204:109–10.

31. Jung JY. Characteristics of Asthma-COPD Overlap according to Various Criteria. Tuberc Respir Dis (Seoul) 2021;84:87–8.

32. Miravitlles M. Diagnosis of asthma-COPD overlap: the five commandments. Eur Respir J 2017;49:1700506.

33. Sin DD, Miravitlles M, Mannino DM, et al. What is asthma-COPD overlap syndrome? Towards a consensus definition from a round table discussion. Eur Respir J 2016;48:664–73.

34. Plaza V, Álvarez F, Calle M, et al. Consensus on the Asthma-COPD Overlap Syndrome (ACOS) Between the Spanish COPD Guidelines (GesEPOC) and the Spanish Guidelines on the Management of Asthma (GEMA). Arch Bronconeumol 2017;53:443–9.

35. Soler-Cataluña JJ, Cosío B, Izquierdo JL, et al. Consensus document on the overlap phenotype COPD-asthmna in COPD. Arch Bronconeumol 2012;48:331–7.
36. Mekov E, Nuñez A, Sin DD, et al. Update on Asthma-COPD Overlap (ACO): a narrative review. Int J Chron Obstruct Pulmon Dis 2021;16:1783–99.
37. Gibson PG, McDonald VM. Asthma-COPD overlap 2015: now we are six. Thorax 2015;70:683–91.
38. Thomson NC. Asthma and smoking-induced airway disease without spirometric COPD. Eur Respir J 2017;49(5).
39. Price D, Crockett A, Arne M, et al. Spirometry in primary care case-identification, diagnosis and management of COPD. Prim Care Respir J 2009;18:216–23.
40. Boulet LP, Boulay MÈ, Dérival JL, et al. Asthma-COPD Overlap Phenotypes and Smoking: Comparative features of asthma in smoking or non-smoking patients with an incomplete reversibility of airway obstruction. COPD 2018;15:130–8.
41. St-Laurent J, Bergeron C, Page N, et al. Influence of smoking on airway inflammation and remodelling in asthma. Clin Exp Allergy 2008;38:1582–9.
42. Lange P, Celli B, Agustí A, et al. Lung-Function Trajectories Leading to Chronic Obstructive Pulmonary Disease. N Engl J Med 2015;373(2):111–22.
43. Agusti A, Bel E, Thomas M, et al. Treatable traits: toward precision medicine of chronic airway diseases. Eur Respir J 2016;47:410–9.
44. Pavord ID, Beasley R, Agusti A, et al. After asthma: redefining airways diseases. Lancet 2018;391:350–400.
45. Miravitlles M. Asthma-COPD Overlap (ACO) PRO-CON Debate. ACO: Call Me by My Name. COPD 2020;17:471–3.
46. Lemiere C, Boulet LP. Cigarette smoking and asthma: a dangerous mix. Can Respir J 2005;12:79–80.
47. Thomson NC, Chaudhuri R. Asthma in smokers: challenges and opportunities. Curr Opin Pulm Med 2009;15:39–45.
48. Thomson NC, Chaudhuri R, Heaney LG, et al. Clinical outcomes, and inflammatory biomarkers in current smokers and exsmokers with severe asthma. J Allergy Clin Immunol 2013;131:1008–16.
49. ten Brinke A. Risk factors associated with irreversible airflow limitation in asthma. Curr Opin Allergy Clin Immunol 2008;8:63–9.
50. Boulet LP. Irreversible airway obstruction in asthma. Curr Allergy Asthma Rep 2009;9:168–73.
51. Boulet LP, Boulay ME, Coxson H, et al. Asthma with irreversible airway obstruction in smokers and non-smokers: links between airway inflammation and structural changes. Respiration 2020;99:1090–100.
52. Morissette M, Godbout K, Côté A, et al. Asthma COPD overlap: Insights into cellular and molecular mechanisms. Mol Aspects Med 2021;85:101021.
53. Hall NJ, Stanton MP. Long-term outcomes of congenital lung malformations. Semin Pediatr Surg 2017;26:311–6.
54. Sprio AE, Ciprandi G, Riccardi E, et al. The influence of smoking on asthma in the real-life. Respir Med 2020;170:106066.
55. Perret JL, Dharmage SC, Matheson MC, et al. The interplay between the effects of lifetime asthma, smoking, and atopy on fixed airflow obstruction in middle age. Am J Respir Crit Care Med 2013;187:42–8.
56. Assad NA, Balmes J, Mehta S, et al. Chronic obstructive pulmonary disease secondary to household air pollution. Sem Resp Crit Care Med 2015;36:408–21.
57. To T, Zhu J, Larsen K, et al. Progression from asthma to chronic obstructive pulmonary disease. is air pollution a risk factor? Am J Respir Crit Care Med 2016; 194:429–38.

58. Tan WC, Sin DD, Bourbeau J, et al. Characteristics of COPD in never-smokers and ever-smokers in the general population: results from the CanCOLD study. Thorax 2015;70:822–9.
59. Tomlinson JEM, McMahon AD, Chaudhuri R, et al. Efficacy of low and high dose inhaled corticosteroid in smokers versus non-smokers with mild asthma. Thorax 2005;60:282–7.
60. Thomson NC. Challenges in the management of asthma associated with smoking-induced airway diseases. Expert Opin Pharmacother 2018;19:1565–79.
61. Pedersen SE, Bateman ED, Bousquet J, et al. Determinants of response to fluticasone propionate and salmeterol/fluticasone propionate combination in the Gaining Optimal Asthma control study. J Allergy Clin Immunol 2007;120:1036–42.
62. Kondo M, Tamaoki J. Therapeutic approaches of asthma and COPD overlap. Allergol Int 2018;67:187–90.
63. Bacharier LB, Mori A, Kita H. Advances in asthma, asthma-COPD overlap, and related biologics in 2018. J Allergy Clin Immunol 2019;144:906–19.

Genetic Determinants in Airways Obstructive Diseases: The Case of Asthma Chronic Obstructive Pulmonary Disease Overlap

Aabida Saferali, PhD[a,b], Craig P. Hersh, MD, MPH[a,b,c],*

KEYWORDS

- Asthma • Chronic obstructive pulmonary disease • Genome-wide association study
- Single-nucleotide polymorphism • RNA-Sequencing • Whole-genome sequencing

KEY POINTS

- There have been multiple genome-wide association studies (GWAS) for asthma and chronic obstructive pulmonary disease (COPD) separately, with well-replicated results.
- GWAS of asthma–COPD overlap (ACO) have not yielded replicated results due to small sample sizes and inconsistent definitions of ACO.
- Studies of ACO using other genomic methods, such as gene expression profiling, have been feasible with smaller sample sizes.
- GWAS in COPD studies using objective measurements of airway reactivity or allergic biomarkers may provide more reliable outcomes.
- Future genetic studies of ACO will require the collection of multiple biospecimens from large, multi-racial populations with clearly defined disease definitions.

INTRODUCTION

Chronic obstructive pulmonary disease (COPD) and asthma are both complex diseases with genetic and environmental risk factors. Genetic studies of COPD and asthma individually have been performed with varying degrees of success over the past 25 years. Early genetic studies focused on finding shared regions of the genome among affected relatives using linkage analysis[1,2]; however, this method was largely ineffective in complex diseases such as COPD and asthma. In addition, candidate gene studies were performed by selecting genes based on what was then known or suspected about disease pathobiology; yet these studies were mostly unreproducible

a Channing Division of Network Medicine, Brigham and Women's Hospital, Boston, MA, USA;
b Harvard Medical School, Boston, MA, USA; c Division of Pulmonary and Critical Care Medicine, Brigham and Women's Hospital, Boston, MA, USA
* Corresponding author. 181 Longwood Avenue, Boston, MA 02115.
E-mail address: craig.hersh@channing.harvard.edu

Immunol Allergy Clin N Am 42 (2022) 559–573
https://doi.org/10.1016/j.iac.2022.03.003
immunology.theclinics.com
0889-8561/22/© 2022 Elsevier Inc. All rights reserved.

due to small sample sizes and inadequate adjustment for multiple comparisons.[3,4] These were followed by the era of genome-wide association studies (GWAS), initially using genotyping chips to assess hundreds of thousands of genetic variants across the genome, which can be expanded to millions of variants using statistical imputation.[5] These chips have been supplanted first by whole-exome sequencing and now by whole-genome sequencing, which allows for direct measurement of millions of common and rare genetic variants.[6] Furthermore, advances have been made in other 'omics methodologies such as transcriptomics, metabolomics, and epigenetics, which can be studied using an integrated approach to provide a comprehensive view of disease.[7,8] GWAS studies are conducted by assembling large populations of study subjects, most commonly cases and controls, although population-based or family-based studies can also be performed.

GENOME-WIDE ASSOCIATION STUDIES OF ASTHMA, CHRONIC OBSTRUCTIVE PULMONARY DISEASE, AND THEIR OVERLAP
Asthma

The first GWAS for asthma was conducted in 2007 by Moffat and colleagues.[9] This study included 994 asthmatics and 1243 controls and included a replication sample of 5261 subjects. Subsequently, numerous GWAS studies of asthma and related traits have been conducted, leading to the identification of 38 genetic loci associated with asthma.[10] The GABRIEL consortium included 10,367 individuals with clinically diagnosed asthma and 16,110 unaffected individuals.[11] Along with replicating previously identified associations such as that of chromosome 17q12 which contains Gasdermin B (*GSDMB*) and orosomucoid-like protein 3 (*ORMDL3*), the GABRIEL study identified additional asthma associations including genetic variants in or near *IL1RL1/IL18R1*, *HLA-DQ*, *IL33*, *SMAD3*, and *IL2RB*.[11]

At least 6 separate asthma GWAS have been published using subjects from United Kingdom (UK) Biobank, a large general population sample with detailed health information.[12] Ferreira and colleagues[13] studied subjects with self-report of doctor diagnosis of asthma, dividing them into 13,962 subjects with childhood-onset asthma (diagnosed at age <19) and 26,582 with adult-onset asthma (age ≥20), identifying 123 genetic loci for childhood-onset asthma and 56 for adult-onset asthma, with 37 overlapping loci. Pividori and colleagues[14] defined childhood-onset asthma at age less than 12 (n = 9433) and adult-onset asthma at age greater than 25 (n = 21,564) and found 23 childhood specific loci, 1 adult-specific locus, and 37 shared loci. Johansson and colleagues[15] analyzed 41,934 white subjects with self-reported asthma and found 75 loci, 15 of which had not been identified in prior asthma GWAS. Valette and colleagues[16] defined 56,167 white subjects with self-reported or medical record diagnosis code for asthma and found 72 loci. Han and colleagues[17] analyzed 64,538 asthma cases (based on doctor's diagnosis, ICD-10 codes, or self-report) and 329,321 controls, finding 145 significant loci. They then performed a meta-analysis of the UK Biobank and the Trans-National Asthma Genetic Consortium,[18] for a total of 88,486 asthma cases and 447,859 controls, which yielded 167 genetic loci, most of which overlapped with their UK Biobank results. In the Global Biobank Meta-analysis Initiative (GBMI), Tsuo and colleagues[19] aggregated data from more than 150,000 asthma cases and 1.6 million controls across 18 biobanks from across the world, including the UK Biobank, finding 180 loci for asthma, 49 of which were novel. The genetic loci across these UK Biobank studies were largely overlapping; however, the differences in genetic regions found in each study highlight the effects of even subtle changes in case definition and sample size.

Chronic Obstructive Pulmonary Disease

To date, several GWAS of COPD have been reported, with the first being published in 2009. In this study, Pillai and colleagues[20] identified the genome-wide significant association (p < 5 × 10^{-8}) of a locus on chromosome 15q25 including genes *CHRNA3*, *CHRNA5*, and *IREB2*, in addition to the near significant association of the *HHIP* region. *HHIP* was also found to be associated with FEV$_1$/FVC in a concurrently published GWAS from the Framingham Heart Study.[21] The association of *HHIP* with FEV$_1$/FVC has subsequently been replicated in several large studies.[22,23] Additional loci identified in early GWAS studies include the *FAM13A* locus which was found to be associated with FEV$_1$/FVC and COPD susceptibility. A subsequent GWAS of the COPDGene Study of 10,192 smokers combined in a meta-analysis with 3 additional studies identified the RIN2 region to be associated.[24] The International COPD Genetic Consortium (ICGC) GWAS included COPD cases with airflow obstruction and controls with normal spirometry from 26 cohorts resulting in a total of more than 83,000 subjects being included in a two-stage analysis followed by a meta-analysis.[25] This led to the discovery of 22 genome-wide significant loci, including 9 which had been previously identified in COPD GWAS studies, 9 which had been previously described in studies of lung function, and 4 novel loci. A subsequent GWAS which included 257,811 subjects from 25 studies including ICGC and the UK Biobank resulted in the identification of 82 loci associated with COPD with genome-wide significance, 47 of which were previously described, with 35 novel associations.[26]

Shared Genetic Loci between Chronic Obstructive Pulmonary Disease and Asthma

The "Dutch Hypothesis," formulated in 1961 by Orie, proposed that asthma and COPD are 2 manifestations of the same disease caused by the interaction of genetic susceptibility and environmental factors including viral infection, air pollution, cigarette smoking, and exposure to allergens.[27] It was hypothesized that the timing of exposure would influence whether the resulting disease was asthma, COPD, or displayed features of both. Smolonska and colleagues[28] searched for common underlying genetic factors for asthma and COPD by performing GWAS for both asthma and COPD and combining the results in a meta-analysis. They identified 3 loci, containing the *DDX1, COMMD10,* and *GNG5P5* genes, with evidence of association with both diseases; however, no single-nucleotide polymorphisms (SNPs) reached genome-wide significance, usually considered as a *P*-value<5 × 10^{-8}. An SNP in *GNG5P5* was genome-wide significant (*P* = 9.96 × 10^{-9}) in the initial, but not secondary replication. The authors suggest that their findings indicated that there is either no common genetic component involved in asthma and COPD or that the environmental components are the dominant susceptibility factors that obscure any shared genetic contribution.

Several recent large GWAS of COPD (ICGC and ICGC + UK Biobank, described above) have identified susceptibility loci for COPD and have compared these results to asthma GWAS findings.[25,26] The ICGC COPD GWAS found that there was no overlap between genome-wide significant associations in COPD when compared with the GABRIEL asthma study,[11] and no asthma or COPD loci had a significant association with the other disease when *P*-values were adjusted for the number of look-ups.[25] However, linkage disequilibrium (LD) score regression revealed a significant genetic correlation between COPD and asthma ($r_{genetic}$ = 0.38, *P* = 6.2 × 10^{-5}) in subjects of European-ancestry, which supports the existence of shared genetic etiology. The ICGC and UK Biobank COPD GWAS found that for 9 of the 82 COPD associated loci (*ID2, ZBTB38, C5orf56, MICA, AGER, HLA-DQB1, ITGB8, CLEC16 A,* and *THRA*), the lead COPD GWAS variant was in LD with an asthma associated variant with a correlation $r^2 > 0.2$.[26] Furthermore, a Bayesian method of overlap analysis[29] identified 9 shared genome segments between COPD and previous asthma GWAS studies (**Table 1**). In addition to asthma, the GBMI analyzed more than 81,000 COPD cases (based on diagnosis codes) and 1.3 million controls.[19] COPD had a high genetic correlation with asthma ($r_{genetic} = 0.67$, $P = 1.55 \times 10^{-226}$). Of the 46 genetic variants associated with COPD, 12 were also significantly associated with asthma (see **Table 1**). However, when asthma and COPD genes were annotated to biological pathways, there were no overlapping pathways between asthma and COPD.

Asthma–Chronic Obstructive Pulmonary Disease Overlap

Several GWAS studies have been performed specifically for ACO, with mixed results (**Table 2**). The first GWAS was published in 2015 by Hardin and colleagues[30] and included 450 subjects with ACO, defined as FEV_1/FVC less than 0.7 with FEV_1 less than 80% predicted (corresponding to Global Initiative for Chronic Obstructive Lung Disease [GOLD] stage 2–4 COPD) with self-report of a doctor's diagnosis of asthma before age 40,[31] who were compared with 3120 subjects with COPD; all subjects were current or former smokers. While there were no SNPs that reached the genome-wide significance threshold of $p < 5 \times 10^{-8}$, a meta-analysis of non-Hispanic white and African American subjects revealed that the SNPs located in or near the G protein-coupled receptor 65 (*GPR65*) on chromosome 14 had suggestive evidence of association ($P = 1.18 \times 10^{-7}$); *GPR65* is involved in airway eosinophilia.[32] The top genes in white subjects, *CSMD1* and *SOX5*, showed suggestive association as well. *SOX5* has been associated with COPD and abnormal lung development.[33] Subsequently, a study in Korean subjects defined ACO (N = 228) more specifically by selecting subjects with positive bronchodilator response or airway hyperresponsiveness (AHR) on methacholine provocation tests in 2 consecutive visits measured at least 3 months apart in addition to having a FEV_1/FVC less than 0.7; 63% were ever-smokers.[34] The GWAS failed to identify significant associations. These 2 GWAS in ACO were likely underpowered to detect significant associations.

More recently, a large GWAS in the UK Biobank included 8068 subjects with ACO, defined by self-reported asthma and spirometry demonstrating airflow obstruction ($FEV_1/FVC<0.7$ with $FEV_1<80\%$ predicted, corresponding to GOLD stages 2–4) and 40,360 healthy controls without asthma or COPD.[35] Only 54% of ACO subjects were ever smokers, so this case definition likely includes a combination of smoking-related COPD, nonsmoking COPD, and asthma with fixed airflow obstruction. Twelve

Table 1
Overlapping genetic loci found in genome-wide association studies (GWAS) of asthma and COPD

Study	Asthma GWAS	COPD GWAS	Overlapping Loci – Nearest Gene(s)
Sakonsakolpat et al,[26] 2019	Trans-National Asthma Genetic Consortium[18]	International COPD Genetics Consortium + UK Biobank	*ADAM19, BTN3A3, LINC01012, ZBED9, OR14J1, FLOT1, ARMC2, ELAVL2, STAT6*
Tsuo et al,[19] 2021	Global Biobank Meta-analysis Initiative	Global Biobank Meta-analysis Initiative	*GSDMB, HLA-DQA1, IL18R1, LINC02676, IRF1-AS1, EMSY, SMAD3, NPNT, ENSG00000285783, LINC01997, FAM227B, PBX3*

Table 2
Genome-wide association studies of asthma–COPD overlap (ACO)

Study	ACO Definition	Comparison Group	Top Genes
Hardin et al,[30] 2014	GOLD 2–4 with doctor's diagnosis of asthma before age 40. 100% ever- smokers. N = 450	GOLD 2–4 without asthma. N = 3120	GPR65[a], CSMD1[a], SOX5[a]
Park et al,[34] 2018	FEV$_1$/FVC<0.7 with AHR or BDR. 63% ever-smokers. N = 228	Asthma: FEV$_1$/FVC $\geq$0.7 with AHR or BDR. N = 731	MSRA[a], RNF144A[a], TAF4B[a], LINC01135[a]
John et al,[35] 2022	GOLD 2–4 with self-report of asthma. 54% ever-smokers. N = 8068	No asthma or COPD. N = 40,360	LOC100289230[b], GLB1[b], FAM105A[b], PHB[b], TSLP[b], IL17RD[b], HLA-DQB1[b], C5orf56[b]

Abbreviations: AHR, airway hyperresponsiveness; BDR, bronchodilator response; GOLD, global initiative for chronic obstructive lung disease.
[a] Suggestive association p < 1 × 10^{-5}.
[b] Significant association p < 5 × 10^{-8}.

additional studies were used for validation, including 4301 ACO subjects and 48,609 controls. Using LD score regression, this study confirmed that there is genetic correlation between ACO and COPD ($r_{genetic}$ = 0.83, P = 3.19 × 10^{-299}) and ACO and asthma ($r_{genetic}$ = 0.74, P = 6.18 × 10^{-44}). GWAS revealed 8 genome-wide significant associations for ACO in a meta-analysis of the two-stage study design (**Fig. 1**). None of these loci overlapped with the previous ACO GWAS, yet most had been previously associated with asthma, COPD, and/or lung function.

OTHER OMICS TECHNIQUES IN ASTHMA–CHRONIC OBSTRUCTIVE PULMONARY DISEASE OVERLAP
Comparison of other Omics Versus Genome-Wide Association Studies

The studies above have all tested associations between germline genetic variants and phenotypes of asthma, COPD, and their overlap. DNA is relatively stable, with

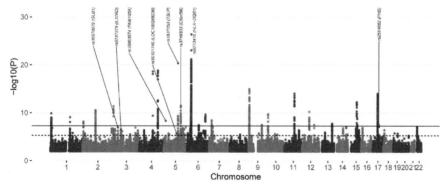

Fig. 1. Results of genome-wide association study of asthma–COPD overlap in the UK Biobank. In the "Manhattan" plot, the x-axis displays the genomic location by chromosome, and the y-axis the –log$_{10}$(P-value) for association testing. Points above the solid horizontal line are considered genome-wide significant (p < 5 × 10^{-8}). The 8 top signals from a joint analysis in additional cohorts are labeled. (*From* John C, Guyatt AL, Shrine N, et al. Genetic Associations and Architecture of Asthma-COPD Overlap [published online ahead of print, 2022 Jan 31]. *Chest.* 2022;S0012-3692(22)00198-2.)

straightforward protocols for collection, transport, storage, and genotyping, which has allowed for the ever-enlarging sample sizes.[36] However, the effects of genetic variants on clinical outcomes can be small, which has necessitated these large sample sizes.[5] Furthermore, variation is largely fixed at conception, and does not respond to events throughout the life course such as aging, environmental exposures, or disease. In contrast, other 'omics measurements, such as gene expression or metabolomics, are more dependent on factors such as the tissue of origin, endogenous or exogenous exposures, and disease status.[6] Therefore, these other molecules may provide complementary information and may have larger effects on clinical phenotypes, allowing for human studies with smaller sample sizes. Yet each of these 'omics technologies will have specific protocols for sample collection and assay, which may be more difficult and costly than DNA genotyping.[37,38]

RNA Sequencing

Whole transcriptome profiling, using microarrays or RNA sequencing can be applied to individual tissue types to identify causal biological pathways and clinically relevant biomarkers. Christenson and colleagues[39] performed microarray gene expression profiling in bronchial epithelial brushings in 2 COPD case-control studies totaling more than 400 subjects. Expanding on their previous definition of a 3-gene signature for T helper type 2 (Th2) high asthma,[40] they developed a 100-gene score of Th2 gene expression using asthma microarray datasets. In the COPD samples, the Th2 score was associated with lower lung function but did not correlate with asthma history. In bronchial biopsies from the GLUCOLD study,[41] the Th2 score was associated with blood and airway eosinophil counts and reduction in hyperinflation with inhaled corticosteroid (ICS) treatment, but no clinical history of asthma.[39] This finding is of significant value as it identifies a distinguishing feature which may identify subjects more likely to benefit from asthma therapeutics including ICS. However, as bronchoscopy is not part of the routine management of COPD, identifying Th2 related gene expression in COPD whole blood is important.

This led to our work, which took advantage of the large sample size of COPDGene to characterize blood gene expression in ACO (n = 120), COPD (n = 793), and current or former smoker controls (n = 962).[42] While there was a minimal differential expression in ACO when compared with COPD (15 differentially expressed genes at false discovery rate<0.1), the comparison of ACO to smoking controls identified 1692 differentially expressed genes that were not altered in COPD subjects compared with smoking controls. These genes were enriched for pathways including Taste transduction, Hematopoietic cell lineage, Huntington's disease, and Oxidative phosphorylation. Of particular note, the altered genes in the taste transduction pathway include several members of the bitter taste receptor (TAST2R) gene family, which are expressed in multiple airway cell types and have been shown to be involved in airway smooth muscle relaxation, contraction, and proliferation.[43]

We found that 53 of the one hundred genes from the bronchial epithelial Th2 score developed by Christenson and colleagues[39] were detectable in whole blood. The blood Th2 score could distinguish ACO, with ACO subjects having a significantly elevated score compared with asthmatics, usual COPD, and smoking controls (**Fig. 2**). Furthermore, the expression score was associated with decreased lung function, higher blood eosinophils, and increased exacerbation frequency. Hierarchical clustering of gene expression values of the genes included in the gene set revealed 5 distinct groups which were not distinguishable by disease status, suggesting that there is a subset of patients with a Th2 immune response who cannot be identified by asthma history alone. This suggests that molecular phenotypes may be

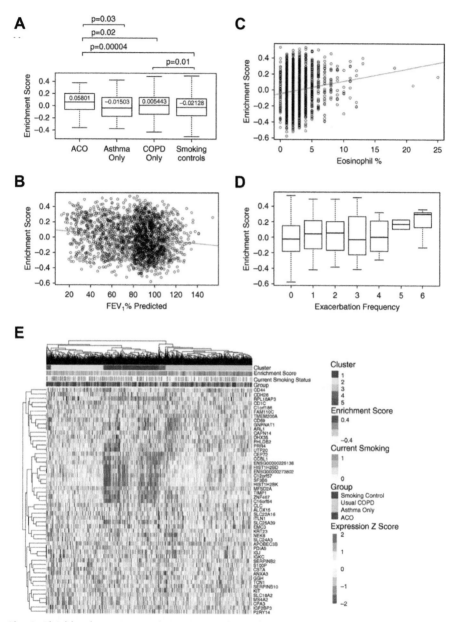

Fig. 2. Th2 blood gene expression scores in the COPDGene Study. (*A*) Higher Th2 scores in asthma–COPD overlap (ACO) compared with COPD or controls (*B–D*) Associations of higher Th2 scores with reduced FEV$_1$, greater blood eosinophils, and increased exacerbation frequency. (*E*) Heatmap of Th2 score gene expression shows 3 predominant subject clusters, which do not correspond to groups defined by COPD, asthma, ACO, or controls. (*Reprinted with permission* of the American Thoracic Society. Copyright © 2022 American Thoracic Society. All rights reserved. Saferali A, et al. Transcriptomic Signature of Asthma-Chronic Obstructive Pulmonary Disease Overlap in Whole Blood. *Am J Respir Cell Mol Biol.* 2021;64(2):268-271. The American Journal of Respiratory Cell and Molecular Biology is an official journal of the American Thoracic Society.)

instrumental in identifying specific COPD subtypes that may differ in clinical characteristics and therapeutic response.

MicroRNA

MicroRNAs (miRNAs) are short noncoding regulatory RNA molecules that can post-transcriptionally regulate gene expression by binding to or degrading target mRNAs.[44] A single miRNA can target several messenger RNAs, often within the same pathway, and thus altered the expression of miRNAs can have significant downstream effects on hundreds of mRNA processes.[45] There is evidence that miRNA expression can be altered in disease, and therefore may be considered as biomarkers. Increasing evidence suggests that miRNAs play an important role in lung development and homeostasis, and miRNAs have been shown to be involved in respiratory diseases including asthma, COPD, sarcoidosis, and lung cancer.[46] To investigate miRNAs in ACO, Hirai and colleagues[47] used an array to profile expression of 84 miRNAs detectable in plasma in 6 asthma and 6 ACO subjects, defined by different criteria in subjects with a primary diagnosis of asthma versus COPD. They identified 9 miRNA with decreased expression in ACO. In a replication of the cohort which included 30 subjects each with ACO, asthma, and usual COPD, 5 miRNA with altered expression in ACO compared with asthma or COPD were identified. In particular, they found that miR-15b-5p can distinguish ACO subjects with an area under the receiver operating curve of 0.71.

Metabolomics

Several studies have previously identified inflammatory biomarkers that are affected in ACO.[48,49] Altered immune response and inflammation can result in a shift in tissue metabolism as a result of the recruitment and activity of inflammatory cells.[50,51] Metabolomic profiling allows for the large-scale investigation of a range of metabolites. Ghosh and colleagues[52] performed global metabolomic profiling with gas chromatography-mass spectrometry in individuals with asthma, COPD, ACO and healthy controls (n = 132 in the discovery set, 104 in the validation set). The ACO definition included airflow obstruction, smoking history, asthma history, or extreme bronchodilator response, as well as minor criteria related to atopy. They identified 11 metabolites that were significantly altered in ACO compared with asthma and COPD: serine, threonine, ethanolamine, glucose, cholesterol, 2-palmitoylglycerol, stearic acid, lactic acid, linoleic acid, D-mannose, and succinic acid.

Epigenetics

Epigenetics describes a mechanism through which DNA modifications can modulate gene expression without altering the DNA sequence. One form of epigenetic modifications is DNA methylation, whereby a methyl group is added to the 5' position of the pyrimidine ring of a cytosine present in a CpG dinucleotide sequence.[53] DNA methylation is associated with gene expression, with gene promoter methylation often resulting in transcriptional repression and gene body methylation resulting in higher gene expression. Studies have found that while aberrant DNA methylation changes can be found in asthma and COPD individually,[54,55] they can also be found in ACO.[56] Chen and colleagues[56] studied whole-genome DNA methylation profiles in peripheral blood mononuclear cells from a discovery cohort of 12 patients with ACO and 6 healthy nonsmokers; ACO was defined by COPD with bronchodilator responsiveness and atopy. They identified 404 differentially methylated loci including 125 hypermethylated and 279 hypomethylated loci. Of these, 19 loci overlapped with asthma-related differentially methylated loci, including hypermethylated loci at *TNRC6B* and *MET* and hypomethylated probes at *DHX30*, *SFXN*, *C19orf28*, and *CLCN7*, while there was no overlap with previous COPD-related findings. In a validation cohort including 22 ACO subjects, 48 usual COPD, and 10 healthy smokers, the *PDE9A*, *SEPT8*, and *ZNF323* genes showed the most significant associations with ACO, with the *PDE9A* and *ZNF323* genes being hypermethylated in ACO compared with COPD and healthy controls, and *SEPT8* being hypomethylated.

Genetics and Omics of Related Phenotypes

The limitations of current definitions of asthma–COPD overlap related to research and clinical care are detailed in other articles in this issue. The previous genetics studies have been hampered by inconsistent definitions as well (see **Table 2**). A common strategy in complex trait genetics is to study intermediate phenotypes, which are quantitative measures related to the condition of interest, such as FEV_1 in COPD or body mass index in obesity.[57,58] This approach has been applied to the genetics of ACO as well. The traits analyzed have generally fallen into 2 categories: airway reactivity and markers of allergy.

Airway Reactivity

Airway reactivity is considered a hallmark of asthma, though testing for AHR is not routinely performed in COPD and therefore does not factor into most ACO definitions. The Lung Health Study showed that methacholine reactivity was associated with subsequent lung function decline in smokers with mild to moderate COPD.[59] Hansel and colleagues[60] performed a GWAS of methacholine response in more than 2800 Lung Health Study subjects. A locus on chromosome 9 ($\sim$900kb from *LINGO2* gene) was significantly associated with AHR; 3 other loci showed suggestive evidence of association. Expression quantitative trait locus (eQTL) analysis showed that 2 of these 4 loci affected the expression of nearby genes in lung tissue[61]: sarcoglycan delta (*SGCD*) on chromosome 5 and myosin heavy chain 15 (*MYH15*) on chromosome 3. Immunohistochemistry in human lung samples showed SGCD to be found in airway smooth muscle and MYH15 in airway epithelium, vascular endothelium, and inflammatory cells.

Our group performed GWAS of bronchodilator response to albuterol in nearly 5800 current or former smokers with COPD from 4 studies. In a meta-analysis, no genes met the strict threshold for genome-wide significance. However, SNPs near 2 potassium channel genes, *KCNK1* (Potassium Two Pore Domain Channel Subfamily K Member 1) and *KCNJ2* (Potassium Inwardly Rectifying Channel Subfamily K Member 2), showed suggestive association ($p \sim 10^{-7}$). In the analysis restricted to African Americans, 3 loci were genome-wide significant, including Cadherin 13 (*CDH13*) and *SGCD*. The latter is the same gene found associated with AHR by Hansel and colleagues[60]; however, each study found different genetic variants.

Markers of Allergy/Th2 Inflammation

In contrast to these 2 GWAS of airway reactivity outcomes, gene expression analysis has been the primary method to study allergy phenotypes in COPD. As opposed to genetic variation, gene expression analysis is specific to the target tissue studied. The study by Christenson and colleagues[39] of a 100 gene bronchial epithelial Th2 expression signature, as well as our application of this score to blood RNA-sequencing in the COPDGene Study,[42] is described above.

In COPDGene, we also showed that COPD exacerbation risk increased linearly with increasing blood eosinophil counts.[62] Receiver operating characteristic curve analysis determined that 300 cells/μl was the optimal threshold, with an incidence rate ratio for exacerbations of 1.32 (95% CI 1.10–1.63). In COPDGene and the ECLIPSE study, subjects with eosinophilic COPD were overrepresented in those with asthma–COPD overlap, using our previous definition of self-report of a doctor's diagnosis of asthma before age 40[31]; however, the actual number of overlapping subjects was low. Using the whole blood RNA-sequencing data, we compared 49 subjects with eosinophilic COPD to 182 with noneosinophilic COPD, finding 505 differentially expressed genes at the false discovery rate less than 0.05, including genes known to be expressed in eosinophils.[63] The 505 genes significantly overlapped with eosinophilic asthma genes from 2 studies,[64,65] including genes predictive of response to lebrikizumab (anti-IL13)[64] along with genes differentially expressed in patients with COPD treated with benralizumab.[66] These shared gene signatures point to common mechanisms with eosinophilic asthma and the potential for targeted therapies in eosinophilic COPD.

Asensio and colleagues[67] performed serum microarray profiling of miRNAs in 40 subjects with airflow obstruction, 10 each with eosinophilic COPD ($\geq$200 cells/μl), non-eosinophilic COPD, smoking asthma (akin to asthma–COPD overlap) and nonsmoking asthma. They found 29 miRNAs and 1 small nucleolar RNA differentially expressed in the comparisons of eosinophilic COPD to each other group. Only 2 miRNAs, miR-619-5p and miR-4486, were consistent in the 3 comparisons, both downregulated.

These 'omics studies of T2 inflammation and eosinophilic COPD have demonstrated some more consistent overlaps in gene expression compared with asthma–COPD overlap, but still limited overlaps in clinical phenotypes. In 2870 COPDGene subjects from the initial study visit, we showed that measurements of total and allergen-specific Immunoglobulin E may distinguish a subgroup of atopic asthma–COPD overlap.[68] In the COPDGene whole blood RNA-sequencing study at the 5-year study visit, we measured total IgE levels in 691 subjects including 76 with ACO.[42] There were 61 genes associated with IgE levels, including *IL1RL1* (IL-1 receptor-like 1), a highly replicated asthma susceptibility gene.[69] Based on total IgE greater than 100 IU/mL, we identified 35 subjects with atopic ACO. Compared with 142 nonatopic COPD subjects, there were no differences in gene expression, likely due to the small sample size.

GWAS for allergic traits including eosinophil counts and IgE levels have been performed in general population cohorts and in asthma studies.[11,70–72] GWAS for these traits have not been specifically conducted in COPD studies. However, whole-genome sequencing from nearly 10,000 subjects in COPDGene has been completed through the National Heart Lung and Blood Institute Trans-Omics in Precision Medicine (TOPMed) program.[73] Genome-wide analyses of total IgE[74] and eosinophil counts[75] have been performed in TOPMed. Several of the significant loci in these studies overlap with asthma GWAS loci, but none overlap with the results of ACO genetics studies.

SUMMARY

Thus far, there are few consistent results across the published genetics studies of asthma–COPD overlap and no genes that can be tied definitively to the clinical phenotype. Genetic analysis has been hindered by the lack of a universal definition of ACO that can be widely applied in large cohort studies. Each study has defined ACO differently and compared ACO subjects to varying reference groups. Most of the studies have been further limited by small sample sizes, though more recent GWAS have included larger numbers. Future genetics and 'omics studies in ACO may serve multiple purposes. Several have already clustered subjects using their gene expression patterns.[39,42] These clusters can be correlated to clinical measurements, allowing iterative refinement of ACO definitions, and potentially a genomic biomarker for disease, in line with the concept of precision medicine.[76] With improvements in ACO diagnosis derived from epidemiology studies and clinical populations, genetic and 'omics studies will be able to identify genes involved in ACO pathobiology, which could improve our understanding of disease mechanisms and propose new therapeutic targets for existing or novel drugs. Multiple 'omics datasets can be combined in network analyses, as genes do not act in isolation to influence clinical outcomes.[7] To realize this potential will require large sample sizes of well-characterized subjects across the spectrum of airway disease, with appropriate biospecimen collection. Similar to the broader field of human genetics, most of the ACO genetics studies have included primarily subjects of European descent.[77,78] As ACO is prevalent worldwide, future genetic studies will need to include individuals of multiple racial and ethnic backgrounds to fully understand the condition.

CLINICS CARE POINTS

- Alpha-1 antitrypsin deficiency (AATD) is a known genetic subtype of chronic obstructive pulmonary disease (COPD).
- Testing for AATD is recommended in all patients with COPD or asthma with incompletely reversible airflow obstruction.[79,80]
- Testing includes the measurement of alpha-1 antitrypsin levels coupled with genotyping or protein phenotyping.

DISCLOSURE OF POTENTIAL CONFLICT OF INTEREST

A. Saferali does not have any conflicts of interest to disclose. C.P. Hersh has received grants from Bayer, Boehringer-Ingelheim, Novartis and Vertex, and consulting fees from AstraZeneca and Takeda.

FUNDING SOURCES:

NIH grants R01HL130512, R01HL157879, P01HL114501, K01HL157613.

REFERENCES

1. Silverman EK, Mosley JD, Palmer LJ, et al. Genome-wide linkage analysis of severe, early-onset chronic obstructive pulmonary disease: airflow obstruction and chronic bronchitis phenotypes. Hum Mol Genet 2002;11(6):623–32.
2. Denham S, Koppelman GH, Blakey J, et al. Meta-analysis of genome-wide linkage studies of asthma and related traits. Respir Res 2008;9:38.
3. Hersh CP, Demeo DL, Lange C, et al. Attempted replication of reported chronic obstructive pulmonary disease candidate gene associations. Am J Respir Cell Mol Biol 2005;33(1):71–8.
4. Hirschhorn JN, Altshuler D. Once and again-issues surrounding replication in genetic association studies. J Clin Endocrinol Metab 2002;87(10):4438–41.
5. Visscher PM, Wray NR, Zhang Q, et al. 10 Years of GWAS DISCOVERY: biology, function, and translation. Am J Hum Genet 2017;101(1):5–22.
6. Hersh CP, Adcock IM, Celedon JC, et al. High-throughput sequencing in respiratory, critical care, and sleep medicine research. an official american thoracic society workshop report. Ann Am Thorac Soc 2019;16(1):1–16.

7. Silverman EK, Loscalzo J. Network medicine approaches to the genetics of complex diseases. Discov Med 2012;14(75):143–52.

8. Hobbs BD, Hersh CP. Integrative genomics of chronic obstructive pulmonary disease. Biochem Biophys Res Commun 2014;452(2):276–86.

9. Moffatt MF, Kabesch M, Liang L, et al. Genetic variants regulating ORMDL3 expression contribute to the risk of childhood asthma. Nature 2007;448(7152):470–3.

10. Bansal M, Garg M, Agrawal A. Advances in asthma genetics. Adv Genet 2021;107:1–32.

11. Moffatt MF, Gut IG, Demenais F, et al. A large-scale, consortium-based genome-wide association study of asthma. N Engl J Med 2010;363(13):1211–21.

12. Collins R. What makes UK Biobank special? Lancet 2012;379(9822):1173–4.

13. Ferreira MAR, Mathur R, Vonk JM, et al. Genetic architectures of childhood- and adult-onset asthma are partly distinct. Am J Hum Genet 2019;104(4):665–84.

14. Pividori M, Schoettler N, Nicolae DL, et al. Shared and distinct genetic risk factors for childhood-onset and adult-onset asthma: genome-wide and transcriptome-wide studies. Lancet Respir Med 2019;7(6):509–22.

15. Johansson A, Rask-Andersen M, Karlsson T, et al. Genome-wide association analysis of 350 000 Caucasians from the UK Biobank identifies novel loci for asthma, hay fever and eczema. Hum Mol Genet 2019;28(23):4022–41.

16. Valette K, Li Z, Bon-Baret V, et al. Prioritization of candidate causal genes for asthma in susceptibility loci derived from UK Biobank. Commun Biol 2021;4(1):700.

17. Han Y, Jia Q, Jahani PS, et al. Genome-wide analysis highlights contribution of immune system pathways to the genetic architecture of asthma. Nat Commun 2020;11(1):1776.

18. Demenais F, Margaritte-Jeannin P, Barnes KC, et al. Multiancestry association study identifies new asthma risk loci that colocalize with immune-cell enhancer marks. Nat Genet 2018;50(1):42–53.

19. Tsuo K, Zhou W, Wang Y, et al. Multi-ancestry meta-analysis of asthma identifies novel associations and highlights the value of increased power and diversity. medRxiv 2021;2021.2011.2030.21267108.

20. Pillai SG, Ge D, Zhu G, et al. A genome-wide association study in chronic obstructive pulmonary disease (COPD): identification of two major susceptibility loci. PLoS Genet 2009;5(3):e1000421.

21. Wilk JB, Chen TH, Gottlieb DJ, et al. A genome-wide association study of pulmonary function measures in the Framingham Heart Study. PLoS Genet 2009;5(3):e1000429.

22. Hancock DB, Eijgelsheim M, Wilk JB, et al. Meta-analyses of genome-wide association studies identify multiple loci associated with pulmonary function. Nat Genet 2010;42(1):45–52.

23. Repapi E, Sayers I, Wain LV, et al. Genome-wide association study identifies five loci associated with lung function. Nat Genet 2010;42(1):36–44.

24. Cho MH, McDonald ML, Zhou X, et al. Risk loci for chronic obstructive pulmonary disease: a genome-wide association study and meta-analysis. Lancet Respir Med 2014;2(3):214–25.

25. Hobbs BD, de Jong K, Lamontagne M, et al. Genetic loci associated with chronic obstructive pulmonary disease overlap with loci for lung function and pulmonary fibrosis. Nat Genet 2017;49(3):426–32.

26. Sakornsakolpat P, Prokopenko D, Lamontagne M, et al. Genetic landscape of chronic obstructive pulmonary disease identifies heterogeneous cell-type and phenotype associations. Nat Genet 2019;51(3):494–505.

27. Orie NGM. The host factor in bronchitis. Bronchitis Int Symp 1961.

28. Smolonska J, Koppelman GH, Wijmenga C, et al. Common genes underlying asthma and COPD? Genome-wide analysis on the Dutch hypothesis. Eur Respir J 2014;44(4):860–72.

29. Pickrell JK, Berisa T, Liu JZ, et al. Detection and interpretation of shared genetic influences on 42 human traits. Nat Genet 2016;48(7):709–17.

30. Hardin M, Cho M, McDonald ML, et al. The clinical and genetic features of COPD-asthma overlap syndrome. Eur Respir J 2014;44(2):341–50.

31. Hardin M, Silverman EK, Barr RG, et al. The clinical features of the overlap between COPD and asthma. Respir Res 2011;12(1):127.

32. Kottyan LC, Collier AR, Cao KH, et al. Eosinophil viability is increased by acidic pH in a cAMP- and GPR65-dependent manner. Blood 2009;114(13):2774–82.

33. Hersh CP, Silverman EK, Gascon J, et al. SOX5 is a candidate gene for chronic obstructive pulmonary disease susceptibility and is necessary for lung development. Am J Respir Crit Care Med 2011;183(11):1482–9.

34. Park SY, Jung H, Kim JH, et al. Longitudinal analysis to better characterize Asthma-COPD overlap syndrome: Findings from an adult asthma cohort in Korea (COREA). Clin Exp Allergy 2019;49(5):603–14.

35. John C, Guyatt AL, Shrine N, et al. Genetic associations and architecture of asthma-chronic obstructive pulmonary disease overlap. Chest 2022. epub ahead of print.

36. Olson JE, Ryu E, Johnson KJ, et al. The Mayo Clinic Biobank: a building block for individualized medicine. Mayo Clin Proc 2013;88(9):952–62.

37. GTEx Consortium. The Genotype-Tissue Expression (GTEx) project. Nat Genet 2013;45(6):580–5.

38. Chetwynd AJ, Dunn WB, Rodriguez-Blanco G. Collection and preparation of clinical samples for metabolomics. Adv Exp Med Biol 2017;965:19–44.

39. Christenson SA, Steiling K, van den Berge M, et al. Asthma-COPD overlap. Clinical relevance of genomic signatures of type 2 inflammation in chronic obstructive pulmonary disease. Am J Respir Crit Care Med 2015;191(7):758–66.

40. Woodruff PG, Boushey HA, Dolganov GM, et al. Genome-wide profiling identifies epithelial cell genes associated with asthma and with treatment response to corticosteroids. Proc Natl Acad Sci U S A 2007;104(40):15858–63.

41. van den Berge M, Steiling K, Timens W, et al. Airway gene expression in COPD is dynamic with inhaled corticosteroid treatment and reflects biological pathways associated with disease activity. Thorax 2014;69(1):14–23.

42. Saferali A, Yun JH, Lee S, et al. Transcriptomic signature of asthma-chronic obstructive pulmonary disease overlap in whole blood. Am J Respir Cell Mol Biol 2021;64(2):268–71.

43. Nayak AP, Shah SD, Michael JV, et al. Bitter taste receptors for asthma therapeutics. Front Physiol 2019;10:884.

44. Bartel DP. MicroRNAs: genomics, biogenesis, mechanism, and function. Cell 2004;116(2):281–97.

45. Pritchard CC, Cheng HH, Tewari M. MicroRNA profiling: approaches and considerations. Nat Rev Genet 2012;13(5):358–69.

46. Alipoor SD, Adcock IM, Garssen J, et al. The roles of miRNAs as potential biomarkers in lung diseases. Eur J Pharmacol 2016;791:395–404.

47. Hirai K, Shirai T, Shimoshikiryo T, et al. Circulating microRNA-15b-5p as a biomarker for asthma-COPD overlap. Allergy 2021;76(3):766–74.

48. Gao J, Iwamoto H, Koskela J, et al. Characterization of sputum biomarkers for asthma-COPD overlap syndrome. Int J Chron Obstruct Pulmon Dis 2016;11:2457–65.

49. de Llano LP, Cosio BG, Iglesias A, et al. Mixed Th2 and non-Th2 inflammatory pattern in the asthma-COPD overlap: a network approach. Int J Chron Obstruct Pulmon Dis 2018;13:591–601.

50. Kominsky DJ, Campbell EL, Colgan SP. Metabolic shifts in immunity and inflammation. J Immunol 2010;184(8):4062–8.

51. Larsen GL, Holt PG. The concept of airway inflammation. Am J Respir Crit Care Med 2000;162(2 Pt 2):S2–6.

52. Ghosh N, Choudhury P, Kaushik SR, et al. Metabolomic fingerprinting and systemic inflammatory profiling of asthma COPD overlap (ACO). Respir Res 2020;21(1):126.

53. Laird PW. Principles and challenges of genomewide DNA methylation analysis. Nat Rev Genet 2010;11(3):191–203.

54. Edris A, den Dekker HT, Melen E, et al. Epigenome-wide association studies in asthma: a systematic review. Clin Exp Allergy 2019;49(7):953–68.

55. Qiu W, Baccarelli A, Carey VJ, et al. Variable DNA methylation is associated with chronic obstructive pulmonary disease and lung function. Am J Respir Crit Care Med 2012;185(4):373–81.

56. Chen YC, Tsai YH, Wang CC, et al. Epigenome-wide association study on asthma and chronic obstructive pulmonary disease overlap reveals aberrant DNA methylations related to clinical phenotypes. Sci Rep 2021;11(1):5022.

57. Shrine N, Guyatt AL, Erzurumluoglu AM, et al. New genetic signals for lung function highlight pathways and chronic obstructive pulmonary disease associations across multiple ancestries. Nat Genet 2019;51(3):481–93.

58. Yengo L, Sidorenko J, Kemper KE, et al. Meta-analysis of genome-wide association studies for height and body mass index in approximately 700000 individuals of European ancestry. Hum Mol Genet 2018;27(20):3641–9.

59. Tashkin DP, Altose MD, Connett JE, et al. Methacholine reactivity predicts changes in lung function over time in smokers with early chronic obstructive pulmonary disease. The Lung Health Study Research Group. Am J Respir Crit Care Med 1996;153(6 Pt 1):1802–11.

60. Hansel NN, Pare PD, Rafaels N, et al. Genome-wide association study identification of novel loci associated with airway responsiveness in chronic obstructive pulmonary disease. Am J Respir Cell Mol Biol 2015;53(2):226–34.

61. Hao K, Bosse Y, Nickle DC, et al. Lung eQTLs to help reveal the molecular underpinnings of asthma. PLoS Genet 2012;8(11):e1003029.

62. Yun JH, Lamb A, Chase R, et al. Blood eosinophil count thresholds and exacerbations in patients with chronic obstructive pulmonary disease. J Allergy Clin Immunol 2018;141(6):2037–2047 e2010.

63. Yun JH, Chase R, Parker MM, et al. Peripheral blood gene expression signatures of eosinophilic chronic obstructive pulmonary disease. Am J Respir Cell Mol Biol 2019;61(3):398–401.

64. Choy DF, Jia G, Abbas AR, et al. Peripheral blood gene expression predicts clinical benefit from anti-IL-13 in asthma. J Allergy Clin Immunol 2016;138(4):1230–1233 e1238.

65. Barnig C, Alsaleh G, Jung N, et al. Circulating human eosinophils share a similar transcriptional profile in asthma and other hypereosinophilic disorders. PLoS One 2015;10(11):e0141740.

66. Sridhar S, Liu H, Pham TH, et al. Modulation of blood inflammatory markers by benralizumab in patients with eosinophilic airway diseases. Respir Res 2019; 20(1):14.

67. Asensio VJ, Tomas A, Iglesias A, et al. Eosinophilic COPD patients display a distinctive serum miRNA profile from asthma and non-eosinophilic COPD. Arch Bronconeumol (Engl Ed) 2020;56(4):234–41.

68. Hersh CP, Zacharia S, Prakash Arivu Chelvan R, et al. Immunoglobulin E as a biomarker for the overlap of atopic asthma and chronic obstructive pulmonary disease. Chronic Obstr Pulm Dis 2020;7(1):1–12.

69. Portelli MA, Dijk FN, Ketelaar ME, et al. Phenotypic and functional translation of IL1RL1 locus polymorphisms in lung tissue and asthmatic airway epithelium. JCI Insight 2020;5(8):e132446.

70. Granada M, Wilk JB, Tuzova M, et al. A genome-wide association study of plasma total IgE concentrations in the framingham heart study. J Allergy Clin Immunol 2012;129(3):840–845 e821.

71. Astle WJ, Elding H, Jiang T, et al. The allelic landscape of human blood cell trait variation and links to common complex disease. Cell 2016;167(5):1415–1429 e1419.

72. Chen MH, Raffield LM, Mousas A, et al. Trans-ethnic and ancestry-specific blood-cell genetics in 746,667 individuals from 5 global populations. Cell 2020;182(5): 1198–1213 e1114.

73. Taliun D, Harris DN, Kessler MD, et al. Sequencing of 53,831 diverse genomes from the NHLBI TOPMed program. Nature 2021;590(7845):290–9.

74. Daya M, Cox C, Acevedo N, et al. Multiethnic genome-wide and HLA association study of total serum IgE level. J Allergy Clin Immunol 2021;148(6):1589–95.

75. Mikhaylova AV, McHugh CP, Polfus LM, et al. Whole-genome sequencing in diverse subjects identifies genetic correlates of leukocyte traits: the NHLBI TOPMed program. Am J Hum Genet 2021;108(10):1836–51.

76. Jameson JL, Longo DL. Precision medicine–personalized, problematic, and promising. N Engl J Med 2015;372(23):2229–34.

77. Martin AR, Kanai M, Kamatani Y, et al. Clinical use of current polygenic risk scores may exacerbate health disparities. Nat Genet 2019;51(4):584–91.

78. Fatumo S, Chikowore T, Choudhury A, et al. A roadmap to increase diversity in genomic studies. Nat Med 2022;28(2):243–50.

79. Sandhaus RA, Turino G, Brantly ML, et al. The diagnosis and management of alpha-1 antitrypsin deficiency in the adult. Chronic Obstr Pulm Dis 2016;3(3): 668–82.

80. Miravitlles M, Dirksen A, Ferrarotti I, et al. European respiratory society statement: diagnosis and treatment of pulmonary disease in alpha1-antitrypsin deficiency. Eur Respir J 2017;50(5):1700610.

The Physiology of Asthma-Chronic Obstructive Pulmonary Disease Overlap

David A. Kaminsky, MD[a],*, Charles G. Irvin, PhD[b]

KEYWORDS

- Asthma • COPD • Asthma-COPD overlap • Physiology • Pulmonary function tests

KEY POINTS

- Asthma and chronic obstructive pulmonary disease (COPD) share the common feature of airway obstruction and some other clinical and physiologic manifestations, but they are distinct in many ways.
- When asthma and COPD overlap, it is difficult to distinguish overlap from the individual components.
- Spirometry and the response to bronchodilator are the key tests to help diagnose asthma, COPD, and asthma-COPD overlap.
- Other tests, including lung volumes, diffusing capacity for carbon monoxide, response to bronchial challenge, and oscillometry, may help distinguish asthma, COPD, and asthma-COPD overlap.

INTRODUCTION

Asthma and chronic obstructive pulmonary disease (COPD) are both characterized by airway obstruction, which is defined by spirometry as a low ratio of forced expiratory volume in one second (FEV_1)/forced vital capacity (FVC) or FEV_1/FVC. Besides this common physiologic abnormality, both diseases can exhibit the same respiratory symptoms, which include cough, shortness of breath, chest tightness, wheezing, and dyspnea on exertion. However, asthma and COPD differ in many respects related to underlying causes, mechanism of airway obstruction, pattern and progression of symptoms, and response to therapy. It remains unclear whether there is a unique physiologic phenotype for the patient when both diseases coexist. To better understand asthma, COPD, and then the overlap of the two, the authors describe the

[a] Pulmonary and Critical Care Medicine, University of Vermont Larner College of Medicine, Given D213, 89 Beaumont Avenue, Burlington, VT 05405, USA; [b] Pulmonary and Critical Care Medicine, University of Vermont Larner College of Medicine, HSRF 226, 149 Beaumont Avenue, Burlington, VT 05405, USA
* Corresponding author.
E-mail address: David.kaminsky@med.uvm.edu

Immunol Allergy Clin N Am 42 (2022) 575–589
https://doi.org/10.1016/j.iac.2022.04.001
0889-8561/22/© 2022 Elsevier Inc. All rights reserved.
immunology.theclinics.com

physiologic features of asthma and COPD and highlight what is currently known about lung physiology when asthma and COPD overlap in an individual patient (**Table 1**).

DISCUSSION
Asthma

Asthma is a lung disease characterized by airway inflammation that results in airway narrowing and airways hyperresponsiveness (AHR), with resulting episodic symptoms of cough, wheezing, shortness of breath, or chest tightness.[1] The airway narrowing of asthma is related to both bronchial constriction from airway smooth muscle contraction as well as airway lumen narrowing from airway wall inflammation, remodeling, and edema.[2,3] Airway smooth muscle constriction is usually responsive to bronchodilator therapy such that asthma is classically described as having "reversible" airway obstruction. Although people with asthma typically have a significant bronchodilator response (BDR),[4] they may or may not fully reverse the underlying obstruction, especially if the disease is severe, long-standing, or suboptimally managed.[5,6] When measured by spirometry, airway obstruction in asthma is demonstrated by FEV_1/FVC below the lower limit of normal for the corresponding healthy reference population.[7] A significant BDR is defined as a postbronchodilator increase over baseline in either FEV_1 or FVC by 12% and 200 mL.[7] Another pathophysiological feature of airway obstruction, when present and especially as the disease progresses, is air trapping as measured by an elevated residual volume (RV) and hyperinflation as measured by an elevated functional residual capacity (FRC).[8] Total lung capacity (TLC) in asthma is usually normal, although it may be elevated in some circumstances. Gas exchange in asthma may be altered, but this is usually due to problems with matching of ventilation and perfusion and not due to alveolar-capillary membrane dysfunction[9]; hence, the diffusing capacity of the lung for carbon monoxide (D_LCO) is usually normal. Occasionally the D_LCO in asthma is reported to be elevated,[10] which may relate to shifts of intrathoracic blood volume.[11] Important details related to these general physiologic findings in asthma are discussed later.

The meaning of a low forced expiratory volume in one second

A common misconception is that a low FEV_1 is solely the result of airway narrowing. In fact, the fall in FEV_1 is largely the result of the fall in FVC due to an increase in RV, which is reflected by the tight correlation of FVC and FEV_1 in asthma, that is, as the FEV1 decreases, so too does the FVC.[12,13] As patients with asthma often display a significant BDR, this suggests that the improvement in FEV1 is due to not only relaxation of airway smooth muscle, but also a decrease in RV from less overall obstruction, which allows for better lung emptying on exhalation. Those patients who manifest a predominant decrease in RV after bronchodilator have been termed volume responders, whereas those who respond with changes in FEV_1 or the FEV_1/FVC have been referred to as flow responders.[14] Patients who exhibit a volume response (decrease in FVC) are likely to be obese, more severe, and require oral steroid therapy.[15,16]

Determinants of maximal expiratory flow

Maximal expiratory airflow is most commonly thought to be related to underlying increased airway resistance, but it is also determined by the static elastic recoil driving pressure for airflow.[3] Elastic recoil in patients with asthma is usually reported as being normal, but several studies have demonstrated that some patients with asthma exhibit reduced recoil[17,18] and, moreover, can experience a rapid decrease in driving pressure.[19–21] Decreased elastic recoil would explain decreases in maximal airflow and, in such a case, is similar to COPD (see later discussion). Although decreased elastic

Table 1
Physiologic features of asthma, chronic obstructive pulmonary disease, and asthma-chronic obstructive pulmonary disease overlap

Physiologic Assessment	Asthma	COPD	ACO
Airflow Obstruction	+ (variable)	+	+ (by definition)
Bronchodilator responsiveness	+/−	+/−	+ (by definition)
Airway hyperresponsiveness	++	+	+
Hyperinflation	+	++	+ to ++
Loss of elastic recoil	(sometimes)	+ (emphysema)	?
Ventilation heterogeneity	+	+	?
DLCO	Normal or ↑	Normal or ↓ (emphysema)	Normal or ↓
Abnormal oscillometry	+	+	?

+, usually present; ++, prominent; +/−, variably present; −, absent; ?, unknown.
Modified from Irvin CG, Kaminsky DA. Chapter 5: Pathophysiology of Asthma, COPD and the Overlap. In: Bernstein JA, Boulet LP, Wechsler ME, eds. Asthma, COPD, and Overlap: A Case-Based Overview of Similarities and Differences. 1st ed. CRC Press; 2018. p,58.

recoil can be significant, it is usually not as profound, especially at high lung volumes (TLC), as the decrease in recoil observed in patients with emphysema.[4] Even some healthy individuals have been found to have intrinsically low elastic recoil,[21] but how this affects acquisition of a low and/or unresponsive FEV_1 is unknown.

Bronchodilator responsiveness

Not all people with asthma have a significant BDR; this may be due in part to remodeling of the airway[22] or reduced elastic recoil described in some patients with persistent airflow obstruction and asthma.[17] Defining a significant BDR and relating it to relevant clinical manifestations of asthma is unclear,[23] but a higher BDR generally correlates with worse asthma control.[24–26]

Airway hyperresponsiveness

AHR was at one time considered to be the *sine qua non* for asthma.[27] AHR is an exaggerated response to a specific (eg, allergen and others) or nonspecific trigger (eg, cold, exercise, and so forth) that normally would not worsen lung function and explains much of the variation in asthma symptoms.[15] AHR is classified either as direct, meaning acting directly on airway smooth muscle (ASM) (eg, using methacholine), or indirect, meaning indirectly stimulating ASM through an inflammatory mechanism (eg, using exercise or mannitol).[28] Direct challenges are thought to be more sensitive but less specific for asthma, as AHR due to bronchoconstriction of ASM can be seen in situations other than asthma (eg, atopy). Several studies have shown that AHR is not a stable phenotype because it is responsive to treatment and exhibits substantial variability, which especially depends on exposure to irritant and/or antigenic triggers.[29–31] Nevertheless, clinical studies that target AHR as an outcome measure have demonstrated that this approach can be more effective than traditional methods for assessing asthma improvement.[15,32] One interesting phenomenon is that not all asthmatics are hyperresponsive to all bronchial challenge modalities (eg, direct vs indirect challenges), suggesting AHR can be used for more detailed phenotyping.[15,30]

Ventilation heterogeneity

An important physiologic abnormality in asthma is ventilation heterogeneity, reflecting the unevenness of time constants throughout the lung.[3] This finding is thought to be due to uneven airway narrowing, particularly in the more peripheral airways, from heterogenous airway constriction, inflammation, and remodeling in both an axial and parallel distribution. Ventilation heterogeneity contributes to AHR[33–36] and poor quality of life[37] and thus is an important mechanism of symptoms in asthma.[3]

Variability of lung function over time

Periodicity of airflow limitation and symptoms are defining asthma characteristics and represent the periodic/effervescent nature of the disease. Patients demonstrate marked variability in lung function (eg, peak flow) that can fluctuate hour-to-hour, day to night, in response to triggers, and by season, making diagnosis and investigations of the mechanisms difficult. Further complicating the problem, patients can have little or no detectable functional abnormalities between bouts of asthma.[38] Longer term trends in fluctuation of lung function over time may be useful for predicting the course of asthma.[39] Unfortunately, there is no consensus as to how best to measure periodicity of airflow limitation.[32] This one feature is perhaps the most distinctive aspect of the patient with asthma. Whether or not patients with asthma-chronic obstructive pulmonary disease overlap (ACO) exhibit this degree of variability has not been studied.

Chronic Obstructive Pulmonary Disease

COPD has many similarities to asthma but some significant differences.[13] Airway obstruction forms a central part of the diagnosis and assessment of the patient with COPD.[40,41] The current definition of airflow obstruction in COPD is based on the Global Initiative for Chronic Obstructive Lung Disease (GOLD) statement that defines airflow obstruction as a postbronchodilator FEV_1/FVC of less than 0.70.[42] However, it is important to point out that although this is the current definition of airway obstruction in the context of COPD, airway obstruction per se may be more accurately defined by FEV_1/FVC less than the lower limit of normal, which is conventionally defined as the fifth percentile and corresponds to a z-score of -1.64 (where the z-score represents the number of standard deviations a value is from the mean).[7] Using this definition takes into account that $FEV1_1/FVC$ naturally decreases with age, thus avoiding overdiagnosis of airway obstruction in older people (>50 year old) and underdiagnosis of airway obstruction in younger people (<40 year old).[43] This may be particularly relevant to diagnosing obstruction in patients with asthma, who tend to be younger and therefore may be missed if using only a fixed cutoff of 0.70 for FEV_1/FVC to diagnose airflow obstruction.

The meaning of a low forced expiratory volume in one second

Similar to asthma, a decrease in FEV_1 in a patient with COPD is not pathognomonic for any specific physiologic alterations, and the decrease in FEV_1 is associated with the decrease in FVC.[44–46] The decrease in FEV_1 in a patient with COPD reflects airway obstruction, especially in the case of bronchitis where there is a loss of lung volume, and dynamic closure of airways, as the transmural pressure increases during expiration.[47,48] Pathologically there is a loss of parenchymal structure adjacent to the airway with resultant loss of anatomic connections between airways and surrounding lung parenchyma, particularly evident in the lung periphery.[49] The resulting loss of elastic recoil in these regions contributes to airway obstruction by reducing the tethering forces that maintain airway patency, thus allowing enhanced narrowing of the airway during exhalation. This dynamic collapse of the airways in some patients with COPD can be quite striking. The loss of airflow during progression of COPD is a mixed process of airway occlusion, loss of communicating volume, air trapping, and loss of static elastic recoil.[50] Without careful, detailed lung function assessments that include placement of an esophageal balloon, which is beyond the capabilities of all but a few laboratories, the exact nature of the loss of lung function remains unclear.[50]

Changes in lung volumes

As with asthma, airway obstruction results in similar physiologic changes in lung volumes including air trapping (elevated RV) and hyperinflation (elevated FRC). Unlike in asthma, patients with COPD who have a substantial component of emphysema may demonstrate a significantly elevated TLC, which reflects lung overdistention from loss of elastic recoil allowing inspiratory muscle force to achieve an overall higher lung volume at peak inspiration.[4]

Bronchodilator responsiveness

Bronchodilator responsiveness in patients with COPD is much more common than typically appreciated and may be seen in up to 50% of people with COPD[51–53] and as with asthma, can be variable over time.[54] The situation is complicated by the fact that there is little consensus on the best approach to determine bronchodilator responsiveness.[23] A BDR is often small and usually less than 100 mL even with combined therapies.[55,56] Moreover, there is little agreement on the minimal clinically important difference for FEV_1, which ranges from 75 mL[47] to 200 mL.[32] In one study, the presence of a significant BDR in FEV_1 in patients with COPD has been associated with improved exercise tolerance, less dyspnea, better quality of life, and fewer exacerbations,[57] although when defined by a combined FEV_1 and FVC BDR in another study, patients with COPD had more frequent and severe exacerbations, although less emphysema and lower mortality.[58] Bronchodilator responsiveness in FVC is more common in more advanced COPD and, in one study, correlated with the extent of emphysema and small airways disease.[59]

Airway hyperresponsiveness

AHR is also observed in patients with COPD, and is more common in women,[60] associated with air-trapping and airway inflammation,[61] and predictive of declines in FEV_1, disease-specific mortality, and all-cause mortality.[51–53,62] The mode of testing for AHR is important, as the type of provocation (eg, direct vs indirect) used to assess AHR will result in an outcome that is not the same in all patients.[15]

Ventilation heterogeneity

Similar to asthma, the pathologic process of COPD begins in the smaller, peripheral airways (<2 mm in diameter). But unlike asthma, the lung in COPD is characterized by neutrophilic infiltration and the gradual destruction of peripheral airways and alveolar sacs.[63] As the destruction is usually inhomogeneous, this leads to ventilatory inhomogeneity. For example, patients with mild COPD or asymptomatic smokers demonstrate airway flow inhomogeneity,[64–66] much the same as an asthmatic. Indeed peripheral resistance in both patients with mild forms of asthma[67] and COPD[68] is 4- to 10-fold higher than normal and involves larger and more proximal airways as the disease progresses. A recent and intriguing report[69] identified patients with current or former smoking history with significant symptoms and exacerbations but preserved lung function. These patients had slightly lower FEV_1 and FVC, computed tomography (CT) evidence of airways disease, and limited exercise capacity; as such, the physiology resembled a patient with mild asthma between asthma attacks and implicates physiologic abnormalities of the lung periphery. Ventilation heterogeneity is associated with neutrophil inflammation of the lung periphery and exacerbation frequency in COPD.[70] As for patients with asthma, increased ventilation heterogeneity is associated with poor quality of life in patients with COPD,[37] but unlike in asthma, ventilation heterogeneity does not seem to be associated with AHR in COPD.[35]

Variability of lung function over time

Lung function varies over time in COPD as it does in asthma. Detrended fluctuation analysis of peak flow variability has been found to predict COPD exacerbation,[71] similar to data found in asthma.

Low diffusing capacity

One defining characteristic of the pathophysiology of patients with COPD, and specifically in emphysema, is the prevalence of low D_LCO. Patients with mild asthma or bronchitis have a D_LCO that is within normal limits, whereas patients with emphysema show a reduced D_LCO[4] that correlates to emphysematous structural changes assessed by pathology or CT scans. As stated earlier, patients with asthma have also been described with an elevated D_LCO.[10,11]

In many cases, a battery of lung function tests, which includes spirometry with flow volume loops, lung volumes, DLCO, bronchodilator responsiveness, and bronchial challenge tests, coupled with a CT scan and a careful history, results in a clear picture of the distinction between asthma and COPD. The difficulty occurs when features of both asthma and COPD coexist.

Physiologic Features of Patients with Asthma-Chronic Obstructive Pulmomary Disease Overlap

It is important to emphasize the fact that there is no universally accepted definition, criteria, or even terminology for describing patients with an asthma-COPD overlap presentation. Moreover, the most recent GOLD guidelines no longer recognize a specific entity of asthma-COPD overlap.[72] Instead, GOLD 2021 now states that "...instead we emphasize that asthma and COPD are different disorders, although they may share some common traits and clinical features...."[72] The new GOLD 2021 recommends a personalized approach to diagnosing and treating the patient who presents with respiratory symptoms, fully recognizing that a patient with COPD may have some features of asthma. In such cases, the treatment paradigm should be one that follows current asthma guidelines with an emphasis on early use of inhaled corticosteroids.[73] All definitions of ACO include persistent airflow obstruction defined by low FEV_1/FVC and some degree of BDR,[74–81] so these aspects of lung function, by definition, will be present in all patients with ACO. It has long been recognized that asthma and COPD share many physiologic characteristics,[82] so recognizing ACO as a distinct physiologic entity is difficult. For the purposes of this section and given the heterogeneity of overlap patients, we will consider the following pathophysiologic manifestations of ACO (see **Table 1**). The major limitation to any discussion of ACO is the paucity of studies that were specifically designed to assess ACO and studies investigating ACO patients that contain lung function measurements that extend beyond basic spirometry.

The meaning of a low forced expiratory volume in one second

The FEV_1 in patients with ACO is typically less than in those with asthma but greater than or similar to those with COPD.[77,83] As previously reviewed,[84] the FEV_1 of patients who are either asthmatics or asthmatics with COPD features shows a remarkable consistency of spirometric impairment, ranging from 60% to 66% predicted and most report a long duration of asthma or asthmalike symptoms. It is well appreciated that poorly controlled and poorly treated asthma leads to fixed airflow limitation.[85,86] The most common assumption is that chronic uncontrolled asthma leads to airway remodeling that is the root cause for the permanent decreases of FEV_1.[2,22] Alternatively, the loss or persistent loss of elastic recoil, especially if coupled with airway fibrosis, would contribute to the significant loss of FEV_1 in this group in some, in a yet, undefined synergistic fashion. Loss of recoil despite no apparent emphysema on CT imaging has been described in one small study of patients with ACO.[87]

Could ACO be related to early life severe asthma? Children with severe asthma in early life often have reduced lung function at adulthood that does not respond to bronchodilators. Indeed, early life asthma leads to a profound increase in the odds (35-fold) for COPD.[88] Early onset asthma also leads to accelerated decline in lung function, which in time would manifest as ACO, as the patient would be expected to present with fixed airflow limitation.[89] Some studies have shown similar rates of decline in lung function over time in asthma, COPD, and ACO.[90,91] Other studies have demonstrated a slower rate of decline in lung function (FEV_1) in patients with ACO[92] or early onset asthma and ACO[93] compared with those with COPD; however, in data from the Copenhagen Heart study, the greatest decline was seen in patients with late-onset asthma and ACO compared with those with early onset asthma and ACO and those with COPD or healthy lungs.[93]

Could ACO be related to accelerated loss of lung function with age? Lung function declines with age but it does so in a variable fashion.[94] Moreover, in a patient with an overlay of asthma and COPD there is an acceleration of this decrease with age.[95–97] Interestingly, although most studies of ACO report that patients are older than those with asthma (but younger than those with COPD[74]), surprisingly little is known about the confounding effects of aging on the lung in the context of disease other than the resultant fixed loss of FEV_1 that fails to respond to treatment.[98]

Bronchodilator responsiveness

The most frequently used criteria used for BDR are 12% and 200 mL but it must be recognized that this standard was a compromise between 10% and 15%.[7] A BDR of 400 mL is considered a major criterion of the ACO definition from a recent consensus opinion document.[99] BDR was more common, as was a lower D_LCO, in patients with ACO than in patients with adult-onset asthma.[100] It should be stressed that BDR is not helpful in distinguishing asthma from COPD nor is BDR even reproducible in patients with COPD.[55] As expected, the prevalence of ACO in any population being examined will vary considerably with the definition of BDR used.[101] A lack of a BDR was the most common reason that patients with COPD only, or with asthma and COPD, did not meet the definition of ACO.[102] Nevertheless, BDR remains a central feature of the patient with ACO.

Airways hyperresponsiveness

When measured, AHR is a common feature of the patient with ACO,[103] which should come as no surprise, given that AHR is reported in patients with either asthma or COPD. As there are many mechanisms that cause AHR,[15] those involved in ACO may be driven by mechanisms that cause AHR in either asthma or COPD or something completely different. It is not known whether the patient with ACO will have a positive response to all forms of bronchial challenge. Only one study investigating ACO patients taken from an asthma cohort reported this group to be hyperresponsive to both mannitol and methacholine.[104] The response to mannitol might not be positive in an ACO group that is derived from a COPD cohort, but when measured, several studies of patients with ACO show AHR to methacholine.[104,105] In the study by De Marco and colleagues,[105] there was a greater prevalence of AHR to methacholine among patients with ACO compared with those with asthma or COPD alone. Further investigation of the prevalence and type (direct vs indirect) of AHR among patients with ACO is warranted.

Diffusing capacity

Similar to FEV_1, D_LCO in ACO is commonly lower than that of patients with asthma but higher than that of patients with COPD,[106,107] but the D_LCO in ACO has also been reported to not be different from that in COPD.[108]

Other measures of lung function

Patients with ACO have hyperinflation in line with those with COPD[106] but sometimes exceeding that associated with asthma and COPD.[101,104] Parameters from body plethysmography (eg, ΔsGeff, change in specific effective conductance, a measure of airway resistance, and ΔFRC) have been shown to be more sensitive to detecting a BDR compared with spirometry in asthma, COPD, and ACO.[109] Asthma and COPD have been shown to be distinguished by oscillometry,[110] and one study has now demonstrated that oscillometry might be able to distinguish ACO as well,[111] although another study was unable to find features of oscillometry specific to patients with ACO.[106] However, Lu and colleagues[112] have shown that combining a small airway imaging parameter from CT (relative volume change between HU −856 to −950) with an oscillometry parameter (difference in resistance between 5 and 20 Hz, R5–R20) had a good predictive value for ACO. Oscillometry parameters correlated well with FEV_1 in measuring the rate of decline of lung function in ACO as well as asthma and COPD.[113] Clearly more work needs to be done to determine whether oscillometry may distinguish asthma, COPD, and ACO. Beyond measurement of static lung volumes and oscillometry, exercise capacity as measured by 6-minute walk distance has been compared between patients with COPD and ACO and found to not differ significantly between the two.[114–116]

SUMMARY

Although asthma and COPD share a fundamental underlying pathophysiology of airflow obstruction and similar clinical manifestations, the distinct mechanisms involved and associated physiologic abnormalities may be different. However, when asthma and COPD overlap, it becomes difficult to define a unique physiologic signature indicating ACO (see **Table 1**). What is clear is that relying on spirometry and BDR is not sufficient to distinguish ACO from its components of asthma and COPD. However, further investigation of lung volumes, D_LCO, and AHR, with potential additional studies of ventilation heterogeneity and variability of lung function over time, may give further insight into distinguishing physiologic features of ACO. The relatively new technique of oscillometry may also hold promise in defining ACO as a possibly unique entity. Additional future research into the nature of AHR (direct vs indirect) and structure-function correlations using lung function testing and CT imaging are needed to better define the physiologic signature of ACO. Given the poor quality of life in patients with ACO,[116] and potential implications for diagnosis and targeted therapy, further characterization and detailed physiologic investigation is clearly warranted.

CLINICS CARE POINTS

- Always measure spirometry with BDR in any patient with shortness of breath or other symptoms suspected of having asthma or COPD.
- Consider measuring other lung function tests including lung volumes, DLCO, bronchial challenge to determine AHR, and oscillometry to further characterize lung function to help distinguish patients with asthma from those with COPD and potentially those with ACO.

- The physiologic definition of ACO is not standardized but always includes evidence of fixed airflow obstruction and some degree of response to bronchodilator.
- Measures of FEV_1 and D_LCO in patients with ACO tend to decrease in between the classic abnormalities found in patients with either asthma or COPD, with air trapping in ACO being more in line with that in COPD, but there is currently wide variation in these findings.

DISCLOSURE

Dr D.A. Kaminsky has research funding support from American Lung Association and National Institutes of Health, is a speaker for MGC Diagnostics, Inc., is a consultant for Olympus Corp., and is a contributor to UptoDate, Inc. Dr C.G. Irvin has research funding support from American Lung Association and National Institutes of Health, is on the Scientific Advisory Board for MGC Diagnostics, Inc., and is a contributor to Upto-Date, Inc.

REFERENCES

1. Reddel HK, Bacharier LB, Bateman ED, et al. Global initiative for asthma strategy 2021: executive summary and rationale for key changes. Am J Respir Crit Care Med 2022;205:17–35.
2. Bossé Y, Riesenfeld EP, Paré PD, et al. It's not all smooth muscle: non-smooth-muscle elements in control of resistance to airflow. Annu Rev Physiol 2010;72: 437–62.
3. Kaminsky DA, Chapman DG. Asthma and Lung Mechanics. Compr Physiol 2020;10:975–1007.
4. Irvin CG. Pulmonary physiology. In: Barnes P, Drazen J, Rennard S, et al, editors. Asthma and COPD. 2nd edition. Boston, MA: Elsevier Academic Press; 2009.
5. Bennett GH, Carpenter L, Hao W, et al. Risk factors and clinical outcomes associated with fixed airflow obstruction in older adults with asthma. Ann Allergy Asthma Immunol 2018;120:164–8.e161.
6. Ulrik CS, Backer V. Nonreversible airflow obstruction in life-long nonsmokers with moderate to severe asthma. Eur Respir J 1999;14:892–6.
7. Pellegrino R, Viegi G, Brusasco V, et al. Interpretative strategies for lung function tests. Eur Respir J 2005;26:948–68.
8. Pellegrino R, Brusasco V. On the causes of lung hyperinflation during broncho-constriction. Eur Respir J 1997;10:468–75.
9. Young IH, Bye PT. Gas exchange in disease: asthma, chronic obstructive pulmonary disease, cystic fibrosis, and interstitial lung disease. Compr Physiol 2011;1:663–97.
10. Saydain G, Beck KC, Decker PA, et al. Clinical significance of elevated diffusing capacity. Chest 2004;125:446–52.
11. Collard P, Njinou B, Nejadnik B, et al. Single breath diffusing capacity for carbon monoxide in stable asthma. Chest 1994;105:1426–9.
12. Brown RH, Pearse DB, Pyrgos G, et al. The structural basis of airways hyperresponsiveness in asthma. J Appl Physiol (1985) 2006;101:30–9.
13. Irvin CG. Lessons from structure-function studies in asthma: myths and truths about what we teach. J Appl Physiol (1985) 2006;101:7–9.
14. Paré PD, Lawson LM, Brooks LA. Patterns of response to inhaled bronchodilators in asthmatics. Am Rev Respir Dis 1983;127:680–5.

15. Chapman DG, Irvin CG. Mechanisms of airway hyper-responsiveness in asthma: the past, present and yet to come. Clin Exp Allergy 2015;45:706–19.

16. Gibbons WJ, Sharma A, Lougheed D, et al. Detection of excessive bronchoconstriction in asthma. Am J Respir Crit Care Med 1996;153:582–9.

17. Gelb AF, Licuanan J, Shinar CM, et al. Unsuspected loss of lung elastic recoil in chronic persistent asthma. Chest 2002;121:715–21.

18. Tonga KO, Chapman DG, Farah CS, et al. Reduced lung elastic recoil and fixed airflow obstruction in asthma. Respirology 2020;25:613–9.

19. Mansell A, Dubrawsky C, Levison H, et al. Lung mechanics in antigen-induced asthma. J Appl Physiol 1974;37:297–301.

20. McCarthy DS, Sigurdson M. Lung elastic recoil and reduced airflow in clinically stable asthma. Thorax 1980;35:298–302.

21. Woolcock AJ, Vincent NJ, Macklem PT. Frequency dependence of compliance as a test for obstruction in the small airways. J Clin Invest 1969;48:1097–106.

22. Kaminska M, Foley S, Maghni K, et al. Airway remodeling in subjects with severe asthma with or without chronic persistent airflow obstruction. J Allergy Clin Immunol 2009;124:45–51.e41-44.

23. Kaminsky DA. What Is a significant bronchodilator response? Ann Am Thorac Soc 2019;16:1495–7.

24. Busse WW, Holgate ST, Wenzel SW, et al. Biomarker profiles in asthma with high vs low airway reversibility and poor disease control. Chest 2015;148:1489–96.

25. Heffler E, Crimi C, Campisi R, et al. Bronchodilator response as a marker of poor asthma control. Respir Med 2016;112:45–50.

26. Kuo CR, Chan R, Lipworth B. Impulse oscillometry bronchodilator response and asthma control. J Allergy Clin Immunol Pract 2020;8:3610–2.

27. Nair P, Martin JG, Cockcroft DC, et al. Airway hyperresponsiveness in asthma: measurement and clinical relevance. J Allergy Clin Immunol Pract 2017;5:649–59.e642.

28. Brannan JD, Lougheed MD. Airway hyperresponsiveness in asthma: mechanisms, clinical significance, and treatment. Front Physiol 2012;3:460.

29. Cartier A, Thomson NC, Frith PA, et al. Allergen-induced increase in bronchial responsiveness to histamine: relationship to the late asthmatic response and change in airway caliber. J Allergy Clin Immunol 1982;70:170–7.

30. Sumino K, Sugar EA, Irvin CG, et al. Methacholine challenge test: diagnostic characteristics in asthmatic patients receiving controller medications. J Allergy Clin Immunol 2012;130:69–75.e66.

31. Sumino K, Sugar EA, Irvin CG, et al. Variability of methacholine bronchoprovocation and the effect of inhaled corticosteroids in mild asthma. Ann Allergy Asthma Immunol 2014;112:354–60.e351.

32. Tepper RS, Wise RS, Covar R, et al. Asthma outcomes: pulmonary physiology. J Allergy Clin Immunol 2012;129:S65–87.

33. Chapman DG, Berend N, Horlyck KR, et al. Does increased baseline ventilation heterogeneity following chest wall strapping predispose to airway hyperresponsiveness? J Appl Physiol (1985) 2012;113:25–30.

34. Downie SR, Salome CM, Verbanck S, et al. Ventilation heterogeneity is a major determinant of airway hyperresponsiveness in asthma, independent of airway inflammation. Thorax 2007;62:684–9.

35. Hardaker KM, Downie SR, Kermode JA, et al. Ventilation heterogeneity is associated with airway responsiveness in asthma but not COPD. Respir Physiol Neurobiol 2013;189:106–11.

36. Lui JK, Parameswaran H, Albert MS, et al. Linking Ventilation Heterogeneity Quantified via Hyperpolarized 3He MRI to Dynamic Lung Mechanics and Airway Hyperresponsiveness. PLoS One 2015;10:e0142738.

37. Young HM, Guo F, Eddy RL, et al. Oscillometry and pulmonary MRI measurements of ventilation heterogeneity in obstructive lung disease: relationship to quality of life and disease control. J Appl Physiol (1985) 2018;125:73–85.

38. Reddel HK. Peak flow monitoring in clinical practice and clinical asthma trials. Curr Opin Pulm Med 2006;12:75–81.

39. Kaminsky DA, Wang LL, Bates JH, et al. Fluctuation Analysis of Peak Expiratory Flow and Its Association with Treatment Failure in Asthma. Am J Respir Crit Care Med 2017;195:993–9.

40. Burgel PR, Paillasseur JL, Janssens W, et al. A simple algorithm for the identification of clinical COPD phenotypes. Eur Respir J 2017;50:1701034.

41. Han MK, Agusti A, Calverley PM, et al. Chronic obstructive pulmonary disease phenotypes: the future of COPD. Am J Respir Crit Care Med 2010;182:598–604.

42. Available at: https://goldcopd.org/wp-content/uploads/2020/11/GOLD-REPORT-2021-v1.1-25Nov20_WMV.pdf. Accessed December 08, 2021.

43. Roberts SD, Farber MO, Knox KS, et al. FEV1/FVC ratio of 70% misclassifies patients with obstruction at the extremes of age. Chest 2006;130:200–6.

44. Coton S, Vollmer WM, Bateman E, et al. Severity of Airflow Obstruction in Chronic Obstructive Pulmonary Disease (COPD): Proposal for a New Classification. Copd 2017;14:469–75.

45. Deesomchok A, Webb KA, Forkert L, et al. Lung hyperinflation and its reversibility in patients with airway obstruction of varying severity. Copd 2010;7: 428–37.

46. Irvin CG. Classifying the Severity of COPD: Are We There Yet? Editorial for "Coton, S. et al. Severity of Airflow Obstruction in Chronic Obstructive Pulmonary Disease (COPD): Proposal for a New Classification". Copd 2017;14:463–4.

47. Leaver DG, Tatterfield AE, Pride NB. Contributions of loss of lung recoil and of enhanced airways collapsibility to the airflow obstruction of chronic bronchitis and emphysema. J Clin Invest 1973;52:2117–28.

48. Tiddens HA, Bogaard JM, de Jongste JC, et al. Physiological and morphological determinants of maximal expiratory flow in chronic obstructive lung disease. Eur Respir J 1996;9:1785–94.

49. Hogg JC, Paré PD, Hackett TL. The Contribution of Small Airway Obstruction to the Pathogenesis of Chronic Obstructive Pulmonary Disease. Physiol Rev 2017; 97:529–52.

50. Pride NB, Ingram RH Jr, Lim TK. Interaction between parenchyma and airways in chronic obstructive pulmonary disease and in asthma. Am Rev Respir Dis 1991;143:1446–9.

51. Postma DS, Kerstjens HA. Characteristics of airway hyperresponsiveness in asthma and chronic obstructive pulmonary disease. Am J Respir Crit Care Med 1998;158:S187–92.

52. Rijcken B, Schouten JP, Mensinga TT, et al. Factors associated with bronchial responsiveness to histamine in a population sample of adults. Am Rev Respir Dis 1993;147:1447–53.

53. Tashkin DP, Celli B, Decramer M, et al. Bronchodilator responsiveness in patients with COPD. Eur Respir J 2008;31:742–50.

54. Albert P, Agusti A, Edwards L, et al. Bronchodilator responsiveness as a phenotypic characteristic of established chronic obstructive pulmonary disease. Thorax 2012;67:701–8.

55. Calverley PM, Burge PS, Spencer S, et al. Bronchodilator reversibility testing in chronic obstructive pulmonary disease. Thorax 2003;58:659–64.

56. Calzetta L, Rogliani P, Ora J, et al. LABA/LAMA combination in COPD: a meta-analysis on the duration of treatment. Eur Respir Rev 2017;26.

57. Hansen JE, Dilektasli AG, Porszasz J, et al. A New Bronchodilator Response Grading Strategy Identifies Distinct Patient Populations. Ann Am Thorac Soc 2019;16:1504–17.

58. Fortis S, Comellas A, Make BJ, et al. Combined Forced Expiratory Volume in 1 Second and Forced Vital Capacity Bronchodilator Response, Exacerbations, and Mortality in Chronic Obstructive Pulmonary Disease. Ann Am Thorac Soc 2019;16:826–35.

59. Barjaktarevic IZ, Buhr RG, Wang X, et al. Clinical Significance of Bronchodilator Responsiveness Evaluated by Forced Vital Capacity in COPD: SPIROMICS Cohort Analysis. Int J Chron Obstruct Pulmon Dis 2019;14:2927–38.

60. Tashkin DP, Altose MD, Connett JE, et al. Methacholine reactivity predicts changes in lung function over time in smokers with early chronic obstructive pulmonary disease. The Lung Health Study Research Group. Am J Respir Crit Care Med 1996;153:1802–11.

61. van den Berge M, Vonk JM, Gosman M, et al. Clinical and inflammatory determinants of bronchial hyperresponsiveness in COPD. Eur Respir J 2012;40: 1098–105.

62. Scichilone N, Battaglia S, La Sala A, et al. Clinical implications of airway hyper-responsiveness in COPD. Int J Chron Obstruct Pulmon Dis 2006;1:49–60.

63. Agustí A, Hogg JC. Update on the Pathogenesis of Chronic Obstructive Pulmonary Disease. N Engl J Med 2019;381:1248–56.

64. Buist AS, Vollmer WM, Johnson LR, et al. Does the single-breath N2 test identify the smoker who will develop chronic airflow limitation? Am Rev Respir Dis 1988; 137:293–301.

65. Coe CI, Watson A, Joyce H, et al. Effects of smoking on changes in respiratory resistance with increasing age. Clin Sci (Lond) 1989;76:487–94.

66. Cosio M, Ghezzo H, Hogg JC, et al. The relations between structural changes in small airways and pulmonary-function tests. N Engl J Med 1978;298:1277–81.

67. Kaminsky DA, Irvin CG, Gurka DA, et al. Peripheral airways responsiveness to cool, dry air in normal and asthmatic individuals. Am J Respir Crit Care Med 1995;152:1784–90.

68. Yanai M, Sekizawa K, Ohrui T, et al. Site of airway obstruction in pulmonary disease: direct measurement of intrabronchial pressure. J Appl Physiol (1985) 1992;72:1016–23.

69. Woodruff PG, Barr RG, Bleecker E, et al. Clinical Significance of Symptoms in Smokers with Preserved Pulmonary Function. N Engl J Med 2016;374:1811–21.

70. Day K, Ostridge K, Conway J, et al. Interrelationships Among Small Airways Dysfunction, Neutrophilic Inflammation, and Exacerbation Frequency in COPD. Chest 2021;159:1391–9.

71. Donaldson GC, Seemungal TA, Hurst JR, et al. Detrended fluctuation analysis of peak expiratory flow and exacerbation frequency in COPD. Eur Respir J 2012; 40:1123–9.

72. Roman-Rodriguez M, Kaplan A. GOLD 2021 Strategy Report: Implications for Asthma-COPD Overlap. Int J Chron Obstruct Pulmon Dis 2021;16:1709–15.

73. Rodrigues A, de Oliveira JM, Furlanetto KC, et al. Are the Effects of High-Intensity Exercise Training Different in Patients with COPD Versus COPD+Asthma Overlap? Lung 2020;198:135–41.

74. Alshabanat A, Zafari Z, Albanyan O, et al. Asthma and COPD Overlap Syndrome (ACOS): A Systematic Review and Meta Analysis. PLoS One 2015;10: e0136065.

75. Leung C, Sin DD. Asthma-COPD Overlap: What Are the Important Questions? Chest 2022;161:330–44.

76. Mart MF, Peebles RS Jr. Asthma-chronic obstructive pulmonary disease overlap syndrome. Curr Opin Immunol 2020;66:161–6.

77. Mekov E, Nuñez A, Sin DD, et al. Update on asthma-COPD Overlap (ACO): a narrative review. Int J Chron Obstruct Pulmon Dis 2021;16:1783–99.

78. Milne S, Mannino D, Sin DD. Asthma-COPD overlap and chronic airflow obstruction: definitions, management, and unanswered questions. J Allergy Clin Immunol Pract 2020;8:483–95.

79. Romem A, Rokach A, Bohadana A, et al. Identification of asthma-COPD overlap, ASTHMA, AND CHRonic obstructive pulmonary disease phenotypes in patients with airway obstruction: influence on treatment approach. Respiration 2020;99: 35–42.

80. Sharma S, Khurana S, Federman AD, et al. Asthma-chronic obstructive pulmonary disease overlap. Immunol Allergy Clin North Am 2020;40:565–73.

81. Venkata AN. Asthma-COPD overlap: review of diagnosis and management. Curr Opin Pulm Med 2020;26:155–61.

82. Sciurba FC. Physiologic similarities and differences between COPD and asthma. Chest 2004;126:117S–24S [discussion: 159S-161S].

83. Backer V, Klein DK, Bodtger U, et al. Clinical characteristics of the BREATHE cohort - a real-life study on patients with asthma and COPD. Eur Clin Respir J 2020;7:1736934.

84. Gibson PG, McDonald VM. Asthma-COPD overlap 2015: now we are six. Thorax 2015;70:683–91.

85. Dixon AE, Irvin CG. Early intervention of therapy in asthma. Curr Opin Pulm Med 2005;11:51–5.

86. Stern DA, Morgan WJ, Wright AL, et al. Poor airway function in early infancy and lung function by age 22 years: a non-selective longitudinal cohort study. Lancet 2007;370:758–64.

87. Gelb AF, Yamamoto A, Verbeken EK, et al. Unraveling the Pathophysiology of the Asthma-COPD Overlap Syndrome: Unsuspected Mild Centrilobular Emphysema Is Responsible for Loss of Lung Elastic Recoil in Never Smokers With Asthma With Persistent Expiratory Airflow Limitation. Chest 2015;148:313–20.

88. Tai A, Tran H, Roberts M, et al. The association between childhood asthma and adult chronic obstructive pulmonary disease. Thorax 2014;69:805–10.

89. James AL, Palmer LJ, Kicic E, et al. Decline in lung function in the Busselton Health Study: the effects of asthma and cigarette smoking. Am J Respir Crit Care Med 2005;171:109–14.

90. Brzostek D, Kokot M. Asthma-chronic obstructive pulmonary disease overlap syndrome in Poland. Findings of an epidemiological study. Postepy Dermatol Alergol 2014;31:372–9.

91. Pleasants RA, Ohar JA, Croft JB, et al. Chronic obstructive pulmonary disease and asthma-patient characteristics and health impairment. Copd 2014;11: 256–66.

92. Park HY, Lee SY, Kang D, et al. Favorable longitudinal change of lung function in patients with asthma-COPD overlap from a COPD cohort. Respir Res 2018; 19:36.

93. Lange P, Çolak Y, Ingebrigtsen TS, et al. Long-term prognosis of asthma, chronic obstructive pulmonary disease, and asthma-chronic obstructive pulmonary disease overlap in the Copenhagen City Heart study: a prospective population-based analysis. Lancet Respir Med 2016;4:454–62.
94. Janssens JP. Aging of the respiratory system: impact on pulmonary function tests and adaptation to exertion. Clin Chest Med 2005;26:469–84, vi-vii.
95. de Marco R, Pesce G, Marcon A, et al. The coexistence of asthma and chronic obstructive pulmonary disease (COPD): prevalence and risk factors in young, middle-aged and elderly people from the general population. PLoS One 2013; 8:e62985.
96. MacNee W. Is Chronic Obstructive Pulmonary Disease an Accelerated Aging Disease? Ann Am Thorac Soc 2016;13(Suppl 5):S429–37.
97. Silva GE, Sherrill DL, Guerra S, et al. Asthma as a risk factor for COPD in a longitudinal study. Chest 2004;126:59–65.
98. Hanania NA, King MJ, Braman SS, et al. Asthma in the elderly: Current understanding and future research needs–a report of a National Institute on Aging (NIA) workshop. J Allergy Clin Immunol 2011;128:S4–24.
99. Sin DD, Miravitlles M, Mannino DM, et al. What is asthma-COPD overlap syndrome? Towards a consensus definition from a round table discussion. Eur Respir J 2016;48:664–73.
100. Tommola M, Ilmarinen P, Tuomisto LE, et al. Differences between asthma-COPD overlap syndrome and adult-onset asthma. Eur Respir J 2017;49:1602383.
101. Barrecheguren M, Pinto L, Mostafavi-Pour-Manshadi SM, et al. Identification and definition of asthma-COPD overlap: The CanCOLD study. Respirology 2020;25: 836–49.
102. Krishnan JA, Nibber A, Chisholm A, et al. Prevalence and characteristics of asthma-chronic obstructive pulmonary disease overlap in routine primary care practices. Ann Am Thorac Soc 2019;16:1143–50.
103. Tkacova R, Dai DLY, Vonk JM, et al. Airway hyperresponsiveness in chronic obstructive pulmonary disease: a marker of asthma-chronic obstructive pulmonary disease overlap syndrome? J Allergy Clin Immunol 2016;138: 1571–9.e1510.
104. Lee HY, Kang JY, Yoon HK, et al. Clinical characteristics of asthma combined with COPD feature. Yonsei Med J 2014;55:980–6.
105. de Marco R, Marcon A, Rossi A, et al. Asthma, COPD and overlap syndrome: a longitudinal study in young European adults. Eur Respir J 2015;46:671–9.
106. Kitaguchi Y, Yasuo M, Hanaoka M. Comparison of pulmonary function in patients with COPD, asthma-COPD overlap syndrome, and asthma with airflow limitation. Int J Chron Obstruct Pulmon Dis 2016;11:991–7.
107. Suzuki T, Tada Y, Kawata N, et al. Clinical, physiological, and radiological features of asthma-chronic obstructive pulmonary disease overlap syndrome. Int J Chron Obstruct Pulmon Dis 2015;10:947–54.
108. Cosio BG, Soriano JB, López-Campos JL, et al. Defining the Asthma-COPD Overlap Syndrome in a COPD Cohort. Chest 2016;149:45–52.
109. Kraemer R, Smith HJ, Gardin F, et al. Bronchodilator Response in Patients with COPD, Asthma-COPD-Overlap (ACO) and Asthma, Evaluated by Plethysmographic and Spirometric z-Score Target Parameters. Int J Chron Obstruct Pulmon Dis 2021;16:2487–500.
110. Paredi P, Goldman M, Alamen A, et al. Comparison of inspiratory and expiratory resistance and reactance in patients with asthma and chronic obstructive pulmonary disease. Thorax 2010;65:263–7.

111. Shirai T, Hirai K, Gon Y, et al. Forced oscillation technique may identify asthma-COPD overlap. Allergol Int 2019;68:385–7.
112. Lu D, Chen L, Fan C, et al. The value of impulse oscillometric parameters and quantitative hrct parameters in differentiating asthma-COPD overlap from COPD. Int J Chron Obstruct Pulmon Dis 2021;16:2883–94.
113. Tanaka Y, Hirai K, Nakayasu H, et al. Annual changes in forced oscillation technique parameters correlate with FEV1 decline in patients with asthma, COPD, and asthma-COPD overlap. Allergol Int 2020;69:626–7.
114. Fu JJ, Gibson PG, Simpson JL, et al. Longitudinal changes in clinical outcomes in older patients with asthma, COPD and asthma-COPD overlap syndrome. Respiration 2014;87:63–74.
115. Hardin M, Silverman EK, Barr RG, et al. The clinical features of the overlap between COPD and asthma. Respir Res 2011;12:127.
116. Miravitlles M, Soriano JB, Ancochea J, et al. Characterisation of the overlap COPD-asthma phenotype. Focus on physical activity and health status. Respir Med 2013;107:1053–60.

Asthma-Chronic Obstructive Pulmonary Disease Overlap
The Role for Allergy

Kasey M. Shao[a], Jonathan A. Bernstein, MD[b],*

KEYWORDS

- Asthma • COPD • ACOS • Inflammatory response • Th2 cytokines

KEY POINTS

- Asthma-chronic obstructive pulmonary disease overlap (ACO) is a distinct disease with increased exacerbations, hospitalizations, and higher morbidity and mortality compared with asthma and COPD alone.
- ACO pathophysiology is complex, involving T2 and non-T2 inflammatory mechanisms.
- Patients with ACO are more likely to have a component of T2 inflammation and have allergic comorbid conditions such as allergic rhinitis.
- ACO shares risk factors and clinical characteristics with subjects with asthma alone, especially in patients younger than 40 years.

INTRODUCTION

Asthma and chronic obstructive pulmonary disease (COPD) are the 2 most common chronic respiratory diseases. In general, asthma and COPD are considered 2 distinct diseases. Asthma is a heterogenous disease often associated with chronic eosinophilic airway inflammation with reduced lung function that significantly improves after bronchodilation characterized clinically by intermittent or persistent respiratory symptoms, including wheezing, shortness of breath, chest tightness, and cough.[1] In contrast, COPD is defined as an inflammatory lung disease propagated by macrophages, neutrophils, and lymphocytes characterized by progressive airflow obstruction with little to no reversibility to bronchodilators.[2] Recently, overlapping immunologic, physiologic, and clinical manifestation of these 2 respiratory conditions

K.M. Shao has no disclosures. J.A. Bernstein – Principal investigator, consultant and speaker for Sanofi -Regeneron, Astra Zeneca, Novartis, Genentech, GSK; PI – TEVA, BI.

[a] Department of Molecular Biology, Princeton University, 7696 Frist Campus Center, Princeton, NJ 08544, USA; [b] Division of Immunology, Allergy and Rheumatology, Department of Internal Medicine, College of Medicine, University of Cincinnati, 231 Albert Sabin Way, Cincinnati, OH 45267, USA

* Corresponding author.

E-mail address: BERNSTJA@UCMAIL.UC.EDU

Abbreviations	
ACO	asthma-COPD overlap
COPD	chronic obstructive pulmonary disease
GINA	global Initiative for Asthma
IgE	Immunoglobulin E
AHR	airway hyperresponsiveness
FeNO	Fraction of exhaled nitric oxide
LLN	Lower limit of normal values
TNF-α	tumor necrosis factor alpha
BA	bronchial asthma
ADAM33	a distintegrin and metalloprotease domain
ICS	inhaled corticosteroids
LABAs	long-acting$\beta2$ agonists
LAMAs	long-acting muscarinic antagonists
SABAs	short-acting$\beta2$ agonists
SMART	single maintenance and rescue therapy
LTMAs	leukotriene-modifying agents
PROSPERO	Prospective Observational Study to Evaluate Predictors of Clinical Effectiveness in Response to Omalizumab
IL-17	Interleukin-17
GWAS	genome-wide association study

have become increasingly recognized, leading to the proposed phenotype of asthma-COPD overlap (ACO).[3] Overall, about 15% to 55% patients with asthma have clinical features of ACO.[4] Both environmental and genetic determinants are known to contribute to the development ACO. Patients with ACO exhibit higher disease burden with increased exacerbations and hospitalizations, lower quality-of-life scores, and higher morbidity and mortality compared with those with asthma.[5] However, it is often difficult to accurately diagnose ACO in clinical practice, as there are no specific biomarkers that differentiate ACO from asthma. In this review, the authors focus on the role of allergy in the understanding the recent advancements in the pathologic mechanisms, diagnostic criteria, and disease-specific therapeutics for ACO.

DEFINITION AND DIAGNOSIS

The Global Initiative for Chronic Obstructive Lung Disease and Global Initiative for Asthma (GINA) define ACO as persistent airflow limitation with a clinical presentation that is associated with features of both asthma and COPD.[6,7] GINA uses the term ACO, and not ACO syndrome, to reflect the concept that ACO is a combination of symptoms of asthma and COPD.[8] However, there is still no consensus on how to define ACO. Patients with a history of heavy smoking and a long-standing history of asthma with fixed airway obstruction and patients with COPD who also have features of asthma manifested as reversibility of airway obstruction can both be described as having ACO, although these patients can present with different pathologic and clinical characteristics. One of the defining characteristics of individuals with ACO is that they have worse disease severity and quality of life compared with patients with asthma or COPD alone.[9,10]

Guidelines used to define ACO vary between countries. Common criteria include evidence of airway inflammation marked by increased numbers of eosinophils with or without neutrophils; airway hyperresponsiveness, which is more severe than in patients with asthma or COPD alone; the presence of chronic airflow limitation similar to COPD; and symptoms of wheezing and dyspnea more severe than patients with asthma or COPD (**Table 1**). ACO is also commonly associated with a previous

Table 1
Clinical and physiologic characteristics of asthma, chronic obstructive pulmonary disease, and asthma-chronic obstructive pulmonary disease overlap

Features	Asthma	COPD	ACO
Airway inflammation	• Predominantly eosinophilic	• Predominantly neutrophilic	• Eosinophilic and/or neutrophilic
Symptoms	• Circadian variability • Triggered by a variety of stimuli	• Constant with day-to-day variation • Exertional	• More wheezing and dyspnea than asthma or COPD • Conflicting data about cough and phlegm
Past history	• Personal history of allergies • Family history of asthma and atopy	• Exposure to noxious particles or gases • Family history of COPD	• Smoking common and necessary for diagnosis in some studies • Atopy more common than in COPD
Lung function and AHR	• Variable airflow limitation • Hyperresponsiveness	• Chronic airflow limitation	• Chronic airflow limitation similar to COPD • Significant BDR in less than half • AHR very common and more severe than in asthma
Exacerbation and comorbidities	• Exacerbations occur	• Comorbidities and exacerbations contribute to impairment • Systemic inflammation	• Exacerbations more frequent and severe than in asthma and COPD • Systemic inflammation • Comorbidities usually present

Abbreviation: AHR, airway hyperresponsiveness.

smoking history and the presence of atopy. In addition, patients with ACO have more severe exacerbations compared with those with pure asthma or COPD.

The Spanish guidelines for COPD (GesEPOC) in 2012 were the first to propose specific criteria for the diagnosis of ACO (**Table 2**). The major criteria were as follows: a high positive change in forced expiratory volume in the first second of exhalation (FEV1) postbronchodilator administration ($\geq$400 mL and $\geq$ 15% increase in FEV1), sputum eosinophilia, or a previous diagnosis of asthma before the age of 40 years. Minor criteria were high titer of total serum immunoglobulin E (IgE), previous history of atopy, or a positive bronchodilator test ($\geq$200 mL and $\geq$ 12% in FEV1) on at least 2 occasions. Using these guidelines, to be diagnosed with ACO, a patient must fulfill 2 major or 1 major and 2 minor criteria.[11] However, these guidelines did not provide a clear threshold for sputum eosinophilia. Other national guidelines proposed similar criteria for diagnosing ACO (see **Table 2**). The Czech guideline defined COPD as a decrease in the FEV1/FVC ratio less than the lower limit of normal value.[12] These diagnostic criteria for diagnosis of COPD were not specified in the Spanish guideline. In

Table 2
Asthma-chronic obstructive pulmonary disease overlap diagnosis criteria

Spanish	Czech
Definite diagnosis of COPD	
Not specified	$FEV_1/PVC < LLN$
Major criteria	
Very positive bronchodilator test ($FEV_1 \geq 15\%$ and ≥ 400 mL)	Very positive bronchodilator test ($FEV_1 \geq 15\%$ and ≥ 400 mL)
Eosinophilia in sputum (threshold not specified)	Sputum eosinophils $\geq 3\%$ and/or FeNO $\geq 45–50$ ppb
Personal history of asthma before the age of 40 y	Personal history of asthma
	Positive bronchial challenge test
Minor criteria	
Positive bronchodilator test ($FEV_1 \geq 12\%$ and ≥ 200 mL)	Positive bronchodilator test ($FEV_1 \geq 12\%$ and ≥ 200 mL)
High total IgE	High total IgE
Personal history of atopy	Personal history of atopy

Abbreviations: FeNO, fraction of exhaled nitric oxide; LLN, lower limit of normal values.
Data from Refs.[11,12]

addition, Czech guidelines proposed a threshold for sputum eosinophils greater than or equal to 3% and/or FeNO greater than or equal to 45 to 50 ppb for a diagnosis of ACO. A positive bronchial challenge test using indirect provocative stimuli such as methacholine was also included as a diagnostic criterion for the Czech ACO definition. The minor criteria between these 2 guidelines remained the same. The same fulfillment is required for Czech ACO diagnosis.[12]

THE ROLE OF ALLERGY IN ASTHMA-CHRONIC OBSTRUCTIVE PULMONARY DISEASE OVERLAP

Both asthma and COPD are inflammatory airway diseases. Small airway involvement is common. However, asthma typically develops in childhood, whereas COPD usually becomes symptomatic in persons older than 40 years. Some ACO diagnostic criteria emphasize, in addition to a personal history of asthma, a high total IgE, a history of atopy, and the presence of sputum eosinophils (see **Table 2**). Although these are all more common characteristics of ACO and asthma, allergy does not have to be present to make a diagnosis of either condition. Exhaled nitric oxide (FeNO), another diagnostic parameter in the Czech ACO criteria, can serve to establish an asthma component, as this biomarker is not elevated in patients with COPD.[13] Patients with asthma and ACO with a high FeNO level often respond better to corticosteroid treatment. In addition, patients with asthma and ACO more often have associated allergic comorbidities such as allergic rhinitis, and their airway inflammation tends to be more eosinophilic. Furthermore, lung function in ACO patients tend to resemble asthma more closely, as it is associated with more reversibility compared with patients with COPD.[14] Current ACO diagnostic criteria are rather subjective and a simple definition of "coexistence of asthma with COPD in patients with chronic airway obstruction" (Japanese Respiratory Society) is definitely not sufficiently objective or quantitative.[8] In fact, Miravitlles and colleagues[6,15] referred to patients with ACO as "asthmatic smokers with COPD." They argued that a never-smoker patient with asthma who has persistent airflow obstruction cannot be diagnosed with ACO and that such patients should be diagnosed as obstructive asthma.[6] A longitudinal study of ACO in young European adults (age 20–44 years) concluded that ACO in young adults is a form of early onset severe asthma with recurrent exacerbations.[16] In this study, 218 young ACO patients were compared with 941 asthma-alone patients and 166 COPD-alone patients. Patients with ACO were found to share more risk factors and clinical characteristics with the asthma-alone subjects.[16] Furthermore, the initial treatment of ACO is similar to the treatment of asthma-alone patients.

ASTHMA-CHRONIC OBSTRUCTIVE PULMONARY DISEASE OVERLAP CELLULAR AND MOLECULAR MECHANISMS

It is likely the development of ACO involves various environmental factors, such as smoking and airborne allergens. It is also expected that pathologic features that play roles in asthma and COPD affect the same structure and cellular components in the lungs for ACO. Enhanced chemotactic cytokines and eosinophil/neutrophil surface adherence molecules may account for the eosinophilic/neutrophilic inflammation in patients with ACO, especially those with a tobacco smoking history. Most importantly, early predominant mixed neutrophil/eosinophil inflammation often presents as the dominant histologic trait later in life.[17] Interestingly, patients with ACO with acute exacerbations had relatively low levels of eosinophils but higher plasma levels of cytokines and chemokines. Kubysheva and colleagues[18] compared interleukin-17 (IL-17), IL-18, and tumor necrosis factor alpha (TNF-α) cytokine levels in patients with ACO (n = 57), COPD (n = 58), and bronchial asthma (BA; n = 32) and found that increased IL-18 concentration in ACO was associated with decreased FVC and FEV1 values, whereas increased levels of IL-17 and TNF-α were associated with impaired bronchial obstruction in COPD and BA.[18] High titer of serum antigen–specific IgE, driven by skewed Th2 responses, is a common sustained feature in atopic asthma.[17] Smoke exposure may serve as a natural adjuvant to airborne allergens. The smoking-related Th1 and Th17 phenotype have been linked to COPD exacerbation. Increased numbers of CD8 T-cell infiltrates are found in the lungs of patients with COPD.[19] A study composed of 109 ACO, 89 COPD, and 94 asthma patients measured serum cytokines commonly associated with systemic inflammation (ie, IL-6, IL-8, and TNF-α), Th2 markers (ie, periostin, IL-5, and IL-13), and IL-17. They found higher levels of IL-5 in patients with asthma compared with higher IL-8 levels in patients with COPD with an intermediate expression of these cytokines in patients with ACO.[20] Therefore, ACO showed an inflammatory process that overlaps with the inflammatory characteristics of asthma and COPD. Interestingly, in this study, IL-13 played a central role in ACO, asthma, and COPD.[20] Therefore, the interplay of these driving forces in asthma and COPD may determine the overall outcome and heterogeneity of ACO. Taken together, recurrent asthma promotes a T2 airway inflammatory cascade of events. Lung tissue damage occurs because of the proinflammatory responses, which may be secondary to epidermal growth factor receptor activation. Subsequently, IL-17 is secreted that activates the airway epithelium to produce mucous as a protective response. IL-17 also induces IL-8, which helps recruit neutrophils and their activity that subsequently attracts eosinophils, macrophages, and mast cells into the airways. These events along with activation of matrix metalloproteinases lead to anatomic damage to the airways, resulting in physiologic changes manifested as increased AHR.

Genetic association studies have identified several disease susceptibility genes that contribute to the ACO.[21] ADAM33 (a disintegrin and metalloprotease domain), expressed

Table 3
Treatment options for asthma-chronic obstructive pulmonary disease overlap

Domain	Asthma	COPD	ACO
Symptoms	Highly variable with time of day and season	Chronic with little variability except during exacerbations	Persistent and chronic but with variability
FEV1 bronchodilator response	>12% and often >400 mL	May be > or < 12% but not likely >400 mL	Variable but often >12% and >400 mL
Primary adjuvant therapy	ICS	Long-acting bronchodilators	ICS
	Long-acting bronchodilator	Alternative long-acting bronchodilator and/or ICS	Long-acting bronchodilator
Step-down approach	Fundamental and often possible when control is achieved	May be feasible though concern for worsening lung function despite symptoms control	Not well defined

in tracheal smooth muscle and epithelial cells, is involved in airway remodeling by suppressing cell-to-cell and cell-to-matrix interactions. ORMDL3 (orosomucoid-like 3) is another gene revealed by a genome-wide association study (GWAS) involved in asthma.[22] ORMDL3 responds to endoplasmic reticulum stress and activates chemokines and inflammatory cytokines that lead to neutrophil/eosinophil infiltration and immune cell activation, respectively. ORMDL3 expression is enhanced by common stimuli in asthma and COPD, including smoking, allergens, and other activators of IL-4α.[22,23]

A study by Christenson found a significant overlap of airway epithelial gene expression changes in patients with asthma and a subset of patients with COPD. They found a Th2-related gene expression response for these groups, which included specific mast cell markers, CPA3 (a marker for increased intraepithelial mast cells in asthma), KIT (a gene encoding tyrosine kinase protein also known as CD117 or mast cell stem factor) and CCL26 (an eosinophilic chemotactic factor also known as eotaxin-3), which are associated with Th2-high asthma and increasing asthma severity. They concluded that there are similar gene processes leading to airflow obstruction in asthma and a COPD subgroup lending support for an ACO phenotype/endotype. They also suggested that their Th2-related gene expression signatures could serve as biomarkers to predict which patients with COPD will benefit from inhaled corticosteroids (ICS) or other Th2-targeted therapies.[24]

CURRENT TREATMENTS OF ASTHMA-CHRONIC OBSTRUCTIVE PULMONARY DISEASE OVERLAP

Identifying effective therapeutic approaches for patients with ACO remains challenging for physicians due to the heterogeneity of this condition and lack of clinical trials (**Table 3**). ICS decrease inflammatory cytokines and chemokines and the number of eosinophils, mast cells, and T cells.

Treatment of patients with ACO with confirmed atopy should include environmental control measures to reduce the total allergen burden that could be aggravating or worsening their condition. Environmental interventions should be targeted to those allergens they are sensitized. For example, if they are sensitized to dust mites, it is important to keep the indoor humidity between 30% and 50%; vacuum carpets 2 to

3 times a week; and place protective encasements over pillows, mattresses, and box spring to prevent dust mite allergen from permeating through. For pet sensitization, removal of pets from the bedroom, frequent vacuuming of carpets, bedding as for dust mite allergy, and placing an high-efficiency particulate air filter in the bedroom and main activity rooms to reduce airborne allergen may also be effective. For environmental control to be effective, multiple interventions are recommended rather than one single intervention, which have been shown to be less effective (NHLBI EPR 4 2021 guidelines). It is also important to treat comorbid allergic conditions such as allergic rhinitis, which if untreated can lead to poorly controlled asthma or COPD.[25]

Although they are considered first-line controller therapy for persistent asthma, their role in COPD is controversial.[26] Therefore, ICS as a monotherapy is not recommend for patients with ACO. Combined treatment using an ICS with long-acting β_2 agonists (LABAs) has been demonstrated to improve FEV1 in patients with ACO.[27] LABAs are considered a preferred mainstay treatment of patients with COPD and can be used as monotherapy or in combination with long-acting muscarinic antagonists (LAMAs) as COPD maintenance therapy. Data have shown that LAMA monotherapy was as effective as ICS/LABA combined therapy for reducing ACO acute exacerbations.[28] Short-acting β_2 agonists (SABAs) bind to β_2 adrenergic receptors, resulting in bronchial smooth-muscle relaxation, increased mucociliary clearance, and inhibition of mast cell mediator release.[29] SABA has been previously recommended for management of an ACO acute exacerbation. However, with the advent of GINA guideline recommendations for single maintenance and rescue therapy (SMART), it is reasonable to use combination ICS/formoterol as maintenance and reliever therapy in patients with ACO similar to patients with mild to severe persistent asthma (GINA, 2021). Alternatively, if patients with ACO use an SABA for an acute exacerbation, they should be instructed to use an ICS concomitantly. In severe exacerbations where these interventions are not effective, a course of systemic corticosteroids can be prescribed. However, caution should be taken using repeated courses oral corticosteroids due to their short- and long-term cumulative side effects. In these later cases, alternative therapies, including biologics discussed later, should be considered.

Leukotriene-modifying agents (LTMAs), such as montelukast and zafirlukast, have been shown to reduce asthma symptoms and exacerbations but are considered narrow-spectrum therapy and not considered first-line treatment.[30] Therefore, some physicians suggest not prescribing LTMAs routinely to COPD patients unless asthma or ACO is suspected.

Anti-IgE (omalizumab) therapy was first documented in a small cohort of patients with ACO (n = 10).[31] Twelve-month treatment with omalizumab deceased IgE and allergic pulmonary symptoms. Patients also exhibited decreased IL-4 levels.[31] A large-scale, real-world study (the Prospective Observational Study to Evaluate Predictors of Clinical Effectiveness in Response to Omalizumab [PROSPERO] study) included a total of 106 patients with ACO.[5] In this study, patients with ACO treated with omalizumab over 48 weeks experienced significant improvement in asthma outcomes.[5] However, currently there are not enough clinical data to support cytokine and inflammatory pathway blockers such as IL-5, IL-5R, or IL-4α antagonists in patients with ACO.

FUTURE THERAPEUTIC STRATEGIES IN ASTHMA-CHRONIC OBSTRUCTIVE PULMONARY DISEASE OVERLAP

ACO represents a distinct but heterogeneous patient population, as they vary in pathologic and clinical appearance. Currently, gene signatures or GWAS studies of well-defined human ACO cohorts are not available.[9] Personalized medications that target specific inflammatory factors and cellular components, especially eosinophilia, would be ideal. Animal models of ACO would be helpful for elucidating immunopathogenic pathways in this multifactorial condition. However, biased Th1 versus Th2 responses in C57BL/6 versus BALB/c mice have resulted in skewed immune responses in asthma and COPD, limiting the number of animal studies investigating ACO.

In summary, ACO represents a unique subpopulation of patients with asthma. These patients often have increased disease severity and poorer quality of life and exhibit more allergic comorbidities such as allergic rhinitis similar to patients with asthma alone compared with patients with COPD. In this respect, patients with ACO have more T2 inflammation and respond better to ICS and other medications used to treat asthma and allergic comorbidities. If they are atopic, elimination of environmental triggers when feasible should be implemented. Furthermore, there should be consideration for subcutaneous or sublingual allergen immunotherapy, provided their respiratory disease is well controlled and their FEV1 is not too low. Consensus international criteria are urgently needed to better characterize this obstructive lung disease phenotype. As ACO symptoms and presentations are diverse, successful disease management depends on an accurate diagnosis. Relevant animal studies and more clinical trials are required to further understand this condition so targeted therapies improve clinical outcomes and patient quality of life.

CLINICS CARE POINTS

- ACO diagnosis is based on nonspecific clinical and physiologic features that need to be validated to ensure the application.
- Atopy is often a clinical characteristic of ACO and if present should be managed with environmental control measures and treatment of comorbid conditions (ie, allergic rhinitis). Allergen immunotherapy should also be a consideration if their lung disease is stable.
- Combined therapy with ICS and long-acting β2 agonists is recommended for patients with ACO similar to patients with asthma, but no treatment consensus exists.
- Clinical trials are urgently needed to identify optimal therapy for patients with ACO.

REFERENCES

1. Gherasim A, Dao A, Bernstein JA. Confounders of severe asthma: diagnoses to consider when asthma symptoms persist despite optimal therapy. World Allergy Organ J 2018;11:29.
2. Raskin J, Marks T, Miller A. Phenotypes and characterization of COPD: a pulmonary rehabilitation perspective. J Cardiopulm Rehabil Prev 2018;38:43–8.
3. Cosio BG, Dacal D, Perez de Llano L. Asthma-COPD overlap: identification and optimal treatment. Ther Adv Respir Dis 2018;12. 1753466618805662.
4. Sevimli N, Yapar D, Turktas H. The Prevalence of Asthma-COPD Overlap (ACO) Among Patients with Asthma. Turk Thorac J 2019;20:97–102.
5. Hanania NA, Chipps BE, Griffin NM, et al. Omalizumab effectiveness in asthma-COPD overlap: Post hoc analysis of PROSPERO. J Allergy Clin Immunol 2019; 143:1629–16233 e2.
6. Miravitlles M. Diagnosis of asthma-COPD overlap: the five commandments. Eur Respir J 2017;49:1700506.
7. Leung JM, Sin DD. Asthma-COPD overlap syndrome: pathogenesis, clinical features, and therapeutic targets. BMJ 2017;358:j3772.

8. Yanagisawa S, Ichinose M. Definition and diagnosis of asthma-COPD overlap (ACO). Allergol Int 2018;67:172–8.
9. Tu X, Donovan C, Kim RY, et al. Asthma-COPD overlap: current understanding and the utility of experimental models. Eur Respir Rev 2021;30:190185.
10. McDonald VM, Gibson PG. "To define is to limit": perspectives on asthma-COPD overlap syndrome and personalised medicine. Eur Respir J 2017;49:1700336.
11. Miravitlles M, Alvarez-Gutierrez FJ, Calle M, et al. Algorithm for identification of asthma-COPD overlap: consensus between the Spanish COPD and asthma guidelines. Eur Respir J 2017;49:1700068.
12. Koblizek V, Chlumsky J, Zindr V, et al. Chronic Obstructive Pulmonary Disease: official diagnosis and treatment guidelines of the Czech Pneumological and Phthisiological Society; a novel phenotypic approach to COPD with patient-oriented care. Biomed Pap Med Fac Univ Palacky Olomouc Czech Repub 2013;157:189–201.
13. Postma DS, Rabe KF. The Asthma-COPD Overlap Syndrome. N Engl J Med 2015; 373:1241–9.
14. Bujarski S, Parulekar AD, Sharafkhaneh A, et al. The asthma COPD overlap syndrome (ACOS). Curr Allergy Asthma Rep 2015;15:509.
15. Barrecheguren M, Esquinas C, Miravitlles M. The asthma-chronic obstructive pulmonary disease overlap syndrome (ACOS): opportunities and challenges. Curr Opin Pulm Med 2015;21:74–9.
16. de Marco R, Marcon A, Rossi A, et al. Asthma, COPD and overlap syndrome: a longitudinal study in young European adults. Eur Respir J 2015;46:671–9.
17. Morissette M, Godbout K, Cote A, et al. Asthma COPD overlap: Insights into cellular and molecular mechanisms. Mol Aspects Med 2021;85:101021.
18. Kubysheva N, Boldina M, Eliseeva T, et al. Relationship of Serum Levels of IL-17, IL-18, TNF-alpha, and Lung Function Parameters in Patients with COPD, Asthma-COPD Overlap, and Bronchial Asthma. Mediators Inflamm 2020;2020:4652898.
19. Barnes PJ. Inflammatory mechanisms in patients with chronic obstructive pulmonary disease. J Allergy Clin Immunol 2016;138:16–27.
20. de Llano LP, Cosio BG, Iglesias A, et al. Mixed Th2 and non-Th2 inflammatory pattern in the asthma-COPD overlap: a network approach. Int J Chron Obstruct Pulmon Dis 2018;13:591–601.
21. Hikichi M, Hashimoto S, Gon Y. Asthma and COPD overlap pathophysiology of ACO. Allergol Int 2018;67:179–86.
22. Wills-Karp M. At last - linking ORMDL3 polymorphisms, decreased sphingolipid synthesis, and asthma susceptibility. J Clin Invest 2020;130:604–7.
23. James B, Milstien S, Spiegel S. ORMDL3 and allergic asthma: From physiology to pathology. J Allergy Clin Immunol 2019;144:634–40.
24. Christenson SA, Steiling K, van den Berge M, et al. Asthma-COPD overlap. Clinical relevance of genomic signatures of type 2 inflammation in chronic obstructive pulmonary disease. Am J Respir Crit Care Med 2015;191(7):758–66.
25. Singh U, Wangia-Anderson V, Bernstein JA. Chronic rhinitis is a high-risk comorbidity for 30-day hospital readmission of patients with asthma and chronic obstructive pulmonary disease. J Allergy Clin Immunol Pract 2019;7(1):279–85.
26. Singh S, Amin AV, Loke YK. Long-term use of inhaled corticosteroids and the risk of pneumonia in chronic obstructive pulmonary disease: a meta-analysis. Arch Intern Med 2009;169:219–29.
27. Lee SY, Park HY, Kim EK, et al. Combination therapy of inhaled steroids and long-acting beta2-agonists in asthma-COPD overlap syndrome. Int J Chron Obstruct Pulmon Dis 2016;11:2797–803.

28. Su VY, Yang KY, Yang YH, et al. Use of ICS/LABA Combinations or LAMA Is Associated with a Lower Risk of Acute Exacerbation in Patients with Coexistent COPD and Asthma. J Allergy Clin Immunol Pract 2018;6:1927–19235 e3.

29. Johnson M. Beta2-adrenoceptors: mechanisms of action of beta2-agonists. Paediatr Respir Rev 2001;2:57–62.

30. Louie S, Zeki AA, Schivo M, et al. The asthma-chronic obstructive pulmonary disease overlap syndrome: pharmacotherapeutic considerations. Expert Rev Clin Pharmacol 2013;6:197–219.

31. Yalcin AD, Celik B, Yalcin AN. Omalizumab (anti-IgE) therapy in the asthma-COPD overlap syndrome (ACOS) and its effects on circulating cytokine levels. Immunopharmacol Immunotoxicol 2016;38:253–6.

Imaging in Asthma-Chronic Obstructive Pulmonary Disease Overlap

Sarah Svenningsen, PhD[a,b], Miranda Kirby, PhD[c,d],*

KEYWORDS

- Asthma-COPD overlap • Imaging • Computed tomography • Emphysema
- Airway disease

KEY POINTS

- Patients with ACO have evidence of less CT emphysema and vascular pruning, but increased proximal airway remodeling (thicker walls and narrowed lumens) than those with COPD.
- Compared with COPD, expiratory CT gas trapping/hyperinflation is partially reversible and sensitive to bronchodilator treatment in patients with ACO.
- The presence of emphysema on CT may distinguish patients with ACO from those with asthma.

INTRODUCTION

Asthma and chronic obstructive pulmonary disease (COPD) are both common chronic lung diseases with considerable interpatient heterogeneity. The current definition of COPD is persistent airflow obstruction,[1] whereas asthma is characterized by variable airflow obstruction that is partially or fully reversible.[2] Asthma and COPD are typically distinguished based on clinical history and lung function criteria, but patients can also have, or go onto develop, features of both asthma and COPD, which has been termed asthma-COPD overlap (ACO).[3] Compared with patients with asthma or COPD alone, those with features of both diseases tend to have worse symptoms and quality of life[4,5] as well as higher risk of exacerbations and hospitalizations.[4,6] Despite their clinical severity, this patient population has been excluded from pivotal clinical studies

[a] Department of Medicine, Division of Respirology, McMaster University, Hamilton, Canada; [b] Firestone Institute for Respiratory Health, Imaging Research Centre, St Joseph's Healthcare Hamilton, Hamilton, Canada; [c] Department of Physics, Ryerson University, Kerr Hall South Bldg. Room – KHS-344, 350 Victoria Street, Toronto, ON M5B 2K3, Canada; [d] Institute for Biomedical Engineering, Science and Technology (iBEST), St. Michael's Hospital, Unity Health Toronto, Toronto, Canada
* Corresponding author.
E-mail address: Miranda.Kirby@ryerson.ca

Immunol Allergy Clin N Am 42 (2022) 601–614
https://doi.org/10.1016/j.iac.2022.04.003
0889-8561/22/© 2022 Elsevier Inc. All rights reserved.

and therapeutic trials due to their overlapping disease characteristics, and therefore a greater understanding of the pathophysiology of ACO is required.

Imaging studies can objectively quantify the underlying disease characteristics of both COPD and asthma, including airway remodeling/obstruction,[7] airway destruction/loss,[8,9] expiratory gas trapping,[10,11] and emphysema.[12] There are also several studies that have investigated the imaging characteristics that distinguish patients with COPD from those with asthma. For example, computed tomographic (CT) studies show that patients with COPD have a greater extent of emphysema and small airway disease compared with those with asthma,[13] whereas airway walls are thicker and airway lumens are narrower in patients with asthma compared with those with COPD (**Fig. 1**).[14–16] Therefore, there is the potential to identify imaging features that are characteristic to asthma and COPD, as well as those with overlapping diagnoses.

DISCUSSION
Imaging Biomarkers of Asthma and Chronic Obstructive Pulmonary Disease

The past decade has seen the development of chest imaging techniques and biomarkers that offer a comprehensive and quantitative assessment of parenchymal, airway, and vascular pathology (**Fig. 2**). Although modern functional imaging approaches, including xenon-enhanced dual-energy CT and hyperpolarized gas magnetic resonance imaging (MRI), can be applied to regionally visualize and quantify ventilation abnormalities in patients with asthma[17] and COPD[18] alone, CT is the most well-validated imaging approach to evaluate airways disease and emphysema. CT imaging biomarkers relevant to asthma and COPD have been the focus of recent reviews,[17,19] and those that the authors consider applicable to the discussion of their overlap are defined in **Table 1**.

Role of Imaging Biomarkers in Asthma-Chronic Obstructive Pulmonary Disease Overlap

Pathophysiological features that are central to the diagnosis of asthma or COPD, and considered when diagnosing or defining their overlap, include fixed/persistent airflow limitation, bronchodilator reversibility, and airway hyperresponsiveness.[20–23] In clinical practice, the presence or absence of these features is objectively identifiable by well-established spirometry criteria, and imaging is rarely considered.[24] It therefore is not surprising that imaging biomarkers have not appeared in guidelines to inform the definition or diagnosis of ACO. An exception is the recommendation by the Japanese Respiratory Society to consider the presence of low-attenuation areas on CT as an objective metric of emphysema.[25] Researchers, however, are leveraging imaging biomarkers to develop a deeper understanding of ACO.

How has Asthma-Chronic Obstructive Pulmonary Disease Overlap Been Defined in Imaging Studies?

Consistent with the broader literature,[26] the definition of ACO is highly variable across imaging studies (as detailed in **Table 2**). This variability should be considered when interpreting the observations presented in the following discussion, and limits our ability to coalesce observations. It is to be noted that the only objective criterion consistent across all studies is persistent airflow limitation, defined as postbronchodilator force expiratory volume in 1 second (FEV_1)/force vital capacity (FVC) less than 0.70. In a subset of studies, qualitative[27] or quantitative[28] CT evidence of emphysema was considered when defining ACO.

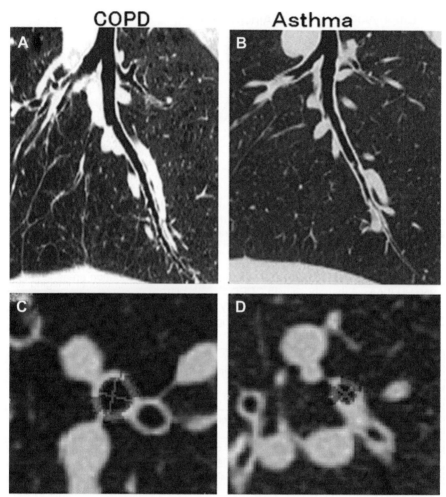

Fig. 1. CT airway dimensions in COPD and asthma. Longitudinal and short-axis images of the right lower posterior bronchus from patients with COPD and asthma. (*A, C*) Longitudinal and short-axis images, respectively, of fourth-generation bronchi of COPD. (*B, D*) Longitudinal and short-axis images, respectively, of fourth-generation bronchi of asthma. (*From* Kurashima K, Hoshi T, Takayanagi N, Takaku Y, Kagiyama N, Ohta C, Fujimura M, Sugita Y. Airway dimensions and pulmonary function in chronic obstructive pulmonary disease and bronchial asthma. Respirology. 2012 Jan; 17 (1):79-86).

Imaging Characteristics in Asthma-Chronic Obstructive Pulmonary Disease Overlap

CT imaging: comparison of asthma-chronic obstructive pulmonary disease overlap with chronic obstructive pulmonary disease and asthma

Previous studies investigating the imaging characteristics associated with ACO have largely focused on identifying the features that distinguish ACO from COPD alone. Although there are some conflicting reports,[29,30] most of these studies report that patients with ACO have less emphysema on CT than those with COPD.[31–33] The most robust study of ACO to date is from the COPDGene investigators.[31] The investigators evaluated more than 3500 participants with ACO and COPD[31] and showed that

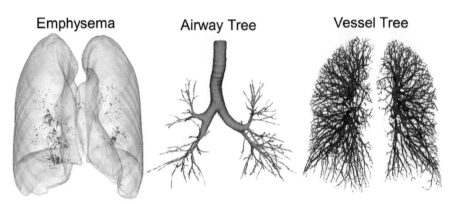

Fig. 2. 3D Reconstructions of CT emphysema, airway, and vessel segmentations. CT lung segmentation with emphysema represented by the low-attenuation areas less than −950 HU are highlighted in red. Segmentations generated by VIDA Diagnostics Inc, (Coralville, IA, USA).

participants with ACO had lower CT percentage of low-attenuation areas less than −950 HU (LAA$_{950}$) than those with COPD.

Another imaging characteristic commonly reported to distinguish ACO from COPD is CT measures of proximal airway remodeling. Patients with ACO have been shown to

Table 1	
Imaging biomarkers of chronic obstructive pulmonary disease and asthma	
Imaging Biomarker	**Definition**
LAA$_{950}$	Percentage of low-attenuation areas less than −950 HU on inspiratory CT images[12]
WT, WA, or WA%	The wall thickness or area of the airway wall or the fraction of the entire airway (lumen and wall) that is airway wall area[57]
Lumen diameter or area	The diameter or area of the airway lumen[57]
Pi10	The Pi10 is the square root of the airway wall area for an idealized airway with a lumen perimeter of 10 mm[58]
LAA$_{856}$	Percentage of voxels in the lung with low-attenuation areas less than −856 HU on expiratory CT images[10]
%CSA<5	Percentage of total cross-sectional area of pulmonary vessels <5 mm[259]
PRM	Inspiration and expiration CT images are registered, and each voxel is classified into normal, emphysema, and small airway disease based on established thresholds for emphysema (−950 HU) and gas trapping (−856 HU) on inspiration and expiration images, resepectively[49]
DPM	Inspiration and expiration CT images are registered, and each voxel is classified into normal, emphysema, or small airway disease based on the continuous probabilities of structural loss and gas trapping, respectively[50]
Mucous score	Each of 20 airway segments are visually scored for the presence or absence of mucous plugs, and then summed[51,52]
TAC	The sum of all airway segments from the segmented airway tree[8,9]

Abbreviations: %CSA, percentage of total cross-sectional area of pulmonary vessels; DPM, disease probability measure; PRM, parametric response map; TAC, total airway count; WA, wall area; WA %, wall area percent; WT, wall thickness.

Table 2
Selected computed tomographic studies reporting imaging characteristics of asthma-chronic obstructive pulmonary disease overlap

Source	Sample Size	ACO Diagnosis	Main CT Findings
Hardin et al,[31] 2014	n = 3120 COPD n = 450 ACO	COPD: GOLD criteria (GOLD stage 2 or greater) ACO: Participants with COPD with a physician's diagnosis of asthma before age 40 years	Patients with ACO had less emphysema and increased airway wall area of segmental airways and subsegmental airways, as well as Pi10, in a multivariable regression model after adjusting for age, sex, race, BMI, and CT scanner type. There was no significant difference in gas trapping between the 2 groups
Niwa et al,[35] 2018	n = 27 Control n = 43 Asthma n = 16 ACO	Asthma: GINA criteria ACO: GINA criteria with >10 pack-year smoking history, and FEV₁/FVC<0.7	The airway wall thickness was significantly greater in both patients with asthma and ACO compared with controls. The airway wall thickness was also significantly greater in patients with ACO than those with asthma
Suzuki et al,[29] 2015	n = 100 COPD n = 40 ACO	COPD: GOLD criteria ACO: GINA/GOLD criteria	There was no significant difference between COPD and ACO for emphysema; however, patients with ACOS had significantly higher WA% and %CSA<5 In treatment-naive patients with ACO, budesonide/formoterol treatment for 12 wk resulted in significantly reduced WA% and %CSA<5
Gao et al,[32] 2016	n = 32 COPD n = 39 ACO	COPD: GOLD criteria ACO: GINA/GOLD criteria	The patients with ACO had less emphysema than patients with COPD, but no differences in gas trapping. The variations in gas trapping were also significantly larger in the ACO group than in COPD group
Kurashima et al,[27] 2012	n = 63 Asthma n = 46 COPD n = 23 Asthma with emphysema n = 61 Control	Asthma: history of asthma without smoking history COPD: GOLD criteria ACO: history of asthma, high serum IgE and airway reversibility, history of smoking (>40 pack-years), and CT emphysema.	The airway inner diameters were narrowed and airway walls were thickened from the third- to the sixth-generation bronchi in asthma (with and without emphysema) compared with controls and COPD

Abbreviations: ACOS, ACO syndrome; BMI, body mass index; FEV1, force expiratory volume in 1 second; FVC, force vital capacity; GINA, Global Initiative for Asthma; GOLD, Global Initiative for Chronic Lung Disease.

have thicker airway walls than those with COPD.[29,31,33,34] Similarly, Niwa and colleagues[35] compared CT airway wall measurements between controls and patients with asthma and those with ACO, and those with ACO had thicker airway walls than controls and those with asthma only. Tanabe and colleagues[36] measured lumen area on ultra-high-resolution CT in a control group of current or former smokers with no history of lung disease, patients with COPD only, and patients with COPD who self-reported a past history of asthma before or after 40 years of age. CT lumen area in the fourth- and fifth-generation airways was smaller in patients with COPD than controls, regardless of age of asthma onset, but only in those with asthma onset before 40 years of age was the lumen area smaller in ACO compared with COPD. Taken together, these findings indicate that patients with ACO have thicker airway walls than both those with asthma and COPD, and greater airway lumen narrowing than COPD, suggesting that proximal airway remodeling may be more prominent in ACO.

Interestingly, despite evidence of increased proximal airway remodeling in ACO, studies report no difference in CT gas trapping measurements between patients with ACO and COPD.[31,32] Gas trapping on CT images acquired at full expiration is thought to reflect remodeling of small airways beyond the resolution limitations of CT.[37] Although COPD is characterized by peripheral airway remodeling/loss, airway remodeling in asthma occurs in both proximal and peripheral airways. Studies show that compared with patients with asthma, those with COPD have increased CT gas trapping.[13,16] The finding that CT gas trapping was not different between ACO and COPD suggests that patients with ACO may have features of small airway disease similar to COPD. Further investigation of small airway disease features in ACO is warranted.

CT pulmonary vascular measurements have also been investigated in patients with ACO and compared to those with COPD. In COPD, reduction in the total cross-sectional area of pulmonary vessels (CSA) less than 5 mm^2 (eg, %CSA<5) is thought to reflect a loss of the peripheral pulmonary vasculature, and is associated with disease severity and CT emphysema.[38] Similarly, in asthma, pruning of the peripheral pulmonary vasculature is associated with asthma severity, control, exacerbations, and eosinophilia, but not with emphysema on CT.[39] Interestingly, Suzuki and colleagues[29] reported that CT %CSA<5 was significantly lower in patients with COPD compared with those with ACO. Although vascular pruning seems to be a feature of both asthma[39] and COPD,[38] this study indicates that patients with ACO have less vascular pruning than those with COPD alone. It is unknown, however, whether patients with ACO have increased vascular pruning compared with those with asthma alone.

The postbronchodilator improvement in gas trapping on expiratory CT imaging has also been investigated in patients with ACO and COPD. Patients with ACO have been shown to have greater reduction in CT LAA$_{856}$ measurements postbronchodilator than patients with COPD.[32] The postbronchodilator improvement in gas trapping in patients with ACO compared with those with COPD has also been measured using sagittal CT reconstructions to quantify various CT measures that reflect lung hyperinflation, such as lung height, anteroposterior lung diameter, and left and right diaphragm height, measured by radiologists.[40] There were no differences in CT measurements between the patients with ACO and COPD prebronchodilator, whereas following bronchodilator administration patients with ACO and COPD showed significantly different sagittal-lung CT measurements.[40] There was also significantly larger improvement in postbronchodilator sagittal-lung CT measurements in patients with ACO than in patients with COPD alone. Taken together, these studies indicate that expiratory airflow limitation and gas trapping/hyperinflation in patients with ACO are, to some extent, partially reversible and sensitive to bronchodilator treatment, whereas in COPD airflow limitation is irreversible.

CT imaging: asthma with emphysema

Although clinical characteristics, such as history of asthma, smoking history, and fixed airflow obstruction, are often considered in defining ACO, there are other features that can potentially be used to characterize patients. For example, unlike COPD in which both airway disease and emphysema contribute to airflow limitation, asthma is predominantly an airway disease. Therefore, the presence of emphysema on CT in patients with asthma could indicate coexisting COPD.

Kurashima and colleagues[27] compared airway dimensions between controls and patients with asthma only, COPD only, and asthma with emphysema on CT. The investigators showed that patients with asthma with or without emphysema had significantly narrowed airways with increased wall area thickness compared with both patients with COPD and controls. Another study by Xie and colleagues[41] showed that while patients with COPD had higher CT emphysema than those with asthma and controls, CT emphysema was also significantly increased in patients with asthma compared with the control group. When the patients with asthma were separated into 2 groups based on extent of CT emphysema, those in the high-CT emphysema subgroup were significantly older, were more likely to be male, had higher pack-years of smoking, had more acute exacerbations, had more upper-zone-predominant emphysema, and had greater airflow limitation than the low-CT emphysema subgroup. A small study of 10 patients with severe asthma with persistent airflow limitation but no smoking history similarly reported higher CT emphysema than controls, and comparable to COPD.[42]

In contrast to the aforementioned studies that used CT emphysema to distinguish ACO from asthma only, Shimizu and colleagues[43] compared CT indices of emphysema in patients with asthma, with and without fixed airflow obstruction, with those in patients with COPD. Independent of smoking history and disease severity, patients with asthma with airflow obstruction showed CT evidence of emphysema that was associated with accelerated lung function decline.[43] Taken together, these findings indicate that emphysema on CT is an important feature in patients with ACO, independent of smoking history, with implications on clinical outcomes that warrant further investigation.

To further investigate the impact of smoking in patients with ACO, Boulet and colleagues[44] investigated patients with asthma with smoking- and nonsmoking-related irreversible airflow limitation using quantitative and qualitative CT, lung function measurements, and inflammatory cell counts on induced sputum. Quantitative CT analysis showed that emphysema and gas trapping were not significantly different between the groups; however, Pi10 was greater in smokers versus nonsmokers. In contrast, the visual emphysema analysis showed higher prevalence of emphysema and higher emphysema score in smokers compared with nonsmokers, but no differences in airway scoring. The analysis also showed that CT airway wall thickness and emphysema were correlated with FEV_1/FVC in the smokers only, whereas gas trapping and FEV_1/FVC were correlated in both groups. This study also showed that neutrophils in the smokers and eosinophils in nonsmokers were associated with CT emphysema and airway structural changes, respectively. These findings indicate that the mechanisms leading to fixed airway obstruction and parenchymal changes may be different between smokers and nonsmokers.

Other imaging modalities

CT has limited resolution, typically ~ 1 mm isotropic resolution, and it cannot provide detailed information related to the components of the airway wall. Furthermore, conventional CT approaches provide no functional information. Therefore, other imaging modalities have been explored to investigate differences between COPD, asthma, and ACO.

Table 3
Summary of computed tomographic imaging characteristics of asthma-chronic obstructive pulmonary disease overlap

Imaging Feature	Asthma	COPD	ACO
Emphysema	No difference relative to controls[60]	Increased relative to controls and asthma[13]	Increased relative to controls,[41] and reduced relative to COPD[31–33]
Proximal airway wall thickening	Increased relative to controls[15,16]	Increased relative to controls,[15,16] decreased relative to asthma[14–16]	Increased relative to controls,[35] asthma,[35] and COPD[29,31,33,34]
Proximal airway lumen	Decreased relative to controls[15,16]	Decreased relative to controls[13] and asthma[13,15]	Decreased relative to controls[27] and COPD[27,36]
Expiratory gas trapping	Increased relative to controls[13,16]	Increased relative to controls and asthma[13,16]	No difference with COPD[31,32]
Pulmonary vasculature pruning	Increased relative to controls[39]	Increased relative to controls[38]	Decreased relative to COPD[29]

Endobronchial ultrasound

Endobronchial ultrasound (EBUS) has been shown to provide useful information in quantifying the thickness of the bronchial walls and their individual layers in patients with asthma and COPD.[45] Unlike CT imaging, EBUS can identify structures within the airway wall, such as the epithelium, submucosa, smooth muscle, and cartilage layers. In a study investigating EBUS airway remodeling measures acquired in the segmental airways in patients with ACO compared with those with severe COPD and asthma, it was shown that the inner layers (ie, epithelium, submucosa, and smooth muscle), which are primarily involved in remodeling, were significantly thicker in patients with ACO than in those with COPD; patients with asthma had thicker inner layers than both those with ACO and COPD.[46] However, a previous CT study[35] showed that patients with ACO had thicker airway walls on CT than those with asthma. CT and EBUS airway wall thickness measurements have been shown to be comparable,[45] and therefore differences may be due to the fact that only patients with severe asthma were included in the EBUS study. It is well known that airway remodeling becomes more pronounced as asthma disease severity increases, which could explain the contradictory results. Nevertheless, more studies are required to compare airway remodeling in ACO with COPD and asthma.

Xenon-ventilation dual-energy CT

Dual-energy CT (DECT) with xenon-ventilation imaging can provide both structural and function information in patients with lung disease. In a study by Hwang and colleagues[30] a visual analysis of the xenon-ventilation patterns was performed and showed that patients with ACO had predominantly wedge/diffuse defects in the periphery of the lung, whereas patients with COPD showed diffuse, heterogeneous defects throughout the lung. Although patients with asthma were not included in this study, the predominant ventilation defect pattern in patients with asthma is the peripheral wedge defect,[47] therefore the findings suggest that the ventilation defect pattern in ACO is more similar to asthma than COPD, and may reflect similar cause. Additional studies that assess the ventilation patterns quantitatively, and perhaps investigating hyperpolarized gas MRI, should be performed to better understand the functional differences in asthma, COPD, and ACO.

FUTURE DIRECTIONS

Imaging Features of Asthma-Chronic Obstructive Pulmonary Disease Overlap: Unanswered Questions

The imaging characteristics of asthma, COPD, and ACO, and their differences, have been summarized in **Table 3**. Although these studies show patients with ACO have more CT emphysema than those with asthma, and more proximal airway remodeling than both those with asthma and COPD, there have been few studies investigating the vasculature and small airways in ACO. For example, studies show less vascular pruning on CT in ACO compared with COPD,[29] but, to the authors' knowledge, no studies have directly compared CT vascular pruning measurements in patients with asthma, COPD, and ACO. Future studies should investigate CT measures of vascular abnormalities, or use dissolved phase xenon-129 MRI,[48] to better understand if abnormal gas transfer is a feature of ACO.

Studies also show that CT gas trapping measurements are not significantly different between patients with ACO and COPD,[31,32] indicating that patients with ACO and COPD have a similar extent of small airway disease. However, it is well-described that quantifying gas trapping on CT expiratory images reflects the contributions of both small airway obstruction and emphysema. Novel approaches, such as parametric response map[49] or disease probability measure[50] measurements, can tease apart the gas trapping contribution that is related to small airway disease. Furthermore, other metrics such as the total airway count[8,9] and the CT mucous score,[51,52] have yet to be investigated in ACO and may provide further insight into small airway remodeling, obstruction, and loss. Future studies should investigate how these novel measures compare in patients with asthma, COPD, and ACO.

Pathways to Asthma-Chronic Obstructive Pulmonary Disease Overlap: Role of Imaging?

There are several proposed mechanistic pathways for the development of ACO that involve the interaction of genetic and environmental factors. One proposed pathway is related to the link between prenatal or early life risk factors and poor lung development or dysanapsis. Dysanapsis, a mismatch of airway tree caliber to lung size, is thought to arise in early life,[53] and poor lung function after birth is associated with worse lung function in adulthood.[54] Importantly, dysanapsis can be quantified using CT imaging, and those with a lower airway caliber relative to lung size are associated with a greater risk of developing COPD.[55] Imaging studies investigating CT dysanapsis could help provide a better understanding of abnormal lung development as a potential risk factor for ACO. For example, such imaging-derived measures could determine whether abnormalities in lung development predispose individuals with asthma to fixed airflow obstruction. However, further development of imaging techniques that provide high-resolution images of the airways without ionizing radiation, such as those derived from ultra-short echo time MRI,[56] may be required to enable long-term monitoring starting in early life.

SUMMARY

ACO represents a unique subset of patients with clinical features of both asthma and COPD. Although there is no consensus on how to diagnose ACO, or if one is required, using the criteria for diagnosis defined by researchers has revealed imaging features that can distinguish patients with ACO from those with asthma or COPD alone. Notably, evidence of increased airway remodeling and emphysema on CT imaging have been observed in those with ACO. However, more clinical research in patients with ACO is required for complete understanding of the disease characteristics, and there are new CT imaging biomarkers reflecting small airway disease, vascular abnormalities, mucous plugging, and abnormal lung development, as well as other non-radiation-based imaging-derived structural/functional quantitative measures, that have yet to be investigated. Although the role of imaging to inform diagnosis and management of these patients is not yet certain, imaging has proven potential to provide a greater understanding of the underlying disease characteristics in ACO, and may therefore identify potential treatable traits to allow for more personalized medicine strategies.

CLINICS CARE POINTS

- Imaging can be used to quantify the underlying disease characteristics of ACO
- Patients with ACO may show increased airway remodeling and reversibility of CT gas trapping/hyperinflation following bronchodilator treatment
- The presence of emphysema on CT may be a distinguishing feature of ACO

DISCLOSURE

M. Kirby acknowledges support from the Natural Sciences and Engineering Research Council of Canada (NSERC) Discovery Grant, the Early Researchers Award Program, and the Canada Research Chair Program (Tier II). S. Svenningsen is supported by the Canada Research Chairs Program (Tier II).

REFERENCES

1. Global Initiative for Chronic Obstructive Lung Disease. Global strategy for the diagnosis, management and prevention of chronic obstructive pulmonary disease. 2021. Available at: https://goldcopd.org. Accessed December 21, 2021.
2. Global Initiative for Asthma. Global strategy for asthma management and prevention. 2021. Available at: https://ginasthma.org. Accessed December 21, 2021.
3. Diagnosis of diseases of chronic airflow limitation: asthma COPD and asthma-COPD overlap syndrome (ACOS) based on the global strategy for asthma management and prevention and the global strategy for the diagnosis, management and prevention of chronic obstructive pulmonary disease. 2014 the global initiative for asthma and the global initiative for chronic. 2014. Available at: www.ginasthma.orgwww.goldcopd.org. Accessed December 8, 2021.
4. Menezes AMB, De Oca MM, Pérez-Padilla R, et al. Increased risk of exacerbation and hospitalization in subjects with an overlap phenotype: COPD-asthma. Chest 2014;145(2):297–304.

5. Kauppi P, Kupiainen H, Lindqvist A, et al. Quality of life and outcomes overlap syndrome of asthma and COPD predicts low quality of life. J Asthma 2011;48: 279–85.

6. Andersén H, Lampela P, Nevanlinna A, et al. High hospital burden in overlap syndrome of asthma and COPD. Clin Respir J 2013;7(4):342–6.

7. Nakano Y, Muller NL, King GG, et al. Quantitative assessment of airway remodeling using high-resolution CT. Chest 2002;122(6 Suppl):271S–5S. Available at: http://www.ncbi.nlm.nih.gov/pubmed/12475796.

8. Kirby M, Tanabe N, Tan WC, et al. Total airway count on computed tomography and the risk of chronic obstructive pulmonary disease progression. findings from a population-based study. Am J Respir Crit Care Med 2018;197(1):56–65.

9. Eddy RL, Svenningsen S, Kirby M, et al. Is computed tomography airway count related to asthma severity and airway structure and function? Am J Respir Crit Care Med 2020;201(8):923–33.

10. Jain N, Covar RA, Gleason MC, et al. Quantitative computed tomography detects peripheral airway disease in asthmatic children. Pediatr Pulmonol 2005;40(3): 211–8.

11. Schroeder JD, McKenzie AS, Zach JA, et al. Relationships between airflow obstruction and quantitative CT measurements of emphysema, air trapping, and airways in subjects with and without chronic obstructive pulmonary disease. Am J Roentgenol 2013;201(3):W460–70.

12. Muller NL, Staples CA, Miller RR, et al. Density mask". An objective method to quantitate emphysema using computed tomography. Chest 1988;94(4):782–7. Available at: http://www.ncbi.nlm.nih.gov/pubmed/3168574.

13. Choi S, Haghighi B, Choi J, et al. Differentiation of quantitative CT imaging phenotypes in asthma versus COPD. BMJ Open Respir Res 2017;4(1):e000252.

14. Kosciuch J, Krenke R, Gorska K, et al. Airway dimensions in asthma and COPD in high resolution computed tomography: can we see the difference? Respir Care 2013;58(8):1335–42.

15. Chen H, Zeng QS, Zhang M, et al. Quantitative low-dose computed tomography of the lung parenchyma and airways for the differentiation between chronic obstructive pulmonary disease and asthma patients. Respiration 2017;94(4): 366–74.

16. Hartley RA, Barker BL, Newby C, et al. Relationship between lung function and quantitative computed tomographic parameters of airway remodeling, air trapping, and emphysema in patients with asthma and chronic obstructive pulmonary disease: A single-center study. J Allergy Clin Immunol 2016;137(5): 1413–1422 e12.

17. Trivedi A, Hall C, Hoffman EA, et al. Using imaging as a biomarker for asthma. J Allergy Clin Immunol 2017;139(1):1.

18. Woods JC, Choong CK, Yablonskiy DA, et al. Hyperpolarized 3He diffusion MRI and histology in pulmonary emphysema. Magn Reson Med 2006;56(6): 1293–300.

19. Bhatt SP, Washko GR, Hoffman EA, et al. State of the art imaging advances in chronic obstructive pulmonary disease insights from the genetic epidemiology of chronic obstructive pulmonary disease. (COPDGene) Study 2019. https://doi.org/10.1164/rccm.201807-1351SO.

20. Sin DD, Miravitlles M, Mannino DM, et al. What is asthma–COPD overlap syndrome? Towards a consensus definition from a round table discussion PERSPECTIVE ASTHMA–COPD OVERLAP SYNDROME. doi:10.1183/13993003.00436-2016

21. Cataldo D, Corhay JL, Derom E, et al. A Belgian survey on the diagnosis of asthma–COPD overlap syndrome. Int J Chron Obstruct Pulmon Dis 2017;12:601.

22. Cosio BG, Soriano JB, López-Campos JL, et al. Defining the Asthma-COPD Overlap Syndrome in a COPD Cohort. Chest 2016;149(1):45–52.

23. Plaza V, Álvarez F, Calle M, et al. Consensus on the Asthma-COPD Overlap Syndrome (ACOS) Between the Spanish COPD Guidelines (GesEPOC) and the Spanish Guidelines on the Management of Asthma (GEMA). Arch Bronconeumol 2017;53(8):443–9.

24. Milne S, Mannino D, Sin DD. Asthma-COPD overlap and chronic airflow obstruction: definitions, management, and unanswered questions. J Allergy Clin Immunol Pract 2020;8(2):483–95.

25. Yanagisawa S, Ichinose M. Definition and diagnosis of asthma–COPD overlap (ACO). Allergol Int 2018;67(2):172–8.

26. Barczyk A, Maskey-Warzęchowska M, Górska K, et al. Asthma-COPD overlap—a discordance between patient populations defined by different diagnostic criteria. J Allergy Clin Immunol Pract 2019;7(7):2326–36.e5.

27. Kurashima K, Hoshi T, Takayanagi N, et al. Airway dimensions and pulmonary function in chronic obstructive pulmonary disease and bronchial asthma. Respirology 2012;17(1):79–86.

28. Cosentino J, Zhao H, Hardin M, et al. Analysis of asthma-chronic obstructive pulmonary disease overlap syndrome defined on the basis of bronchodilator response and degree of emphysema. Ann Am Thorac Soc 2016;13(9):1483–9.

29. Suzuki T, Tada Y, Kawata N, et al. Clinical, physiological, and radiological features of asthma-chronic obstructive pulmonary disease overlap syndrome. Int J Chron Obstruct Pulmon Dis 2015;10:947–54.

30. Hwang HJ, Lee SM, Seo JB, et al. Visual and quantitative assessments of regional xenon-ventilation using dual-energy CT in asthma-chronic obstructive pulmonary disease overlap syndrome: a comparison with chronic obstructive pulmonary disease. Korean J Radiol 2020;21(9):1104–13.

31. Hardin M, Cho M, McDonald M-L, et al. The clinical and genetic features of COPD-asthma overlap syndrome. Eur Respir J 2014;44(2):341–50.

32. Gao Y, Zhai X, Li K, et al. Asthma COPD overlap syndrome on CT densitometry: a distinct phenotype from COPD. COPD 2016;13(4):471–6.

33. Karayama M, Inui N, Yasui H, et al. Physiological and morphological differences of airways between COPD and asthma–COPD overlap. Sci Rep 2019;9(1):7818.

34. Hardin M, Silverman EK, Barr RG, et al. The clinical features of the overlap between COPD and asthma. Respir Res 2011;12(1):127.

35. Niwa M, Fujisawa T, Karayama M, et al. Differences in airway structural changes assessed by 3-dimensional computed tomography in asthma and asthma–chronic obstructive pulmonary disease overlap. Ann Allergy Asthma Immunol 2018;121(6):704–10.e1.

36. Tanabe N, Sato S, Oguma T, et al. Influence of asthma onset on airway dimensions on ultra-high-resolution computed tomography in chronic obstructive pulmonary disease. J Thorac Imaging 2021;36(4):224–30.

37. Vasilescu DM, Martinez FJ, Marchetti N, et al. Noninvasive Imaging Biomarker Identifies Small Airway Damage in Severe Chronic Obstructive Pulmonary Disease. Am J Respir Crit Care Med 2019;200(5):575–81.

38. Estepar RS, Kinney GL, Black-Shinn JL, et al. Computed tomographic measures of pulmonary vascular morphology in smokers and their clinical implications. Am J Respir Crit Care Med 2013;188(2):231–9.

39. Ash SY, Rahaghi FN, Come CE, et al. Pruning of the pulmonary vasculature in asthma the Severe Asthma Research Program (SARP) cohort. Am J Respir Crit Care Med 2018;198(1):39–50.
40. Qu Y, Cao Y, Liao M, et al. Sagittal-lung CT measurements in the evaluation of asthma-COPD overlap syndrome: a distinctive phenotype from COPD alone. Radiol Med 2017;122(7):487–94.
41. Xie M, Wang W, Dou S, et al. Quantitative computed tomography measurements of emphysema for diagnosing asthma-chronic obstructive pulmonary disease overlap syndrome. Int J COPD 2016;11(1):953–61.
42. Obojski A, Patyk M, Zaleska-Dorobisz U. Similarities in quantitative computed tomography imaging of the lung in severe asthma with persistent airflow limitation and chronic obstructive pulmonary disease. J Clin Med 2021;10(21):5058.
43. Shimizu K, Tanabe N, Oguma A, et al. Parenchymal destruction in asthma: Fixed airflow obstruction and lung function trajectory. J Allergy Clin Immunol 2021. https://doi.org/10.1016/J.JACI.2021.07.042.
44. Boulet LP, Boulay ME, Coxson HO, et al. Asthma with irreversible airway obstruction in smokers and nonsmokers: links between airway inflammation and structural changes. Respiration 2020;99(12):1090–100.
45. Gorska K, Korczynski P, Mierzejewski M, et al. Comparison of endobronchial ultrasound and high resolution computed tomography as tools for airway wall imaging in asthma and chronic obstructive pulmonary disease. Respir Med 2016; 117:131–8.
46. Górka K, Gross-Sondej I, Górka J, et al. Assessment of airway remodeling using endobronchial ultrasound in asthma-COPD overlap. J Asthma Allergy 2021; 14:663.
47. Chae EJ, Seo JB, Lee J, et al. Xenon ventilation imaging using dual-energy computed tomography in asthmatics: Initial experience. Invest Radiol 2010; 45(6):354–61.
48. Qing K, Ruppert K, Jiang Y, et al. Regional mapping of gas uptake by blood and tissue in the human lung using hyperpolarized xenon-129 MRI. J Magn Reson Imaging 2014;39(2):346–59.
49. Galban CJ, Han MK, Boes JL, et al. Computed tomography-based biomarker provides unique signature for diagnosis of COPD phenotypes and disease progression. Nat Med 2012;18(11):1711–5.
50. Kirby M, Yin Y, Tschirren J, et al. A novel method of estimating small airway disease using inspiratory-to-expiratory computed tomography. Respiration 2017; 94(4):336–45.
51. Dunican EM, Elicker BM, Gierada DS, et al. Mucus plugs in patients with asthma linked to eosinophilia and airflow obstruction. J Clin Invest 2018;128(3): 997–1009.
52. Okajima Y, Come CE, Nardelli P, et al. Luminal plugging on chest CT scan: association with lung function, quality of life, and COPD clinical phenotypes. Chest 2020;158(1):121–30.
53. Green M, Mead J, Turner JM. Variability of maximum expiratory flow volume curves. J Appl Physiol 1974;37(1):67–74.
54. Stern DA, Morgan WJ, Wright AL, et al. Poor airway function in early infancy and lung function by age 22 years: a non-selective longitudinal cohort study. Lancet 2007;370(9589):758–64.
55. Smith BM, Kirby M, Hoffman EA, et al. Association of dysanapsis with chronic obstructive pulmonary disease among older adults. JAMA 2020;323(22): 2268–80.

56. Dournes G, Menut F, Macey J, et al. Lung morphology assessment of cystic fibrosis using MRI with ultra-short echo time at submillimeter spatial resolution. Eur Radiol 2016;26(11):3811–20.

57. Tschirren J, Hoffman EA, McLennan G, et al. Intrathoracic airway trees: segmentation and airway morphology analysis from low-dose CT scans. IEEE Trans Med Imaging 2005;24(12):1529–39.

58. Grydeland TB, Dirksen A, Coxson HO, et al. Quantitative computed tomography measures of emphysema and airway wall thickness are related to respiratory symptoms. Am J Respir Crit Care Med 2010;181(4):353–9.

59. Matsuoka S, Washko GR, Dransfield MT, et al. Quantitative CT measurement of cross-sectional area of small pulmonary vessel in COPD: correlations with emphysema and airflow limitation. Acad Radiol 2010;17(1):93–9.

60. Kinsella M, Muller NL, Staples C, et al. Hyperinflation in Asthma and Emphysema: Assessment by Pulmonary Function Testing and Computed Tomography. Chest 1988;94(2):286–9.

The Role of Smoking in Asthma and Chronic Obstructive Pulmonary Disease Overlap

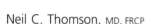

Neil C. Thomson, MD, FRCP

KEYWORDS

- Asthma • Chronic obstructive pulmonary disease
- Asthma–chronic obstructive pulmonary disease overlap • Cigarette smoking
- Smokers with asthma

KEY POINTS

- Exposure to cigarette smoke has a key role in the development, adverse health outcomes, and impaired response to some therapies among individuals with features of asthma and chronic obstructive pulmonary disease overlap (ACO).
- To aid the identification of clinical subtypes, the description of ever smokers with features of asthma and COPD should include data on smoking status, cumulative smoking history, and the phenotype of asthma and smoking-related chronic airway disease.
- Pathogenic mechanisms in smoking-related ACO involve poorly understood, complex interactions between smoking-induced and asthma-induced airway inflammation, corticosteroid insensitivity, and tissue remodeling.
- Evidence for the clinical effectiveness of interventions for adults with smoking-related ACO is limited; management currently involves the identification and targeting of treatable traits such as current smoking, type 2 high eosinophilic inflammation, symptomatic airflow obstruction, and extrapulmonary comorbidities.

INTRODUCTION

In clinical practice, the classification of chronic airways diseases into asthma[1] and COPD[2] is based predominantly on the assessment of symptoms, risk factors, and physiologic variables. The complexities of chronic airway diseases are increasingly recognized, however, with an acknowledgment that some people show characteristics of both asthma and COPD, that susceptibility to risk factors varies between individuals, and that complex biologic processes involving host and environmental factors cause different endotypes of airway disease.[3] The term asthma–COPD overlap (ACO) is currently used to describe patients who exhibit overlapping clinical, physiologic, pathologic, and/or biomarker features associated with asthma and COPD.[4] Several

Institute of Infection, Immunity & Inflammation, University of Glasgow, Glasgow G12 0YN, UK
E-mail address: neil.thomson@glasgow.ac.uk

Immunol Allergy Clin N Am 42 (2022) 615–630
https://doi.org/10.1016/j.iac.2022.03.004
0889-8561/22/© 2022 Elsevier Inc. All rights reserved.

immunology.theclinics.com

clinical phenotypes are described, but due to a lack of consensus on the definition of ACO, it is uncertain whether these phenotypes represent specific endotypes. Some definitions of ACO include a history of heavy cumulative exposure to tobacco smoke or biomass gases as a major diagnostic criterion[5,6] (**Table 1**). ACO is also used to describe individuals with long-standing asthma and persistent airflow obstruction but without a smoking history,[4] although some experts proposed that this subtype should be termed chronic, irreversible asthma, and not ACO.[6] Smoking-related chronic airway diseases, such as chronic bronchitis, emphysema, or small airway disease also develop in patients with ACO and asthmatic individuals with normal spirometry.[7] The term pre-COPD has been proposed to describe current and former smokers with normal spirometry who are at risk of developing COPD ($FEV_1/FVC < 0.7$)[8] and the term also includes some individuals with long-standing asthma and a smoking history.[9]

Exposure to tobacco smoke has a key role in the development, adverse health outcomes, and response to therapies among many individuals with ACO. This article reviews recent data on the prevalence and health burden of cigarette smoking in ACO, cigarette smoking and diagnostic criteria for ACO, cigarette smoking and other risk factors for ACO, and clinical outcomes, pathogenesis, inflammatory biomarkers, and management of smoking-related ACO.

PREVALENCE AND HEALTH BURDEN OF CIGARETTE SMOKING IN ASTHMA–CHRONIC OBSTRUCTIVE PULMONARY DISEASE OVERLAP

Almost 1 billion people are current cigarette smokers worldwide, with higher prevalence rates in men than in women.[10] The World Health Organization projected that by 2025, global tobacco smoking prevalence will decline to 26% among men and to around 5% among women[10] although the total number of cigarette smokers will increase due to population growth. In many countries, the proportion of people with asthma who have a history of smoking is similar to the general population.[11] In developed countries, up to half the adult asthmatic population[12] and most of the people with COPD are current or former cigarette smokers. Current smoking rates among adults more than 40 years with ACO are reported to be either similar[13] or less[14] than those with COPD alone, whereas cumulative exposure to tobacco smoke is lower in ACO.[13,14] Cigarette smoking has a major adverse impact on the health status of people with COPD and asthma,[15] with the health burden greater for those with clinical features of ACO.[16]

Table 1	
Commonly described clinical subtypes of smoking-related asthma–chronic obstructive pulmonary disease overlap (ACO)	
Smoking-Related ACO Subtype	**Description**
Long-standing asthma with a heavy smoking history	Individuals with long-standing asthma, a smoking history (>10 pack-years), and spirometry evidence of persistent airflow obstruction (COPD). In some studies, the term ACO–asthma is used to describe this subgroup.
Smoking-related COPD with "asthma-like" features	Individuals with smoking-related COPD and "asthma-like" features, such as eosinophilia and other markers of type 2 (T2) inflammation, marked bronchodilator reversibility or airway hyperreactivity.[62,65] In some studies, the terms eosinophilic COPD or ACO–COPD are used to describe this subgroup.

CIGARETTE SMOKING AND DIAGNOSTIC CRITERIA FOR ASTHMA–CHRONIC OBSTRUCTIVE PULMONARY DISEASE OVERLAP

In many studies, a heavy smoking history ($\geq$10 pack-years) is a major criterion to define ACO, in addition to spirometry evidence of chronic airflow obstruction (post-bronchodilator FEV_1/FVC <0.7) and either a documented history of asthma before 40 years of age or spirometry COPD associated with biomarkers of type 2 (T2) high inflammation.[5,6] The requirement for a heavy smoking history to diagnose ACO may limit the ability to identify clinical and mechanistic subgroups with lower cumulative lifetime exposure to tobacco smoke.[17] In addition, combining current and former smokers may dilute the adverse clinical effects of current cigarette smoking among adults with asthma or COPD.[18–20] Collectively, these findings suggest that the description of patients with smoking-related ACO should include data on current or former smoking status and cumulative exposure to tobacco smoke. Recently, it has been proposed that rather than using diagnostic labels such as ACO to describe adults with clinical features of asthma and COPD, it is more appropriate to describe individual clinical, physiologic, pathologic, and/or biomarker variables and treatable traits.[21] Future studies should determine whether one or more of the clinical subtypes of smoking-related ACO and asthma correspond to specific endotypes of chronic airway disease.

CIGARETTE SMOKING AND OTHER RISK FACTORS FOR ASTHMA–CHRONIC OBSTRUCTIVE PULMONARY DISEASE OVERLAP

The development and adverse clinical outcomes in adults with ACO are due to multiple risk factors (**Table 2**) and different lung function trajectories. In asthma, cigarette smoking or exposure to biomass fuel smoke can cause an accelerated decline in lung function from maximal levels in early adulthood. Alternatively, a normal decline can occur in adulthood from submaximal levels due to previous severe childhood-onset asthma or other risk factors for suboptimal lung growth from early-life events.[22]

Cigarette smoking variables: A history of current cigarette smoking[23,24] and cumulative exposure to tobacco smoke[17,25,26] are important risk factors for ACO in adults with long-standing asthma, although only a minority develop spirometry COPD.[24] Several longitudinal population-based studies[27–30] reported an accelerated decline in lung function in current smokers with asthma compared with never smokers with asthma, which was associated with higher pack-year history in middle-aged adults with asthma.[31,32]

Asthma phenotype and cigarette smoking: Among current and former smokers with COPD in COPDGene and SPIROMICS (Subpopulations and Intermediate Outcome Measures in COPD) studies, nonatopic asthma was a risk factor for adverse clinical outcomes in the ACO subgroup, whereas the atopic asthma subgroup was at lower risk.[33] In the longitudinal population-based European Community Respiratory Health Survey (ECRHS I), the decline in lung function was increased among cigarette smokers with nonatopic late-onset asthma, but not among cigarette smokers with atopic early-onset or atopic late-onset asthma.[28] Chronic bronchitis, which is a common symptom among cigarette smokers with asthma,[27,34] may contribute to the development of COPD in this subgroup of asthma.[27]

Coexistent risk factors with cigarette smoking: Social and behavioral risk factors associated with smoking, such as educational attainment, poverty, drug, and alcohol abuse,[35] and poor adherence to drug therapies, either alone or in combination, may contribute to the adverse health outcomes found in adults with asthma (see **Table 2**). Lower socioeconomic status is associated with the development and

Table 2
Multiple risk factors for the development, adverse health outcomes, and impaired response to inhaled corticosteroids among individuals with a smoking history and features of asthma and chronic obstructive pulmonary disease overlap (ACO)

Cigarette smoking variables	Smoking status
	    Current smoker
	    Former smoker
	    Ever smoker (current and former smokers)
	Smoking exposure variables
	    Duration (years of smoking)
	    Intensity (cigarettes smoked daily)
	    Cumulative dose (pack-years)
	Nicotine dependence

Asthma phenotypes	Severity Age of onset Asthma associated with chronic bronchitis Inflammatory

Coexistent risk factors
  with cigarette smoking
	Social and behavioral risk factors
	    Lower socioeconomic status
	    Nonadherence with therapies for asthma
	    Alcohol abuse/dependence
	    Drug abuse/dependence
	    Overuse of short-acting beta-agonist
	    Poor asthma management behavior
	    Impaired symptom perception
	Environmental risk factors
	    Indoor and air outdoor pollution
	        including exposure to passive smoke

Additional risk factors	Early life events
	    Early respiratory infections
	    Prematurity/low birth weight
	    Childhood asthma
	    Exposure to maternal smoke
	Other factors
	    Older age
	    Male sex
	    High BMI
	    Genotype

severity of ACO,[17,23,25] although possibly independent of smoking prevalence.[36] A survey of adults aged 40 to 64 year old seen in the pulmonary outpatient clinics of a US university hospital found that current smokers with asthma, COPD, or ACO, were less adherent to medication filling, medication taking, and having yearly vaccinations than nonsmokers.[37] Environmental exposures, such as air pollution[38] or passive smoke[39] increase the risk of developing ACO in adults with asthma and these factors may interact with cigarette smoking.

Additional risk factors: Early life events, such as early respiratory infection, prematurity, low birth weight, poor nutrition, bronchial hyperreactivity, previous severe childhood-onset asthma, family history of asthma, and exposure to maternal smoking are implicated in the development of ACO due to submaximal lung growth[40] (see **Table 2**). Other important risk factors for ACO include older age,[17,23] male sex,[24] high BMI,[17] and genotype.

CLINICAL OUTCOMES IN SMOKING-RELATED ASTHMA–CHRONIC OBSTRUCTIVE PULMONARY DISEASE OVERLAP

Data from numerous observational studies provide sufficient evidence to conclude that current smoking is an important risk factor for worse clinical outcomes in adults with long-standing asthma, including those with and without spirometry COPD.[7] Clinical effects among current smokers with asthma include poor symptom control,[41] lower asthma quality of life,[42] more frequent severe exacerbations,[43,44] greater asthma-related health care utilization, higher prevalence of chronic bronchitis,[27,34] and increased numbers of patients with persistent airflow obstruction compared with never smokers with asthma. Higher cumulative smoking history is associated with frequent hospitalizations in a dose-dependent manner.[45] A Canadian study found that smoking-related ACO–asthma ($\geq$20 pack-years) was associated with worse asthma control and quality of life than nonsmokers with ACO–asthma (<5 pack-years),[46] although the number of exacerbations was similar between groups.[47]

Adults with ACO have a higher burden of self-reported comorbidities than adults aged $\geq$35 years with asthma or COPD alone.[48] In a study of adult-onset asthma, cumulative exposure to cigarette smoke was associated with more comorbidities[45] and was an independent risk factor for cardiovascular disease, anxiety, and depression.[49] A Canadian cross-sectional study found a slightly higher prevalence of psychiatric conditions in heavy smokers with ACO–asthma compared with nonsmokers with ACO.[50] The risk of lung cancer among patients with ACO is similar to those with COPD and higher than smokers with asthma with normal spirometry.[51] Current smoking is an important risk factor for increased all-cause mortality in adults with asthma.[52]

PATHOGENESIS OF SMOKING-RELATED ASTHMA–CHRONIC OBSTRUCTIVE PULMONARY DISEASE OVERLAP

There is limited understanding of the pathogenesis of smoking-related ACO. Mechanisms are extrapolated from data on airway inflammation and remodeling in chronic airway disease due to smoking or asthma[53–55] (**Fig. 1**). In adults with ACO, the airways are exposed to cigarette smoke and to other environmental factors such as allergens, viruses, bacteria, and atmospheric pollutants, which alone and in combination induce airway inflammation.

Cigarette smoke contains high levels of reactive oxygen species (ROS) that activate epithelial cells to produce inflammatory mediators such as interleukin (IL)-6, IL-8, IL-1β, tumor necrosis factor (TNF)α, which recruit and/or activate neutrophils, macrophages and CD8$^+$ cytotoxic T cells (Tc1) cells.[53–55] Oxidative stress and proinflammatory mediators released by activated neutrophils, macrophages, and Tc1 cells in susceptible individuals cause tissue damage resulting in mucus hypersecretion, extracellular matrix changes, small airway dysfunction, emphysema, and which may contribute to corticosteroid insensitivity. In addition, cigarette smoke impairs innate immune responses mediated by epithelial cells, alveolar macrophages, dendritic cells, and natural killer cells, thereby impairing host responses against infections. Exposure to allergens in susceptible people and the release of alarmins such as IL-33, TSLP, IL-25 from injured epithelial cells activate Th2 cells and ILC2s, respectively, to release T2 cytokines IL-4, IL-5, and IL-13.[56] Dendritic cells are involved in processing antigens and are activated by alarmins to initiate immune responses including T2 immunity. IL-4 causes immunoglobulin E (IgE) production from B cells and IL-5 recruits and activates eosinophils. Pro-inflammatory mediators, including IL-13, released from activated eosinophils, Th2 cells, ILC2 cells, and mast cells contribute to mucus hypersecretion, airway hyperreactivity, and tissue remodeling.

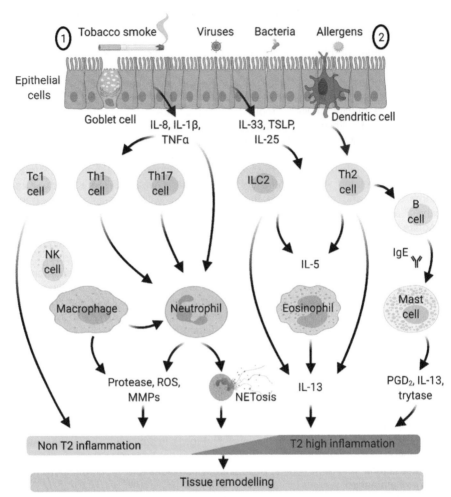

Fig. 1. Schematic diagram illustrating potential inflammatory pathways underlying airway immunopathology of asthma–COPD overlap in adults with a smoking history. In the airways in adults with ACO, cigarette smoke exposure and asthma interact to induce ① smoking-related inflammation and ② asthma-related inflammation involving neutrophils, macrophages, and T2 low inflammation/or T2 high eosinophilic inflammation, respectively, which can result in tissue remodeling. The inflammatory processes are associated with adverse clinical outcomes including worse symptoms, increased risk of exacerbations, development of airflow obstruction, reduced local host defences, and corticosteroid insensitivity. IgE, immunoglobulin E; IL, interleukin; ILC2, type 2 innate lymphoid cell; MMPs, matrix metalloproteinase; NET, neutrophil extracellular trap; NETosis, neutrophil extracellular trap formation; NK, natural killer; PGD_2, prostaglandin D_2; ROS, reactive oxygen species; T2, type 2 inflammation; Tc1, $CD8^+$ cytotoxic T cells; Th2, T helper 2; TNF, tumor necrosis factor; TSLP, thymic stromal lymphopoietin. (Created with BioRender.com.)

Smoking-related corticosteroid insensitivity in some individuals with ACO may result from noneosinophilic airway inflammation. Possible molecular mechanisms include altered glucocorticoid receptor (GR) subtypes, such as increased inactive GRβ and decreased active GRα expression,[57] increased proinflammatory transcription factors activity, such as NF-κB, or reduced histone deacetylase activity (HDAC)2 activity.

In summary, cigarette smoke exposure and asthma interact to induce heterogeneous mechanisms involving non-T2 neutrophilic or paucigranulocytic inflammation and/or T2 high eosinophilic inflammation, which can result in tissue remodeling of airway smooth muscle and extracellular matrix. Inflammatory subgroups of ACO are likely due to differences between individuals in their exposure to risk factors, such as variations in disease severity, as occurs in COPD,[58] the intensity of cigarette smoking, cumulative exposure to tobacco smoke, and other factors (see **Table 2**).

INFLAMMATORY BIOMARKERS IN SMOKING-RELATED ASTHMA–CHRONIC OBSTRUCTIVE PULMONARY DISEASE OVERLAP

Several studies have investigated inflammatory cell phenotypes and T2 inflammation status in current and former smokers with long-standing asthma including adults with ACO.[7] Over one-half had neutrophilic or paucigranulocytic airway inflammation and biomarker evidence of T2 low inflammation,[59,60] which in ACO was associated with a history of higher cumulative exposure to tobacco smoke.[60] Over one-third had eosinophilic inflammation and biomarker evidence of T2 high inflammation, which in ACO was associated with former smoker status and a history of a low to medium cumulative exposure to tobacco smoke.[60,61]

Among individuals with smoking-induced COPD without a history of asthma, approximately one-third have eosinophilic inflammation associated with bronchial[62] and blood[63] T2 high gene expression profiles and corticosteroid responsiveness.[20,62,64] In a study of heavy smokers ($\not\geq$20 pack-years) with ACO, a higher proportion with the ACO–COPD subtype without a history of asthma had T2 high inflammation (49%) than the ACO–asthma subtype (30%),[65] indicating that T2 high inflammation can occur in the absence of a history of asthma. Uncertainties remain on the cut-off value of blood eosinophil to define corticosteroid-responsive eosinophilic COPD and whether smoking-related ACO subtypes differ in clinical characteristics and treatment response.

Low-grade systemic inflammation occurs in current and former smokers with ACO or COPD with similar histories of cumulative exposure to tobacco smoke.[66] Smokers with ACO have similar levels of low-grade systemic inflammation compared with non-smokers with ACO, despite the former group having worse symptom control and poorer quality of life.[46] Whether low-grade systemic inflammation is a causative factor for adverse asthma outcomes in ACO is unknown.

MANAGEMENT

The best approach to the management of smoking-related ACO is uncertain due to limited clinical trial data. In clinical practice, therapies are used that are recommended for asthma and COPD.[1,2] Recently, the identification and targeting of treatable traits were proposed as a strategy to personalize the management of chronic airway diseases including ACO.[67,68] Treatable traits of relevance to the management of smoking-related ACO include pulmonary traits, such as airflow obstruction, chronic bronchitis, and eosinophilic inflammation, extrapulmonary traits, such as comorbidities and risk factor and behavioral traits, such as cigarette smoking, infection risk, and poor adherence with asthma therapies (**Fig. 2**, see **Table 2**). Comprehensive reviews on the treatable trait strategy have been previously published,[67] although to date the strategy has not been validated by randomized clinical trials in patients with features of asthma and COPD.

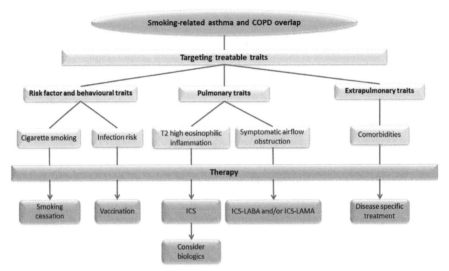

Fig. 2. Management of smoking-related ACO asthma–COPD overlap using components of a treatable trait strategy. The effectiveness of therapies such as azithromycin, as-needed ICS-formoterol, mucolytics, roflumilast, bronchial thermoplasty, and pulmonary rehabilitation are largely untested among patients with smoking-related ACO. ICS, inhaled corticosteroid; LABA, long-acting beta$_2$-agonist; LAMA, long-acting muscarinic antagonist; T2 inflammation, type 2 inflammation

Targeting Risk Factor/Behavioral and Extrapulmonary Traits

Among adults with asthma, quitting smoking is associated with improvements in symptoms,[69–72] asthma-related quality of life,[70] lung function,[72] and airway hyperreactivity[70,71] in several small studies, generally of short duration. Most studies indicate that former smokers with asthma have better levels of symptom control than current smokers. Despite the known adverse effects of active smoking on asthma, data from Canadian Community Health Survey have shown that cigarette smokers with asthma and COPD are no more likely to receive smoking cessation physician counseling and pharmacotherapy compared with the general smoking population.[73] Cigarette smoking quit rates in the general population and patients with smoking-related airway diseases are improved with behavioral counseling in combination with pharmacotherapies, such as nicotine replacement products, varenicline, and bupropion.[74] Implementation of "MPOWER" measures worldwide is a key component of the World Health Organization's (WHO) Framework Convention on Tobacco Control[75] and these measures are relevant to improving outcomes among individuals with smoking-related ACO (**Box 1**).

For patients with smoking-related ACO, infection risk reduction involves annual influenza vaccination[1] and pneumococcal vaccination for patients greater than 65 years.[2] Systemic smoking-associated comorbidities, such as cardiovascular disease and osteoporosis are managed according to international and national recommendations.[2]

Targeting Pulmonary Traits

Data on the effectiveness of pharmacologic and biological interventions for current and former smokers with asthma or ACO are limited due to their exclusion from most large clinical trials.[76,77] The main therapies used to treat T2 high eosinophilic

---

Box 1
WHO MPOWER policy on tobacco control

*M*onitor tobacco use and prevention policies

*P*rotect people from tobacco smoke

*O*ffer help to quit tobacco use

*W*arn about the dangers of tobacco

*E*nforce bans on tobacco advertising promotion and sponsorship

*R*aise taxes on tobacco

From World Health Organization. WHO report on the global tobacco epidemic, 2021: addressing new and emerging products. 2021. https://apps.who.int/iris/bitstream/handle/10665/343287/9789240032095-eng.pdf?sequence=1&isAllowed=y.

---

inflammation are inhaled corticosteroids (ICS) and possibly biologics, and to treat airflow obstruction are long-acting beta-agonists (LABA) and long-acting muscarinic antagonists (LAMA).

Inhaled corticosteroids

Small clinical studies showed that improvements in lung function after low to medium dose ICS for less than 1 month were impaired in current smokers with mild to moderate asthma compared with nonsmokers, but a greater response was shown with high dose ICS after 3 months.[78,79] Observation data suggested that long-term ICS treatment (≥1 year) reduced the decline in lung function among smokers with asthma,[78] but was less effective in preventing severe exacerbations among current smokers compared with never smokers with asthma.[80] Observational studies suggest some clinical benefits from ICS treatment in smoking-related ACO[78] and that blood eosinophil count of greater than 300 predicts decreased exacerbations with ICS.[81] The GINA report advocates treating patients with ACO as asthma, initially with low or medium ICS-containing treatment to reduce the risk of exacerbations. An increase in the dose of ICS is suggested in the GINA report if asthma is poorly controlled among patients exposed to tobacco smoke,[1] although as reported in COPD, a higher dose of ICS might increase the risk of pneumonia.

Inhaled corticosteroids in combination with long-acting bronchodilators

In ACO, LABA and/or LAMA are administered with ICS treatment of symptom control and should not be given alone without ICS.[1] Studies in current smokers with asthma have shown improved clinical outcomes with medium to high dose maintenance ICS-LABA combination treatment compared with ICS alone.[78,80] Data from a population-based study have shown that hospital admission and mortality were reduced by ICS-LABA combination compared with LABA alone in older adults with ACO,[82] findings which were confirmed in a recent systemic review.[83] The ATOMIC (ACO Treatment with Optimal Medications) study, an open-label 48-week randomized trial in 303 Korean patients with ACO treated with ICS-LABA, showed improved lung function with the addition of LAMA, but no difference in exacerbations.[84]

Among patients with COPD, recent data suggest that former smoking status and eosinophilic COPD subtype of ACO predict a beneficial response to add-on ICS to long-acting bronchodilators. In several large clinical trials, the addition of ICS to LABA or LABA and LAMA reduced moderate and severe exacerbations[20,64] and improved lung function[19] to a greater extent in former smokers with COPD compared with current smokers with COPD and ICS benefit was observed in all blood eosinophil counts among former smokers with COPD. Among current smokers, clinical benefits were lacking with lower eosinophil counts (<200/μL), whereas at higher eosinophil counts (>200/μL) exacerbations were reduced.[20,64] Collectively, these studies suggest an impaired therapeutic response to add-on ICS in current smokers with noneosinophil COPD, but that both current and former smokers obtained benefits at higher blood eosinophil counts. The GOLD report recommends add-on ICS for patients with COPD with a blood eosinophil ≥300/μL, hospital admissions, or ≥2 exacerbations/y while treated with LAMA and/or LABA.[2]

Biological agents and other therapies

Data from observational studies suggest that treatment with anti-IgE omalizumab, anti-IL5 mepolizumab, and anti-IL4 receptor α dupilumab may improve clinical outcomes in smoking-related ACO, although the quality of evidence is low.[78] A systematic review of anti-IL5 or anti-IL5Rα in COPD demonstrated that mepolizumab probably reduced moderate to severe exacerbations in patients with blood eosinophil count greater than 150/μL and benralizumab reduced severe exacerbations requiring hospital admission in patients with blood eosinophil count greater than 220/μL.[85]

Overall, published data suggest that therapeutic responses to pharmacologic and biological interventions for smoking-related ACO are influenced by smoking status (current vs former smokers) and by biomarker evidence of T2 high inflammation (raised blood eosinophil count). A flow chart to aid clinicians in the management of smoking-related ACO is outlined in **Fig. 2**, although the recommendations are based on expert opinion and the algorithm has not been validated. Given the high prevalence of tobacco use worldwide, new data from controlled trials and pragmatic trials in real-world populations are required to provide evidence on the effectiveness of drug and biological treatments for smoking-related asthma and ACO.[86,87]

SUMMARY

Exposure to cigarette smoke has a key role in the development, adverse health outcomes, and impaired response to ICS among individuals with features of asthma and chronic obstructive pulmonary disease overlap (ACO). To aid the identification of clinical subtypes, the description of ever smokers with features of asthma and COPD should include data on smoking status, cumulative smoking history, the phenotype of asthma, and smoking-related chronic airway disease. Pathogenic mechanisms in smoking-related ACO involve poorly understood, complex interactions between smoking-induced and asthma-induced airway inflammation, corticosteroid insensitivity, and tissue remodeling. Evidence for the clinical effectiveness of interventions for adults with smoking-related ACO is limited. Management currently involves the identification and targeting of treatable traits such as current smoking, T2 high eosinophilic inflammation, symptomatic airflow obstruction, and extrapulmonary comorbidities.

CLINICS CARE POINTS

- Risk factors for the development and adverse clinical outcomes in adults with smoking-related ACO include smoking status, cumulative exposure to tobacco smoke, the phenotype of asthma such as the age of onset, phenotypes of smoking-related chronic airway diseases, such as chronic bronchitis, emphysema, and small airway disease and inflammatory phenotype, such as T2 inflammation status.

- Adults with smoking-related ACO have poor clinical outcomes, pathogenic mechanisms involving smoking and asthma-associated airway inflammation, corticosteroid insensitivity, and tissue remodeling.
- Management involves identification and targeting treatable traits, such as current smoking, T2 high eosinophilic inflammation, symptomatic airflow obstruction, and extrapulmonary comorbidities, although evidence for the clinical effectiveness of interventions for adults with smoking-related ACO is limited.

DISCLOSURE

The author has no commercial or financial conflicts of interest related to this work.

REFERENCES

1. Global Initiative for Asthma (GINA). 2021. Available at: http://www.ginasthma. org/. Accessed December 12, 2021.
2. Global strategy for the diagnosis, management and prevention of chronic obstructive pulmonary disease. 2021. Available at: http://www.goldcopd.org. Accessed 12th December 2021.
3. Pavord ID, Beasley R, Agusti A, et al. After asthma: redefining airways diseases. Lancet 2018;391(10118):350–400.
4. Woodruff P, van den Berge M, Boucher R, et al. American Thoracic Society/National Heart, Lung, and Blood Institute Asthma–Chronic Obstructive Pulmonary Disease Overlap Workshop Report. Am J Respir Crit Care Med 2017;196(3):375–81.
5. Sin DD, Miravitlles M, Mannino DM, et al. What is asthma–COPD overlap syndrome? Towards a consensus definition from a round table discussion. Eur Respir J 2016;48:664–73.
6. Mekov E, Nuñez A, Sin DD, et al. Update on Asthma-COPD Overlap (ACO): A Narrative Review. Int J Chron Obstruct Pulmon Dis 2021;16:1783–99.
7. Thomson NC. Asthma and smoking-induced airway disease without spirometric COPD. Eur Respir J 2017;49(5):1602061.
8. Han MK, Agusti A, Celli BR, et al. From GOLD 0 to Pre-COPD. Am J Respir Crit Care Med 2021;203(4):414–23.
9. Thomson NC. Asthma with a Smoking History and Pre–Chronic Obstructive Pulmonary Disease. Am J Respir Crit Care Med 2021;204(1):109–10.
10. WHO global report on trends in prevalence of tobacco use 2000-2025. 4th edition. Geneva (Switzerland): World Health Organization; 2021. Available at: https://www.who.int/publications/i/item/9789240039322. Accessed December 12, 2021.
11. To T, Stanojevic S, Moores G, et al. Global asthma prevalence in adults: findings from the cross-sectional world health survey. BMC Public Health 2012;12(1):204.
12. Nissen F, Douglas IJ, Müllerová H, et al. Clinical profile of predefined asthma phenotypes in a large cohort of UK primary care patients (Clinical Practice Research Datalink). J Asthma Allergy 2019;12:7–19.
13. Alshabanat A, Zafari Z, Albanyan O, et al. Asthma and COPD Overlap Syndrome (ACOS): A Systematic Review and Meta Analysis. PLoS One 2015;10(9):e0136065.
14. Marcon A, Locatelli F, Dharmage SC, et al. The coexistence of asthma and COPD: risk factors, clinical history and lung function trajectories. Eur Respir J 2021;58(5):2004656.
15. Soriano JB, Kendrick PJ, Paulson KR, et al. Prevalence and attributable health burden of chronic respiratory diseases, 1990–2017: a systematic analysis for

the Global Burden of Disease Study 2017. Lancet Respir Med 2020;8(6): 585–96.

16. Sadatsafavi M, Tavakoli H, Kendzerska T, et al. History of asthma in patients with chronic obstructive pulmonary disease. a comparative study of economic burden. Ann Am Thorac Soc 2016;13(2):188–96.

17. To T, Zhu J, Gray N, et al. Asthma and chronic obstructive pulmonary disease overlap in women. incidence and risk factors. Ann Am Thorac Soc 2018; 15(11):1304–10.

18. Clatworthy J, Price D, Ryan D, et al. The value of self-report assessment of adherence, rhinitis and smoking in relation to asthma control. Prim Care Resp J 2009; 18(4):300–5.

19. Bhatt SP, Anderson JA, Brook RD, et al. Cigarette smoking and response to inhaled corticosteroids in COPD. Eur Respir J 2018;51(1):1701393.

20. Pascoe S, Barnes N, Brusselle G, et al. Blood eosinophils and treatment response with triple and dual combination therapy in chronic obstructive pulmonary disease: analysis of the IMPACT trial. Lancet Respir Med 2019;7:745–56.

21. Papi A. Asthma COPD Overlap PRO-CON Debate. ACO: The Mistaken Term. COPD 2020;17(5):474–6.

22. Lange P, Celli B, Agustí A, et al. Lung-Function Trajectories Leading to Chronic Obstructive Pulmonary Disease. N Engl J Med 2015;373(2):111–22.

23. Baarnes CB, Andersen ZJ, Tjønneland A, et al. Determinants of incident asthma-COPD overlap: a prospective study of 55,110 middle-aged adults. Clin Epidemiol 2018;10:1275–87.

24. Backman H, Jansson S-A, Stridsman C, et al. Chronic airway obstruction in a population-based adult asthma cohort: Prevalence, incidence and prognostic factors. Respir Med 2018;138:115–22.

25. Morgan BW, Grigsby MR, Siddharthan T, et al. Epidemiology and risk factors of asthma-chronic obstructive pulmonary disease overlap in low- and middle-income countries. J Allergy Clin Immunol 2019;143(4):1598–606.

26. Kiljander T, Helin T, Venho K, et al. Prevalence of asthma–COPD overlap syndrome among primary care asthmatics with a smoking history: a cross-sectional study. NPJ Prim Care Respir Med 2015;25:15047.

27. Lange P, Parner J, Vestbo J, et al. A 15-Year Follow-Up Study of Ventilatory Function in Adults with Asthma. N Engl J Med 1998;339(17):1194–200.

28. Aanerud M, Carsin A-E, Sunyer J, et al. Interaction between asthma and smoking increases the risk of adult airway obstruction. Eur Respir J 2015;45(3):635–43.

29. Perret JL, Dharmage SC, Matheson MC, et al. The Interplay between the Effects of Lifetime Asthma, Smoking, and Atopy on Fixed Airflow Obstruction in Middle Age. Am J Respir Crit Care Med 2013;187(1):42–8.

30. James AL, Palmer LJ, Kicic E, et al. Decline in Lung Function in the Busselton Health Study: The Effects of Asthma and Cigarette Smoking. Am J Respir Crit Care Med 2005;171(2):109–14.

31. Tommola M, Ilmarinen P, Tuomisto LE, et al. The effect of smoking on lung function: a clinical study of adult-onset asthma. Eur Respir J 2016;48(5):1298–306.

32. Backman H, Lindberg A, Hedman L, et al. FEV1 decline in relation to blood eosinophils and neutrophils in a population-based asthma cohort. World Allergy Organ J 2020;13(3):100110.

33. Putcha N, Fawzy A, Matsui EC, et al. Clinical Phenotypes of Atopy and Asthma in COPD: A Meta-analysis of SPIROMICS and COPDGene. Chest 2020;158(6): 2333–45.

34. Thomson N, Chaudhuri R, Messow CM, et al. Chronic cough and sputum production are associated with worse clinical outcomes in stable asthma. Respir Med 2013;107(10):1501–8.
35. Higgins ST, Kurti AN, Redner R, et al. Co-occurring risk factors for current cigarette smoking in a U.S. nationally representative sample. Prevent Med 2016;92: 110–7.
36. To T, Zhu J, Carlsten C, et al. Do community demographics, environmental characteristics and access to care affect risks of developing ACOS and mortality in people with asthma? Eur Respir J 2017;50(3):1700644.
37. Hayes-Watson C, Nuss H, Tseng TS, et al. Self-management practices of smokers with asthma and/or chronic obstructive pulmonary disease: a cross-sectional survey. COPD Res Prac 2017;3(1):3.
38. To T, Zhu J, Larsen K, et al. Progression from asthma to chronic obstructive pulmonary disease. is air pollution a risk factor? Am J Respir Crit Care Med 2016; 194(4):429–38.
39. Eisner MD, Anthonisen N, Coultas D, et al. An Official American Thoracic Society Public Policy Statement: Novel Risk Factors and the Global Burden of Chronic Obstructive Pulmonary Disease. Am J Respir Crit Care Med 2010;182(5): 693–718.
40. Martinez FD. Early-Life Origins of Chronic Obstructive Pulmonary Disease. N Engl J Med 2016;375(9):871–8.
41. Braido F, Brusselle G, Guastalla D, et al. Determinants and impact of suboptimal asthma control in Europe: The INTERNATIONAL CROSS-SECTIONAL AND LONGITUDINAL ASSESSMENT ON ASTHMA CONTROL (LIAISON) study. Respir Res 2016;17(1):51.
42. Upton J, Lewis C, Humphreys E, et al. Asthma-specific health related quality of life of people in Great Britain: A national survey. J Asthma 2016;53(9):975–82.
43. Bloom CI, Nissen F, Douglas IJ, et al. Exacerbation risk and characterisation of the UK's asthma population from infants to old age. Thorax 2018;73(4):313–20.
44. Thomson NC, Chaudhuri R, Heaney LG, et al. Clinical outcomes and inflammatory biomarkers in current smokers and exsmokers with severe asthma. J Allergy Clin Immunol 2013;131(4):1008–16.
45. Tommola M, Ilmarinen P, Tuomisto LE, et al. Cumulative effect of smoking on disease burden and multimorbidity in adult-onset asthma. Eur Respir J 2019;54(3): 1801580.
46. Boulet L-P, Boulay M-È, Dérival J-L, et al. Asthma-COPD Overlap Phenotypes and Smoking :Comparative features of asthma in smoking or non-smoking patients with an incomplete reversibility of airway obstruction. COPD 2018;15(2):130–8.
47. Boulet L-P, Boulay M-E, Milot J, et al. Longitudinal comparison of outcomes in patients with smoking-related asthma-COPD overlap and in non-smoking asthmatics with incomplete reversibility of airway obstruction. Inter J COPD 2019; 14:493–8.
48. Maselli DJ, Hanania NA. Asthma COPD overlap: Impact of associated comorbidities. Pulm Pharmacol Ther 2018;52:27–31.
49. Hekking P-PW, Amelink M, Wener RR, et al. Comorbidities in Difficult-to-Control Asthma. J Allergy Clin Immunol Pract 2018;6(1):108–11.
50. Nadeau M, Boulay M-È, Milot J, et al. Comparative prevalence of co-morbidities in smoking and non-smoking asthma patients with incomplete reversibility of airway obstruction, non-smoking asthma patients with complete reversibility of airway obstruction and COPD patients. Respir Med 2017;125:82–8.

51. Charokopos A, Braman SS, Brown SAW, et al. Lung cancer risk among patients with asthma–chronic obstructive pulmonary disease overlap. Ann Am Thorac Soc 2021;18(11):1894–900.

52. Engelkes M, de Ridder M, Svensson E, et al. Multinational cohort study of mortality in patients with asthma and severe asthma. Respir Med 2020;2:105919.

53. Stampfli MR, Anderson GP. How cigarette smoke skews immune responses to promote infection, lung disease and cancer. Nat Rev Immunol 2009;9(5):377–84.

54. Barnes PJ. Inflammatory mechanisms in patients with chronic obstructive pulmonary disease. J Allergy Clin Immunol 2016;138(1):16–27.

55. Strzelak A, Ratajczak A, Adamiec A, et al. Tobacco Smoke Induces and Alters Immune Responses in the Lung Triggering Inflammation, Allergy, Asthma and Other Lung Diseases: A Mechanistic Review. Int J Environ Res Public Health 2018;15(5):1033.

56. Choy DF, Arron JR. Beyond type 2 cytokines in asthma - new insights from old clinical trials. Expert Opin Ther Targets 2020;24(5):463–75.

57. Livingston E, Darroch C, Chaudhuri R, et al. Glucocorticoid receptor alpha to beta ratio in blood mononuclear cells is reduced in cigarette smokers. J Allergy Clin Immunol 2004;114:1475–8.

58. Agustí A, Hogg JC. Update on the Pathogenesis of Chronic Obstructive Pulmonary Disease. N Eng J Med 2019;381(13):1248–56.

59. Pavlidis S, Takahashi K, Ng Kee Kwong F, et al. T2-high" in severe asthma related to blood eosinophil, exhaled nitric oxide and serum periostin. Eur Respir J 2019;53(1):1800938.

60. Konno S, Taniguchi N, Makita H, et al. Distinct Phenotypes of Smokers with Fixed Airflow Limitation Identified by Cluster Analysis of Severe Asthma. Ann Am Thorac Soc 2018;15(1):33–41.

61. Hsiao H-P, Lin M-C, Wu C-C, et al. Sex-Specific Asthma Phenotypes, Inflammatory Patterns, and Asthma Control in a Cluster Analysis. J Allergy Clin Immunol Pract 2019;7(2):556–67.e15.

62. Christenson SA, Steiling K, van den Berge M, et al. Asthma-COPD Overlap: Clinical Relevance of Genomic Signatures of Type 2 Inflammation in COPD. Am J Respir Crit Care Med 2015;191(7):758–66.

63. Saferali A, Yun JH, Lee S, et al. Transcriptomic signature of asthma-chronic obstructive pulmonary disease overlap in whole blood. Am J Respir Cell Mol Biol 2021;64(2):268–71.

64. Bafadhel M, Peterson S, De Blas MA, et al. Predictors of exacerbation risk and response to budesonide in patients with chronic obstructive pulmonary disease: a post-hoc analysis of three randomised trials. Lancet Respir Med 2018;6(2):117–26.

65. Cosío BG, Pérez de Llano L, Lopez Viña A, et al. Th-2 signature in chronic airway diseases: towards the extinction of asthma–COPD overlap syndrome? Eur Respir J 2017;49(5):1602397.

66. Fu J-j, McDonald VM, Gibson PG, et al. Systemic Inflammation in Older Adults With Asthma-COPD Overlap Syndrome. Allergy Asthma Immunol Res 2014;6(4):316–24.

67. McDonald VM, Fingleton J, Agusti A, et al. Treatable traits: a new paradigm for 21st century management of chronic airway diseases: Treatable Traits Down Under International Workshop report. Eur Respir J 2019;53(5):1802058.

68. Pérez de Llano L, Miravitlles M, Golpe R, et al. A Proposed Approach to Chronic Airway Disease (CAD) Using Therapeutic Goals and Treatable Traits: A Look to the Future. Int J Chron Obstruct Pulmon Dis 2020;15:2091–100.

69. To T, Daly C, Feldman R, et al. Results from a community-based program evaluating the effect of changing smoking status on asthma symptom control. BMC Public Health 2012;12(1):293.

70. Tonnesen P, Pisinger C, Hvidberg S, et al. Effects of smoking cessation and reduction in asthmatics. Nicotine Tob Res 2005;7(1):139–48.

71. Westergaard CG, Porsbjerg C, Backer V. The effect of smoking cessation on airway inflammation in young asthma patients. Clin Exp Allergy 2014;44(3): 353–61.

72. Chaudhuri R, Livingston E, McMahon AD, et al. Effects of smoking cessation on lung function and airway inflammation in smokers with asthma. Am J Respir Crit Care Med 2006;174(2):127–33.

73. Vozoris NT, Stanbrook MB. Smoking prevalence, behaviours, and cessation among individuals with COPD or asthma. Respir Med 2011;105(3):477–84.

74. Jiménez-Ruiz CA, Andreas S, Lewis KE, et al. Statement on smoking cessation in COPD and other pulmonary diseases and in smokers with comorbidities who find it difficult to quit. Eur Respir J 2015;46(1):61–79.

75. WHO report on the global tobacco epidemic. Geneva (Switzerland): World Health Organization; 2019. p. 2019. Available at: https://www.who.int/tobacco/global_report/en/ [Accessed December 12, 2021].

76. Travers J, Marsh S, Williams M, et al. External validity of randomised controlled trials in asthma: to whom do the results of the trials apply? Thorax 2007;62(3): 219–23.

77. Akenroye A, Keet C. Underrepresentation of Blacks, Smokers, and Obese patients in Studies of Monoclonal Antibodies for Asthma. J Allergy Clin Immunol Pract 2020;8(2):739–41.

78. Thomson NC. Challenges in the management of asthma associated with smoking-induced airway diseases. Expert Opin Pharmacother 2018;19(14): 1565–79.

79. Tomlinson JEM, McMahon AD, Chaudhuri R, et al. Efficacy of low and high dose inhaled corticosteroid in smokers versus non-smokers with mild asthma. Thorax 2005;60(4):282–7.

80. Pedersen SE, Bateman ED, Bousquet J, et al. Determinants of response to fluticasone propionate and salmeterol/fluticasone propionate combination in the Gaining Optimal Asthma control study. J Allergy Clin Immunol 2007;120(5):1036–42.

81. Jo YS, Hwang YI, Yoo KH, et al. Effect of Inhaled Corticosteroids on Exacerbation of Asthma-COPD Overlap According to Different Diagnostic Criteria. J Allergy Clin Immunol Pract 2020;8(5):1625–33.e6.

82. Gershon AS, Campitelli MA, Croxford R, et al. Combination long-acting β-agonists and inhaled corticosteroids compared with long-acting β-agonists alone in older adults with chronic obstructive pulmonary disease. JAMA 2014;312(11): 1114–21.

83. Amegadzie JE, Gorgui J, Acheampong L, et al. Comparative safety and effectiveness of inhaled bronchodilators and corticosteroids for treating asthma–COPD overlap: a systematic review and meta-analysis. J Asthma 2021;58(3): 344–59.

84. Park S-Y, Kim S, Kim J-H, et al. A Randomized, Noninferiority Trial Comparing ICS + LABA with ICS + LABA + LAMA in Asthma-COPD Overlap (ACO)

Treatment: The ACO Treatment with Optimal Medications (ATOMIC) Study. J Allergy Clin Immunol Pract 2021;9(3):1304–13011.e2.

85. Donovan T, Milan SJ, Wang R, et al. Anti-IL-5 therapies for chronic obstructive pulmonary disease. Cochrane Database Syst Rev 2020;12(12):Cd013432.

86. Roche N, Anzueto A, Bosnic Anticevich S, et al. The importance of real-life research in respiratory medicine: manifesto of the Respiratory Effectiveness Group. Eur Respir J 2019;54(3):1901511.

87. Thomson NC, Spears M. Asthma Guidelines and Smokers; it's time to be inclusive. Chest 2012;141(2):286–8.

Clinical Assessment and Utility of Biomarkers in Asthma-Chronic Obstructive Pulmonary Disease Overlap

Kewu Huang, MD[a,b], Kian Fan Chung, MD, DSc, FRCP[c],*

KEYWORDS

- Asthma-COPD overlap • Eosinophils • Airflow obstruction
- Fractional exhaled nitric oxide • Asthma • Chronic obstructive pulmonary disease

KEY POINTS

- Asthma-COPD overlap is usually defined by the presence of persistent airflow limitation in those aged 40 years or older, a significant history of smoking or biomass exposure, and symptoms related to atopy or asthma.
- Asthma-COPD overlap represents a heterogeneous group of clinical phenotypes because of the inclusion of features such as those found in asthma and COPD, significant beta-agonist bronchodilator response, the presence of allergy, a raised blood eosinophil count or nitric oxide in exhaled breath, or the presence of emphysema.
- Asthma-COPD overlap is characterized by more frequent exacerbations and associated with higher health costs than those with only asthma or only COPD.

INTRODUCTION

Asthma and chronic obstructive pulmonary disease (COPD) are common prevalent chronic obstructive lung diseases, ranking among 23rd (asthma) and 8th (COPD) causes of disease burden as measured by disability-adjusted life years in 2015.[1] Asthma and COPD as defined clearly by the Global Initiative for Asthma (GINA)[2] and the Global Initiative for Chronic Lung Disease (GOLD)[3] are widely considered as 2 distinct airway disorders. However, detailed phenotyping of patients with chronic airway disease reveals that asthma and COPD rarely exist in their pure forms and that it is common for patients to have features of both asthma and COPD,[4] when the term *asthma-COPD overlap* (ACO) is used.

---

[a] Department of Pulmonary and Critical Care Medicine, Beijing Chao-Yang Hospital, Capital Medical University, Beijing, China; [b] Beijing Institute of Respiratory Medicine, Beijing, China; [c] National Heart & Lung Institute, Imperial College London & Royal Brompton & Harefield NHS Trust, Dovehouse Street, London SW3 6LY, UK
* Corresponding author.
E-mail address: f.chung@imperial.ac.uk

Immunol Allergy Clin N Am 42 (2022) 631–643
https://doi.org/10.1016/j.iac.2022.04.004
0889-8561/22/© 2022 Elsevier Inc. All rights reserved.
immunology.theclinics.com

ACO stands apart from asthma or COPD being generally associated with more frequent exacerbations, higher health costs, more hospital admissions, and a higher mortality rate than either asthma or COPD alone.[5,6] ACO may provide a useful framework within which clinicians can operate, such as the idea that ACO is regarded as a subset of COPD that might respond better to inhaled corticosteroids (ICS). However, this increased attention to ACO has not yet translated into major changes in clinical practice due to the lack of a widely accepted definition and lack of high-quality data from the few clinical trials that have involved patients with ACO. This article presents an update of the current understanding of ACO, focusing on the assessment of ACO and biomarkers that may have a role in identifying ACO and guiding its treatment.

ASTHMA-CHRONIC OBSTRUCTIVE PULMONARY DISEASE OVERLAP: A TERM DERIVED FROM OSLERIAN DIAGNOSTIC LABEL

As early as the 1960s, Sluiter and colleagues from the Netherlands presented data relating to the concomitant features of asthma and bronchitis in their patients that indicated such an overlap of clinical features that became the basis for the "Dutch hypothesis" that all airways disease should be considered as different expression of the same disease.[7] In 2009, Gibson and colleagues[8] introduced the term asthma-COPD overlap syndrome (ACOS) with the need to re-evaluate the concept of asthma and COPD as separate conditions, and to consider situations when they may coexist, or when one condition may evolve into the other. Because most clinicians think that this condition does not represent a single discrete disease entity, a document published jointly by GINA and GOLD in 2017 recommended the use of the term asthma-COPD overlap syndrome (ACO) to replace the previous term ACOS.[9] Later, in 2020, GOLD did not refer to ACO, but emphasized that asthma and COPD were different disorders, although they may share some common traits and clinical features.[10]

This evolution of the term ACO is an epitome of the Oslerian paradigm of classifying chronic airway diseases, which was established in the latter part of the nineteenth century by Sir William Osler on the basis of the principal organ system in which symptoms and signs manifest with some physiologic, anatomic, and pathologic correlation[11] allowing for the consideration of asthma and COPD being 2 distinct diseases with different clinical manifestations and underlying mechanisms. Asthma is commonly regarded as an early-onset, allergic, eosinophilic, type 2 (T2)-related airway inflammation disease, whereas COPD is considered to be a neutrophilic, non-T2-related airway inflammatory commonly caused by smoking and occurring after the age of 40 years. However, according to the so-called Dutch hypothesis, asthma and COPD are 2 extreme phenotypes located on the manifestations of a continuum of airway diseases.[4] Thus, when we label a chronic airway disease with continuous characteristics of asthma and COPD, the term ACO is reasonable in theory, located at the intermediate zone of the 2 disease extremes. The asthma, COPD, and ACO paradigm is illustrated in **Fig. 1**.

ASTHMA-CHRONIC OBSTRUCTIVE PULMONARY DISEASE OVERLAP: DESCRIPTIVE TERM WITH NO WIDELY ACCEPTED DEFINITION

Although different definitions of ACO have been put forward, those taken from guideline documents or expert consensus reviews largely agree on the following components or traits as being part of ACO: (1) presence of persistent airflow limitation in adults aged 40 years and older, (2) a significant smoking or biomass exposure history, and (3) a history of atopy or asthma. Others have suggested that, in addition to a combined history of asthma and COPD, objective measures such as a "large"

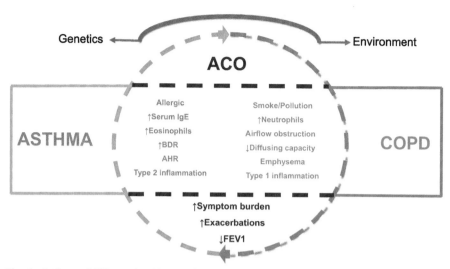

Fig. 1. Asthma, COPD, and ACO paradigm. Asthma and COPD are 2 extreme phenotypes located on the manifestations of a continuum of airway diseases. ACO is located at the intermediate zone of these 2 disease extremes with continuous characteristics of both asthma and COPD. ACO is often distinguished from the extremes by increased symptom and disease burden. AHR, airway hyperresponsiveness; BDR, bronchodilator responsiveness; FEV$_1$, forced expiratory volume in 1 second; IgE, immunoglobulin E.

bronchodilator response, most commonly defined as 200 mL and 12% increase in force expiratory volume in 1 second (FEV$_1$), with sometimes a larger improvement of 400 mL and 15% increase in FEV$_1$; serum IgE levels outside the normal levels with evidence of atopy; and sputum eosinophil counts usually greater than or equal to 2%[4,12,13] or combination with the presence of emphysema on imaging, an attenuated diffusion capacity measurement, or an increased fractional exhaled nitric oxide (FeNO) level.[14]

However, an algorithm for a "syndromic approach" to differentiating asthma, COPD, and ACO, based on the presence or absence of features of both asthma and COPD has been recommended jointly by GINA and GOLD and is widely used to diagnose and assess ACO.[9] These features based on history (age of onset, family history, pattern of symptoms), lung function (bronchodilator responsiveness), and laboratory workup (eosinophil and neutrophil inflammation) are tallied. Clinical features that are particularly favorable toward the diagnosis of asthma include onset before the age of 20 years; symptom variability over minutes, hours, or days; symptom deterioration during the night or early morning; and characteristic triggers (eg, exercise, emotions, dust, or allergen exposure). Conversely, features that particularly suggest a diagnosis of COPD include onset after age 40 years, persistence of symptoms despite treatment, daily symptoms and exertional dyspnea, chronic cough and sputum preceeding dyspnea, heavy smoking history (or biomass fuel exposure), progressive deterioration, limited relief from rapid-acting bronchodilators, and severe hyperinflation on imaging. Patients with more or less equal numbers of these features of asthma and COPD are considered to have ACO. The clinical and diagnostic features for asthma, COPD, and ACO recommended jointly by GINA and GOLD are shown in **Table 1**.

In summary, the first step in diagnosing ACO is to confirm a diagnosis of COPD based on smoking history or other noxious exposure, respiratory symptoms, and

Table 1
Clinical and diagnostic features for asthma, chronic obstructive pulmonary disease, and asthma-chronic obstructive pulmonary disease overlap

Feature	Asthma	COPD	ACO	More Likely to be Asthma if Several of	More Likely to be COPD if Several of
Age of onset	Usually, childhood onset but can commence at any age	Usually, > 40 y of age	Usually age > 40 y, but may have had symptoms in childhood or early adulthood	Onset before 20 y	Onset after 40 y
Pattern of respiratory symptoms	Symptoms may vary over time (day to day, or over longer periods), often limiting activity. Often triggered by exercise, emotions including laughter, dust, or exposure to allergens	Chronic usually continuous symptoms, particularly during exercise, with better and worse days	Respiratory symptoms including exertional dyspnea are persistent, but variability may be prominent	Variable over minutes, hours, or days Worse in night or morning Triggered by exercise, emotions, dust, allergens	Persistence despite treatment Good and bad days but always daily symptoms and exertional dyspnea Chronic cough and sputum preceded onset of dyspnea, unrelated to triggers
Lung function	Current and/or historical variable airflow limitation, for example, bronchodilator reversibility, airway hyperresponsiveness	FEV₁ may be improved by therapy, but post-BD FEV₁/FVC<0.7 persists	Airflow limitation not fully reversible, but often with current or historical variability	Record of variable airflow limitation (spirometry, peak flow)	Record of persistent airflow limitation (post-BD FEV₁/FVC<0.7)
Lung function between symptoms	May be normal between symptoms	Persistent airflow limitation	Persistent airflow limitation	Lung function normal between symptoms	Lung function abnormal between symptoms
Past history or family history	Many patients have allergies and a personal history of asthma in childhood,	History of exposure to noxious particles and gases (mainly	Frequently a history of doctor-diagnosed asthma (current or previous), allergies and a family history of	Previous doctor diagnosis of asthma Family history of asthma, and other allergic conditions	Previous doctor diagnosis of COPD, chronic bronchitis, or emphysema Heavy exposure to a risk

	and/or family history of asthma	tobacco smoking and biomass fuels)	asthma, and/or a history of noxious exposures	(allergic rhinitis or eczema)	factor: tobacco smoke, biomass fuels
Time course	Often improves spontaneously or with treatment, but may result in fixed airflow limitation	Generally, slowly progressive over years despite treatment	Symptoms are partly but significantly reduced by treatment. Progression is usual and treatment needs are high	No worsening of symptoms over time. Symptoms vary either seasonally or from year to year May improve spontaneously or have an immediate response to BD or to ICS over weeks	Symptoms slowly worsening over time (progressive course over years) Rapid-acting BD treatment provides only limited relief
Chest radiograph	Usually, normal	Severe hyperinflation & other changes of COPD	Similar to COPD	Normal	Severe hyperinflation
Exacerbations	Exacerbations occur, but the risk of exacerbations can be reduced by treatment	Exacerbations can be reduced by treatment. If present, comorbidities contribute to impairment	Exacerbations may be more common than in COPD but are reduced by treatment. Comorbidities can contribute to impairment		
Airway inflammation	Eosinophils and/or neutrophils	Neutrophils ± eosinophils in sputum, lymphocytes in airways, may have systemic inflammation	Eosinophils and/or neutrophils in sputum		

Abbreviations: BD, bronchodilator; FVC, force vital capacity.
Reprinted with permission from GINA ©2021 Global initiative for asthma. Available at: www.ginasthma.org.

presence of non–fully reversible airflow obstruction. Then, the diagnosis of asthma should be confirmed by a well-documented history of asthma and/or a current diagnosis of asthma according to guidelines. If the diagnosis of asthma cannot be established, the diagnosis of ACO could be suggested by the identification of asthmatic traits, such as the presence of sputum or blood eosinophilia or elevated levels of FeNO.

ASTHMA-CHRONIC OBSTRUCTIVE PULMONARY DISEASE OVERLAP: CLINICAL FEATURES

The aforementioned approach favored by GINA and GOLD for the diagnosis of ACO obviously would define the clinical features of ACO. Studies of the clinical features of ACO have reported mostly on symptoms of dyspnea particularly on exertion, quality of life, lung function, and exacerbations, symptoms or traits that are particularly relevant to the patient. A higher disease burden for eosinophilic ACO has been reported compared with eosinophilic COPD or asthma.[15] Patients with ACO reported more wheezing and mucous production than patients with asthma or COPD.[16,17] Patients with ACO also scored worse on the Medical Research Council score of dyspnea than those with asthma and COPD.[18–20]

The most consistent feature reported in ACO is the lower FEV_1 compared with asthma, but not dissimilar compared with COPD.[16,20–23] Although 2 studies have reported no difference in FEV_1 decline between ACO, asthma, and COPD,[16,17] a Korean study reported a slower decline in FEV_1 in ACO,[24] whereas the Copenhagen City Heart Study showed a lower decline in ACO with early-onset asthma but a higher decline in ACO with late-onset asthma.[25] However, there is no report of worse exercise capacity in ACO.[22,26] In a systematic study of 11 studies, a higher rate of exacerbations has been reported in ACO compared with asthma and COPD,[27] and these studies confirm this for patients with ACO compared with those with COPD.[18,28,29] The Copenhagen City Heart Study reported a higher risk of exacerbations in patients with ACO associated with late-onset asthma compared with asthma or COPD.[25] Thus, overall, the comparative studies reported so far report a higher symptom burden in ACO, with a higher frequency and likely severity of exacerbations compared with asthma and COPD.

ASTHMA-CHRONIC OBSTRUCTIVE PULMONARY DISEASE OVERLAP: HETEROGENEITY AND CLINICAL PHENOTYPES

Considering that asthma and COPD are heterogeneous diseases, and that ACO is a continuum of airways disease, it is not surprising that ACO can be a heterogeneous disease with various characteristics, which fall into distinct subtypes with different patterns in their quality of life, symptoms, frequency of exacerbation, and degree of airflow obstruction. In the Korean National Health and Nutrition Examination Survey (KNHANES) conducted between 2007 and 2012, subjects with ACO who were 40 years or older and had prebronchodilator FEV_1/force vital capacity (FVC) less than 0.7 were included. Four groups of ACO were distinguished as no wheeze/no smoker, no wheeze/smoker, wheeze/no smoker, and wheeze/smoker, with the latter 2 groups being asthma-predominant ACO and COPD-predominant ACO, respectively. The individuals with asthma-predominant ACO displayed poorer socioeconomic status and quality of life compared with the COPD-predominant ACO group, but it was the COPD-predominant ACO group that displayed more frequent exacerbations and had greater medical costs.[30]

High bronchodilator response ([HBR] defined as a change of >400 mL and >15% in FEV_1) and a high blood eosinophil count (>300 cells/μL) were commonly used as biomarkers for the identification of ACO. In the Spanish MAJORICA cohort of 603 patients with ACO who had (1) age greater than or equal to 40 years, (2) smoking exposure greater than 10 pack-years, (3) postbronchodilator FEV_1/FVC less than 0.7, and (4) at least 1 blood eosinophil count, the prevalence of smoking asthmatics (SA) was 14%, patients with COPD with high bronchodilator response (COPD-HBR) was 1.5%, and patients with eosinophilic COPD (COPD-Eo) was 12%. The SA group used more short-acting β-agonist (SABA), ICS, and oral corticosteroids and made a higher use of health services compared with COPD-HBR and COPD-Eo. This study showed that ACO conferred poorer prognosis in the smoking patients with self-reported wheezing, but the patients with COPD-HBR or COPD-Eo without self-reported wheezing had a better prognosis.[31]

Similar results were also reported by Barrecheguren and colleagues[32] who used 7 different criteria to define ACO in 522 individuals with COPD, and observed that patients with ACO who had atopy and/or physician diagnosis of asthma were more likely to experience frequent exacerbations, whereas those patients with ACO defined by bronchodilator reversibility shared more characteristics with non-ACO COPD. These studies demonstrate that ACO remains an umbrella term that includes diverse conditions with different clinical characteristics and prognosis.

ASTHMA-CHRONIC OBSTRUCTIVE PULMONARY DISEASE OVERLAP: ANY OBJECTIVE LABELS OR BIOMARKERS?

Although ACO does not have a widely accepted definition, there are several objective "labels" or biomarkers that could help in the diagnosis of ACO, which may help in guiding the treatment of ACO.

Airflow obstruction measured by spirometry is an essential or major criterion in all diagnostic algorithms because persistent airflow limitation defined as postbronchodilator FEV_1/FVC ratio of less than 0.7 or the lower limit of normal is a "gold" standard for the diagnosis of COPD. Significant bronchodilator response is considered as physiologic feature of asthma, and there are several guidelines or consensus documents that use the 15% and/or a 400-mL cutoff for distinguishing asthma from COPD[33,34] or for the diagnosis of ACO.[12,35] Although this recommendation is widely used,[31,32,36,37] there is growing evidence that erodes this. First, significant reversibility after bronchodilator administration is commonly observed in patients with COPD.[38] For example, the UPLIFT study showed that more than half of the patients with COPD exhibited bronchodilator reversibility in FEV_1 based on American Thoracic Society criteria.[39] Second, bronchodilator reversibility was not associated with more severe symptom burden, more exacerbations, or impaired health status in patients with COPD,[40] which are considered as clinical characteristic of ACO. Third, a study of fluticasone propionate in subjects with COPD showed that baseline bronchodilator response was not related to airway eosinophilia and did not predict response to ICS.[41] Finally, bronchodilator responsiveness has been shown to be unstable with a large 52% change between visits.[42] All these imply that bronchodilator reversibility may not be an ideal marker of ACO, and its value in predicting response to ICS needs further evaluation.

Eosinophilia in sputum and blood is regarded as a hallmark of allergic asthma,[43] but is also increasingly recognized in patients with COPD.[44] Epidemiologic studies and posthoc analyses of clinical trials of corticosteroid treatment in COPD have shown that the blood eosinophil count is associated with the risk of COPD exacerbations, mortality, decline in FEV_1, and response to both inhaled and systemic corticosteroids.[45,46] However, no difference in blood eosinophil counts between asthma, COPD, and ACO has been reported in the real-world study cohort, NOVELTY, in which the diagnosis of asthma, COPD, and ACO was made by physicians.[47] In the SPIROMICS cohort, stratification by increased sputum eosinophil inflammation, but not blood eosinophil, led to the identification of a subgroup with decreased lung function and more COPD exacerbations.[44] There was no recommendation for or against the use of ICS as an additive therapy to long-acting bronchodilators in patients with COPD and blood eosinophilia, except for those patients with a history of one or more exacerbations in the past year.[48] The benefit of using blood eosinophil counts as a treatment response biomarker in patients with ACO who are considered to be an ICS-responsive group needs to be determined.

In addition, patients with COPD with elevated blood eosinophil count did not show reduction in exacerbations from the addition of benralizumab, an anti-interleukin-5 receptor α monoclonal antibody treatment.[49] Also, mepolizumab, a monoclonal antibody directed against interleukin-5[50] led to a small nonsignificant reduction in exacerbations in a similar group of patients with COPD.

FeNO is a well-recognized biomarker of type 2 airway inflammation used clinically for detecting eosinophilic airway inflammation, monitoring airway inflammation in asthma, and evaluating response to corticosteroid therapy. It was reported that the levels of FeNO were higher in those patients with COPD with a history of allergic rhinitis[51] and that those with a persistently high FeNO level greater than or equal to 20 ppb had a significantly higher risk of acute exacerbations of COPD.[52] In addition, patients with severe COPD who respond to ICS treatment have higher FeNO levels.[53] These studies suggest that patients with ACO would have higher levels of FeNO than patients with COPD because patients with ACO have more exacerbations and may have evidence of eosinophilia and allergic disease. In a meta-analysis of 10 studies that included 1335 participants, FeNO levels were significantly higher in patients with ACO of different definitions compared with patients with COPD alone. The sensitivity and specificity of FeNO in distinguishing ACO from COPD were modest indicating that there is a moderate diagnostic accuracy in differentiating ACO from COPD.[54] However, a cutoff value to differentiate COPD from ACO is not currently possible. The influence of factors such as smoking and treatments with ICS needs to be considered in this analysis. Nevertheless, Li and colleagues,[55] in their study, reported an optimal cutoff value of FeNO of 31.5 ppb in patients with a smoking history for differentiation of ACO from COPD with 70% sensitivity and 89.9% specificity; for those without a history of ICS use, the cutoff value of 39.5 ppb was proposed. However, these need to be prospectively validated.

Serum IgE is a common biomarker representing allergic status. Elevated serum IgE may help identify a subgroup of patients with COPD with asthmalike features. In a cross-sectional observational study conducted in adult populations from New Zealand and China, 2 ACO phenotypes with considerable differences in genetic heritage and environmental exposures were identified, of which cluster 1 was late-onset asthma/COPD overlap with severe obstruction, poor health status, reduced diffusion capacity, and markedly elevated total IgE, whereas the other was early-onset asthma/COPD overlap with moderate airflow obstruction, preserved diffusion capacity, and relatively lower total IgE.[56]

Allergen sensitization is common in the general population,[57] but the association between atopy and asthmalike features in COPD is inconsistent. Results from NHANES III and CODE cohorts showed that individuals with allergic phenotype were more likely to wheeze, experience nocturnal cough, and have an increased risk of COPD exacerbation.[58] Although allergen-specific IgE was found increased in

35% to 36% of subjects with COPD, there was less than 50% overlap between atopic status and asthma. In a meta-analysis, subjects with nonatopic asthma were associated with adverse outcomes and exacerbation risk in those with COPD, whereas groups having atopy alone and atopic asthma had lesser risk.[59] Thus, elevated serum IgE or allergen-specific IgE cannot be used as a marker of asthmalike features in patients with COPD, unless concomitant with other asthmalike features, such as wheezing or elevated FeNO. Similarly, an elevated serum IgE level alone may not be enough as a biomarker to guide the use of ICS.

Although biologic therapy targeting IgE is effective in treating severe allergic asthma, its role in the treatment of ACO is unknown. A posthoc, exploratory analysis of clinical outcomes of adult patients with ACO treated with omalizumab in the PROS-PERO study showed that patients with ACO treated with omalizumab had similar clinical outcomes as patients with asthma without ACO in terms of improvements in exacerbation frequency and asthma control test scores.[60]

Serum periostin, another type 2 biomarker, is reported to be high in patients with ACO as well as in those with asthma but not in patients with COPD, whereas serum YKL-40 level is high in both patients with ACO and COPD, but not in those with asthma.[61] A combined assessment of serum periostin and YKL-40 levels could help in the diagnosis of ACO.

SUMMARY

ACO, representing a group of patients with both features of asthma and COPD, is commonly seen in respiratory clinics and is associated with more frequent exacerbations and higher health costs than pure asthma or pure COPD. Like asthma and COPD, ACO is also a heterogeneous condition. With the lack of a widely accepted definition, an algorithm for a "syndromic approach" to differentiating asthma, COPD, and ACO, based on the presence or absence of the features of both asthma and COPD, is widely used to diagnose and assess the ACO. There are several objective labels or biomarkers suggestive of the diagnosis of ACO, but it is currently uncertain as to whether any biomarkers can assist toward a diagnosis of ACO. A treatable traits approach should be advocated in identifying and managing these chronic airway diseases, with less attention given to the label of asthma or COPD in future.

Future research is needed to understand the underlying mechanisms of the ACO that will lead to a better classification and definition of the disease and hopefully to more targeted treatments. Molecular phenotyping of patients with ACO should be the next step in this direction, and there are currently available cohorts in which this group may be defined and analyzed such as the U-BIOPRED cohort.[62] This approach may determine whether the ACO represents interactions of type 1 and type2 inflammatory processes with other innate and acquired immune responses. Then, the definition, classification, and treatment of airways diseases will arise on the basis of the underlying driving mechanisms.[63]

CLINICS CARE POINTS

- ACO represents a multitude of clinical phenotypes that consists of different mix of treatable traits associated with asthma and COPD and usually indicates greater symptom burden, more greater airflow obstruction, and more frequent exacerbations than asthma or COPD only.

- In the ACO, a diagnosis of COPD is first confirmed based on smoking history or other noxious exposure, presence of respiratory symptoms, and of airflow obstruction, followed by whether there is history of asthma or features of asthmatic traits.
- Biomarkers such as bronchodilator response, blood eosinophil count, nitric oxide in exhaled breath, and serum IgE levels may be useful in the diagnosis and management of ACO in bringing features usually associated with asthma, but there are currently no specific biomarkers for the ACO.
- Management of ACO should focus on the treatable traits manifested by each individual patient.

CONFLICTS OF INTEREST

Dr Huang has nothing to disclose. Dr Chung has received honoraria for participating in Advisory Board meetings of GSK, AstraZeneca, Roche, Novartis, Merck, Boehringer Ingelheim, TEVA, and Shionogi regarding treatments for asthma, chronic obstructive pulmonary disease, and chronic cough and has been remunerated for speaking engagements. He is Emeritus Senior Investigator of the United Kingdom National Institute for Health Research, and he receives funding from United Kingdom Research and Innovation.

REFERENCES

1. Global, regional, and national incidence, prevalence, and years lived with disability for 310 diseases and injuries, 1990-2015: a systematic analysis for the Global Burden of Disease Study 2015. Lancet 2016;388:1545–602.
2. GINA Executive and Science committee. Global strategy for asthma management and prevention. Available at: https://ginasthma.org/wp-content/uploads/2021/05/GINA-Main-Report-2021-V2-WMS.pdf.2021. Accessed December 12, 2021.
3. Global Initiative for Chronic Obstructive Lung Disease. Global strategy for the diagnosis, management, and prevention of chronic obstructive pulmonary disease. Available at: https://goldcopd.org/wp-content/uploads/2020/11/GOLD-REPORT-2021-v1.1-25Nov20_WMV.pdf.2021. Accessed December 12, 2021.
4. Milne S, Mannino D, Sin D. Asthma-COPD overlap and chronic airflow obstruction: definitions, management, and unanswered questions. J Allergy Clin Immunol Pract 2020;8:483–95.
5. Papaiwannou A, Zarogoulidis P, Porpodis K, et al. Asthma-chronic obstructive pulmonary disease overlap syndrome (ACOS): current literature review. J Thorac Dis 2014;S146–51.
6. Alshabanat A, Zafari Z, Albanyan O, et al. Asthma and COPD Overlap Syndrome (ACOS): A Systematic Review and Meta Analysis. PLoS One 2015;10:e0136065.
7. Sluiter H, Koëter G, de Monchy J, et al. The Dutch hypothesis (chronic nonspecific lung disease) revisited. Eur Respir J 1991;4:479–89.
8. Gibson P, Simpson J. The overlap syndrome of asthma and COPD: what are its features and how important is it? Thorax 2009;64:728–35.
9. Global Initiative for Asthma (GINA). Global Initiative for Chronic Obstructive Lung Disease (GOLD). Diagnosis and Initial Treatment of Asthma, COPD, and Asthma–COPD Overlap. 2017. Available at: https://ginasthma.org/wp-content/uploads/2019/11/GINA-GOLD-2017-overlap-pocket-guide-wms-2017-ACO.pdf. Accessed December 12, 2021.

10. Global Initiative for Chronic Obstructive Lung Disease. Global strategy for the diagnosis, management, and prevention of chronic obstructive pulmonary disease. Available at: https://goldcopd.org/wp-content/uploads/2019/12/GOLD-2020-FINAL-ver1.2-03Dec19_WMV.pdf.2020. Accessed December 12, 2021.

11. Vanfleteren LE, Kocks JW, Stone IS, et al. Moving from the Oslerian paradigm to the post-genomic era: are asthma and COPD outdated terms? Thorax 2014;69:72–9.

12. Sin D, Miravitlles M, Mannino D, et al. What is asthma-COPD overlap syndrome? Towards a consensus definition from a round table discussion. Eur Respir J 2016; 48:664–73.

13. Miravitlles M, Calle M, Molina J, et al. Spanish COPD Guidelines (GesEPOC) 2021: updated pharmacological treatment of stable COPD. Arch Bronconeumol 2021. https://doi.org/10.1016/j.arbres.2021.03.005.

14. Yanagisawa S, Ichinose M. Definition and diagnosis of asthma-COPD overlap (ACO). Allergol Int 2018;67:172–8.

15. Hiles SA, Gibson PG, McDonald VM. Disease burden of eosinophilic airway disease: Comparing severe asthma, COPD and asthma-COPD overlap. Respirology 2021;26:52–61.

16. Brzostek D D, Kokot M. Asthma-chronic obstructive pulmonary disease overlap syndrome in Poland. Findings of an epidemiological study. Postepy Dermatol Alergol 2014;31:372–9.

17. Pleasants RA, Ohar JA, Croft JB, et al. Chronic obstructive pulmonary disease and asthma-patient characteristics and health impairment. COPD 2014;11:256–66.

18. Miravitlles M, Soriano JB, Ancochea J, et al. Characterisation of the overlap COPD-asthma phenotype. Focus on physical activity and health status. Respir Med 2013;107:1053–60.

19. de Marco R, Pesce G, Marcon A, et al. The coexistence of asthma and chronic obstructive pulmonary disease (COPD): prevalence and risk factors in young, middle-aged and elderly people from the general population. PLoS one 2013; 8:e62985.

20. Milanese M, Di Marco F, Corsico AG, et al. Asthma control in elderly asthmatics. An Italian observational study. Respir Med 2014;108:1091–9.

21. Kauppi P, Kupiainen H, Lindqvist A, et al. Overlap syndrome of asthma and COPD predicts low quality of life. J Asthma 2011;48:279–85.

22. Fu JJ, Gibson PG, Simpson JL, et al. Longitudinal changes in clinical outcomes in older patients with asthma, COPD and asthma-COPD overlap syndrome. Respiration 2014;87:63–74.

23. Lee H, Kim SH, Kim BK, et al. Characteristics of Specialist-Diagnosed Asthma-COPD Overlap in Severe Asthma: Observations from the Korean Severe Asthma Registry (KoSAR). Allergy 2021;76:223–32.

24. Park H, Lee S, Kang D, et al. Favorable longitudinal change of lung function in patients with asthma-COPD overlap from a COPD cohort. Respir Med 2018; 19:36.

25. Lange P, Çolak Y, Ingebrigtsen TS, et al. Long-term prognosis of asthma, chronic obstructive pulmonary disease, and asthma-chronic obstructive pulmonary disease overlap in the Copenhagen City Heart study: a prospective population-based analysis. Lancet Respir Med 2016;4:454–62.

26. Hardin M, Cho M, McDonald ML, et al. The clinical and genetic features of COPD-asthma overlap syndrome. Eur Respir J 2014;44:341–50.

27. Nielsen M, Bårnes CB, Ulrik CS. Clinical characteristics of the asthma-COPD overlap syndrome–a systematic review. Int J Chron Obstruct Pulmon Dis 2015; 10:1443–54.

28. Kumbhare S, Pleasants R, Ohar J, et al. Characteristics and Prevalence of Asthma/Chronic Obstructive Pulmonary Disease Overlap in the United States. Ann Am Thorac Soc 2016;13:803–10.

29. Menezes AMB, Montes de Oca M, Pérez-Padilla R, et al. Increased risk of exacerbation and hospitalization in subjects with an overlap phenotype: COPD-asthma. Chest 2014;145:297–304.

30. Kim M, Rhee C, Kim K, et al. Heterogeneity of asthma and COPD overlap. Int J Chron Obstruct Pulmon Dis 2018;13:1251–60.

31. Toledo-Pons N, van Boven JFM, Román-Rodríguez M, et al. ACO: Time to move from the description of different phenotypes to the treatable traits. PLoS One 2019;14:e0210915.

32. Barrecheguren M, Pinto L, Mostafavi-Pour-Manshadi S, et al. Identification and definition of asthma-COPD overlap: The CanCOLD study. Respirology 2020;25: 836–49.

33. Llop-Guevara A, Chu DK, Walker TD, et al. A GM-CSF/IL-33 pathway facilitates allergic airway responses to sub-threshold house dust mite exposure. PLoS One 2014;9:e88714.

34. Chronic obstructive pulmonary disease. National clinical guideline on management of chronic obstructive pulmonary disease in adults in primary and secondary care. Thorax 2004;59(Suppl 1):1–232.

35. Plaza V, Álvarez F, Calle M, et al. Consensus on the Asthma-COPD Overlap Syndrome (ACOS) Between the Spanish COPD Guidelines (GesEPOC) and the Spanish Guidelines on the Management of Asthma (GEMA). Arch Bronconeumol 2017;53:443–9.

36. Guerriero M, Caminati M, Viegi G, et al. Prevalence and features of asthma-chronic obstructive pulmonary disease overlap in Northern Italy general population. J Asthma 2019;56:27–33.

37. Barrecheguren M, Román-Rodríguez M, Miravitlles M. Is a previous diagnosis of asthma a reliable criterion for asthma-COPD overlap syndrome in a patient with COPD? Int J Chron Obstruct Pulmon Dis 2015;10:1745–52.

38. Hanania NA, Celli BR, Donohue JF. U. J. Martin. Bronchodilator reversibility in COPD. Chest 2011;140:1055–63.

39. Tashkin DP, Celli B, Decramer M, et al. Bronchodilator responsiveness in patients with COPD. Eur Respir J 2008;31:742–50.

40. Janson C, Malinovschi A, Amaral A, et al. Bronchodilator reversibility in asthma and COPD: findings from three large population studies. Eur Respir J 2019;54. https://doi.org/10.1183/13993003.00561-2019.

41. Reid DW, Wen Y, Johns DP, et al. Bronchodilator reversibility, airway eosinophilia and anti-inflammatory effects of inhaled fluticasone in COPD are not related. Respirology 2008;13:799–809.

42. Calverley PM, Burge PS, Spencer S, et al. Bronchodilator reversibility testing in chronic obstructive pulmonary disease. Thorax 2003;58:659–64.

43. Terl M, Sedlák V, Cap P, et al. Asthma management: a new phenotype-based approach using presence of eosinophilia and allergy. Allergy 2017;72:1279–87.

44. Bafadhel M, Pavord ID, Russell REK. Eosinophils in COPD: just another biomarker? Lancet Respir Med 2017;5:747–59.

45. Singh D, Kolsum U, Brightling C, et al. Eosinophilic inflammation in COPD: prevalence and clinical characteristics. Eur Respir J 2014;44:1697–700.

46. Bafadhel M, McKenna S, Terry S, et al. Blood eosinophils to direct corticosteroid treatment of exacerbations of chronic obstructive pulmonary disease: a randomized placebo-controlled trial. Am J Respir Crit Care Med 2012;186:48–55.

47. Reddel H, Vestbo J, Agustí A, et al. Heterogeneity within and between physician-diagnosed asthma and/or COPD: NOVELTY cohort. Eur Respir J 2021. https://doi.org/10.1183/13993003.03927-2020.

48. Nici L, Mammen M, Charbek E, et al. Pharmacologic Management of Chronic Obstructive Pulmonary Disease. An Official American Thoracic Society Clinical Practice Guideline. Am J Respir Crit Care Med 2020;201:e56–69.

49. Criner GJ, Celli BR, Singh D, et al. Predicting response to benralizumab in chronic obstructive pulmonary disease: analyses of GALATHEA and TERRANOVA studies. Lancet Respir Med 2020;8:158–70.

50. Pavord I, Chanez P, Criner G, et al. Mepolizumab for Eosinophilic Chronic Obstructive Pulmonary Disease. N Engl J Med 2017;377:1613–29.

51. Tamada T, Sugiura H, Takahashi T, et al. Biomarker-based detection of asthma-COPD overlap syndrome in COPD populations. Int J Chron Obstruct Pulmon Dis 2015;10:2169–76.

52. Alcázar-Navarrete B, Ruiz Rodríguez O, Conde Baena P, et al. Persistently elevated exhaled nitric oxide fraction is associated with increased risk of exacerbation in COPD. Eur Respir J 2018;51. https://doi.org/10.1183/13993003.01457-2017.

53. Kunisaki K, Rice K, Janoff E, et al. Exhaled nitric oxide, systemic inflammation, and the spirometric response to inhaled fluticasone propionate in severe chronic obstructive pulmonary disease: a prospective study. Ther Adv Respir Dis 2008;2:55–64.

54. Zhang C, Zhang M, Wang Y, et al. Diagnostic value of fractional exhaled nitric oxide in differentiating the asthma-COPD overlap from COPD: a systematic review and meta-analysis. Expert Rev Respir Med 2021;1–9.

55. Li M, Yang T, He R, et al. The value of inflammatory biomarkers in differentiating asthma-COPD Overlap from COPD. Int J Chron Obstruct Pulmon Dis 2020;15:3025–37.

56. Fingleton J, Huang K, Weatherall M, et al. Phenotypes of symptomatic airways disease in China and New Zealand. Eur Respir J 2017;50. https://doi.org/10.1183/13993003.00957-2017.

57. Bousquet PJ, Castelli C, Daures JP, et al. Assessment of allergen sensitization in a general population-based survey (European Community Respiratory Health Survey I). Ann Epidemiol 2010;20:797–803.

58. Jamieson DB, Matsui EC, Belli A, et al. Effects of allergic phenotype on respiratory symptoms and exacerbations in patients with chronic obstructive pulmonary disease. Am J Respir Crit Care Med 2013;188:187–92.

59. Putcha N, Fawzy A, Matsui E, et al. Clinical Phenotypes of Atopy and Asthma in COPD: A Meta-analysis of SPIROMICS and COPDGene. Chest 2020;158:2333–45.

60. Hanania N, Chipps B, Griffin N, et al. Omalizumab effectiveness in asthma-COPD overlap: Post hoc analysis of PROSPERO. J Allergy Clin Immunol 2019;143:1629–33.e2.

61. Shirai T, Hirai K, Gon Y, et al. Combined Assessment of Serum Periostin and YKL-40 May Identify Asthma-COPD Overlap. J Allergy Clin Immunol Pract 2019;7:134–45.e1.

62. Kuo CS, Pavlidis S, Loza M, et al. T-helper cell type 2 (Th2) and non-Th2 molecular phenotypes of asthma using sputum transcriptomics in U-BIOPRED. Eur Respir J 2017;49:1602135.

63. Chung KF, Adcock IM. Precision medicine for the discovery of treatable mechanisms in severe asthma. Allergy 2019;74:1649–59.

Phenotypes of Asthma–Chronic Obstructive Pulmonary Disease Overlap

Muhammad Adrish, MD, MBA[a],*, Mahesh P. Anand, MBBS[b],
Nicola A. Hanania, MD, MS[a]

KEYWORDS

- Asthma • COPD • Asthma COPD overlap • Phenotype

KEY POINTS

- Physiologic and morphologic differences exist between patients with asthma, chronic obstructive pulmonary disease, and asthma–chronic obstructive pulmonary disease overlap.
- Asthma–chronic obstructive pulmonary disease overlap is a heterogenous disorder with important clinical differences noted between distinct subgroups or phenotypes.
- The identification of distinct phenotypes of asthma–chronic obstructive pulmonary disease overlap is imperative for a more precise approach to its management and use of targeted therapies.

Abbreviations	
COPD	chronic obstructive pulmonary disease

INTRODUCTION

Asthma and chronic obstructive pulmonary disease (COPD) are considered unique diseases with distinct characteristics. However, clinical characteristics of asthma and COPD can coexist in some patients with asthma–COPD overlap (ACO). The prevalence of ACO has been highly variable, ranging from 5.2% to 35.4%. [1,2] Over the years, many researchers have proposed various definitions of this condition; however, no consensus on its definition exists to date. Furthermore, patients with ACO present with varied characteristics. Although there are established guidelines for the management of patients with asthma and COPD, consensus on the appropriate management of ACO is in its infancy. The development of comprehensive treatment strategies for

[a] Section of Pulmonary, Critical Care and Sleep Medicine, Department of Medicine, Baylor College of Medicine, Ben Taub Hospital, 1504 Taub Loop, Houston, TX 77030, USA;
[b] Department of Respiratory Medicine, JSS Medical College, JSSAHER, Mysore, KA, India
* Corresponding author.
E-mail address: Muhammad.Adrish@bcm.edu

Immunol Allergy Clin N Am 42 (2022) 645–655
https://doi.org/10.1016/j.iac.2022.04.009
0889-8561/22/© 2022 Elsevier Inc. All rights reserved.

ACO relies on understanding its underlying pathophysiology and its different subtypes (phenotypes). In this article, we review current knowledge about the phenotypes of ACO and outline future research needs.

WHAT IS A PHENOTYPE?

A phenotype is commonly defined as the observable characteristics of an organism that is the result of the interaction of its genotype with the environment.[3,4] Phenotypes are clustered based on observable properties such as age of onset, triggers, and response to a particular treatment or type of inflammation (eosinophilic or neutrophilic).[4] Phenotypes do not indicate the key pathway involved in a disease. An endotype is a disease condition that is defined by a distinct functional or pathobiological mechanism.[3,4] Molecular phenotyping is related to the identification of specific pathways in a particular phenotype and targeting of the pathway leads to improved disease outcomes.[3] Molecular phenotyping leads to identification of specific endotypes.

DEFINING ASTHMA–CHRONIC OBSTRUCTIVE PULMONARY DISEASE OVERLAP

As mentioned earlier, the exact definition for ACO is yet to be agreed upon. This stems from the fact that ACO has several phenotypes, and it is not easy to encompass all those into a single definition. Several societies and investigators have attempted to define ACO based on clinical features,[5] spirometry,[6] or both.[7]

Gender-Based Phenotypes of Asthma–Chronic Obstructive Pulmonary Disease Overlap

Available evidence suggests that there are significant gender variations among the different identified phenotypes of ACO. Lainez and colleagues[8] classified ACO into 4 phenotypes based on age of onset of symptoms, smoking, and severity of disease. Phenotype A had slight male predominance and phenotypes C and D had a high male predominance. The spectrum of disease severity among male predominant phenotypes varied from less severe (phenotypes C and D) to more severe (phenotype A). Phenotype B was the only phenotype of ACO that had a female predominance and was associated with a late onset of symptoms and more severe disease. Joo and colleagues[9] classified 4 phenotypes of ACO (A, B, C, D) using 2 criteria, namely, pack-years of smoking (<10 [A and B] or >10 pack-years [C and D]) and peripheral blood eosinophil counts (<300 cells/μL [B and D] or $\geq$300 cells/μL [A and C]). Both A and B phenotypes were female predominant, and phenotypes C and D were male predominant. Toledo and colleagues[10] identified 3 phenotypes of ACO, namely, smoking asthmatics with a slight male predominance (56.6%), whereas COPD with a high bronchodilator reversibility (HBR) (>400 mL and 15% improvement in forced expiratory volume in 1 second [FEV_1]) was nearly all males (88.9%) and COPD with eosinophilia had a high male predominance (72.6%).[10]

Age-Based Phenotypes of Asthma–Chronic Obstructive Pulmonary Disease Overlap

Age of symptom onset is another important consideration among various phenotypes of ACO. In a multiple correspondent analysis to identify various phenotypes of ACO, age of onset of respiratory symptoms was identified as an important variable for classification and identified 4 phenotypes.[8] The onset of respiratory symptoms could be early (<40 years, phenotypes A and C) or late (>40 years, phenotypes B and D). The age of onset of symptoms in phenotypes A and C was less than 20 years, whereas the age of onset in phenotypes B and D was greater than 40 years. The other important variables identified as relevant for classification of ACO phenotypes were smoking burden, dyspnea scores, lung function, and body mass index (BMI). Interestingly, the study observed that participants with either an early or late age of onset of respiratory symptoms could have high or low dyspnea scores, high or low lung function, high or low pack-years of smoking, and a high or low BMI. This classification by Lainez that uses age of onset as an important classifying variable is slightly different than the phenotype groups proposed by Rhee,[6] which classifies patients mainly as either asthma predominant or COPD predominant. Toledo and colleagues[10] observed that smoking asthmatics were relatively younger as compared with COPD with HBR and COPD with eosinophilia.

Symptom-Based Phenotypes of Asthma–Chronic Obstructive Pulmonary Disease Overlap

Phenotypes of ACO were observed to be quite heterogeneous in regards of the severity of symptoms. Joo and colleagues[9] observed that phenotype B (smoking <10 pack-years, eosinophils <300 cells/μL) had very low impact, whereas phenotypes A, C, and D had a moderate impact on the patient's quality of life according to the COPD Assessment Test score. According to Toledo and colleagues,[10] smoking asthmatics had the highest symptoms and hospital admissions, whereas COPD with eosinophilia had the least symptoms and hospital admissions among the different phenotypes of ACO. In the Lainez classification of phenotypes of ACO,[8] dyspnea score (modified Medical Research Council score) was an important minor criterion and two of the phenotypes (A and B) had more severe dyspnea.

Spirometry-Based Phenotypes of Asthma–Chronic Obstructive Pulmonary Disease Overlap

The key spirometric characteristics of ACO is the presence of a fixed airflow limitation (FEV_1/forced vital capacity [FVC] of <0.7) and a bronchodilator reversibility of 12% or greater and 200 mL or more.[5] Some researchers have identified that a subset (nearly 10%) of patients with ACO have greater than 15% and greater than 400 mL improvement (HBR) after bronchodilator.[10] A normal FEV_1/forced vital capacity ratio (>0.8) is considered incompatible with the diagnosis of ACO. However, in mild cases of ACO, the postbronchodilator FEV_1 can be greater than 80% predicted. In more severe cases, the FEV_1 is progressively lower and is a good indicator for future risk of exacerbations and early mortality.

Most studies evaluating different phenotypes of ACO have not included spirometry as one of the key features for identifying its various phenotypes. A cluster analysis by Lainez was the only study that used spirometry for classification of ACO.[8] Both phenotypes A and B had an FEV_1 of less than 70% predicted, with high dyspnea scores (modified Medical Research Council of $\geq$2), high BMI (>25 kg/m^2), a high number of pack-years of smoking (>30 pack-years), and were differentiated only by age of symptom onset (phenotype A–early onset; phenotype B–late onset). Phenotypes C and D had an FEV_1 of more than 70% predicted, a BMI of less than 25 kg/m^2, a lower tobacco smoking load (<30 pack-years), and lower dyspnea scores (modified Medical Research Council of <1) and were differentiated from each other with the age of onset of respiratory symptoms (phenotype C–early onset, phenotype D–late onset). Toledo and colleagues[10] observed that smoking asthmatics had the lowest postbronchodilator FEV_1 and COPD with HBR had the highest postbronchodilator FEV_1, although no statistically significant difference could be demonstrated.

PHYSIOLOGIC AND MORPHOLOGIC DIFFERENCES BETWEEN ASTHMA–CHRONIC OBSTRUCTIVE PULMONARY DISEASE OVERLAP AND CHRONIC OBSTRUCTIVE PULMONARY DISEASE

Airflow limitation has been widely used as the marker of severity in both asthma and COPD; however, it has limited usefulness in discriminating these 2 entities. More recently, respiratory impendence has gained attention as an important physiologic test for several respiratory diseases.[11] By measuring resistance and reactance, respiratory impendence can detect small changes in the airways.[12,13] These properties have also been highlighted in healthy smokers who have normal spirometry, but have impaired respiratory impedance suggestive of small airway remodeling.[14] Computed tomography scans, especially 3-dimensional computed tomography scans, can also provide useful information regarding the structural changes seen in the airways of patients with asthma or COPD.[15] These morphologic characteristics were studied by Karayama and colleagues[16] in their patients with COPD and ACO. In this propensity-matched analysis, 86 patients with COPD with comparable smoking histories and airflow limitations were compared with 43 patients with ACO. Patients with ACO were noted to have greater respiratory resistance and reactance during tidal breathing. On 3-dimensional computed tomography analysis, patients with ACO had a higher percentage of wall thickness from third- to sixth-generation bronchi and greater wall thickness adjusted by square root of body surface area (WT/$\sqrt{BSA}$, mm) from third- to fourth-generation bronchi when compared with patients with COPD. Another finding noted by the study authors was the variability in respiratory impendence during inspiratory and expiratory phases. Patients with ACO had greater respiratory resistance and reactance in inspiratory phase, whereas a greater increase in respiratory resistance and reactance in the expiratory phase was noted in COPD. These data suggest that patients with ACO had greater airway narrowing and more severe small airway disease than patients with COPD. The authors also noted fewer emphysematous changes in patients with ACO compared with patients with COPD. Similar findings have also been reported in other studies.[17]

OTHER BIOMARKERS HELPFUL IN PHENOTYPING ASTHMA–CHRONIC OBSTRUCTIVE PULMONARY DISEASE OVERLAP

Among the different phenotypes of ACO in the Toledo classification,[10] COPD with eosinophilia had higher T helper cell type 2 biomarkers (periostin and fractional exhaled nitric oxide [FeNO]) as compared with COPD with HBR and smoking asthmatics. It is possible that FeNO, sputum eosinophilia, T helper cell type 2 biomarkers, and metabolomics are beneficial in further phenotyping of ACO, but current evidence is still lacking.

Metabolomics studies have identified several metabolites that could help to differentiate ACO from COPD or asthma. In one study, levels of eicosanoids from the lipoxygenase pathway were higher in ACO when compared with COPD.[18] In another study, urinary L-histidine was noted to be higher in ACO compared with both COPD and asthma.[19] Several metabolic signatures in ACO are different from COPD and asthma.[20] Sugars such as mannose, succinate, and glucose were lower in ACO as compared with asthma and COPD. The amino acids serine and threonine were lower in ACO as compared with both COPD and asthma. A glycerophospholipid metabolite, ethanolamine, was lower in ACO as compared with asthma and COPD. Cholesterol and 2-palmitoylglycerol were lower in ACO as compared with COPD, but higher in ACO as compared with asthma. Fatty acids such as stearic acid and linoleic acid are higher in ACO as compared with COPD, but lower in ACO as compared with asthma.

Influence of Comorbidities on Asthma–Chronic Obstructive Pulmonary Disease Overlap Phenotypes

Although the prevalence and impact of comorbid conditions have been studied among patients with ACO, it has not been studied among different phenotypes of ACO. Studies have observed that more than 90% of patients with ACO have at least 1 comorbidity and up to two-thirds of these patients may have primary hypertension.[21] Other prevalent disorders include dyslipidemia, diabetes mellitus, obesity, and chronic ischemic heart disease.[22] Allergic rhinitis and other allergic conditions, such as atopic dermatitis and allergic conjunctivitis, are observed among asthma-predominant phenotypes, along with cardiovascular, endocrine, and metabolic comorbidities.[22] Owing to shared risk factors such as smoking, patients with COPD-predominant phenotypes are more likely to suffer from a greater proportion of cardiovascular and musculoskeletal comorbidities, as well as bronchogenic carcinoma, when compared with patients with asthma-predominant phenotypes.[22] Mental health problems such as anxiety and depression are seen among all phenotypes of ACO.[22]

COMPOSITE DETERMINANTS OF ASTHMA–CHRONIC OBSTRUCTIVE PULMONARY DISEASE OVERLAP PHENOTYPES

Several definitions of ACO have been recommended by researchers all over the world.[5,23,24] These definitions assume that ACO is a homogenous disorder, regardless of whether the patient is an asthmatic who smokes or the patient has COPD with clinical features of asthma. Recent studies have demonstrated that ACO is a heterogeneous disorder with important clinical differences noted between distinct subgroups or phenotypes.[25,26] A recent study from Spain suggested to consider ACO in 3 distinct groups of patients with COPD namely smoking asthmatics, COPD with eosinophilia and COPD with an HBR.[27] These phenotypic cohorts were further studied by Toledo-Pons and colleagues.[10] As discussed elsewhere in this article, smoking asthmatics were younger and had a higher use of rescue bronchodilators, steroids, and health care resources. In contrast, COPD with eosinophilia phenotype patients were older, were frequently treated with corticosteroids, and had lower use of health care resources. Patients with HBR were included within the group of patients with eosinophilia and COPD. The smoking asthmatic group was further studied by Boulet and colleagues[28] in a cross-sectional study on asthmatic patients with incomplete reversibility of the airway obstruction. Patients were divided into 2 subgroups based on their smoking history. ACO group was defined as patients with a 20 pack-year or greater smoking history. The second group was defined as nonsmoker. These patients had incomplete reversibility of the airway obstruction and had less than 5 pack-year smoking history. Patients with ACO were more likely to be females (60% vs 38%), had poorer asthma control, and poor asthma-related quality of life. Patients with ACO were also noted to have higher residual volumes and a lower diffusion capacity corrected for alveolar volume, suggesting additional changes to asthma pathophysiology caused by smoking.

Rhee[6] purposed a phenotypic classification based on underlying disease mechanism. Four phenotypic subclasses (A–D) were suggested based on a combination of features that are typically seen in asthma (eosinophilic lung disease and allergies) and COPD (smoking and emphysema). Patients with the allergic asthma-predominant phenotype were classified as phenotype A. Phenotype B was characterized by severe noneosinophilic asthma. It is noteworthy here that both phenotypes A and B include patients with no smoking history. Although exposure to smoking has been identified by guidelines as one of the criteria required to fulfill the diagnosis of

ACO,[23] patients with ACO are inevitably heterogenous and several other factors have been shown to contribute to development of irreversible obstruction in the absence of smoking history. Lange and colleagues[29] used data from the Copenhagen City Heart Study to evaluate changes in the FEV_1 over time in adults with and without asthma. Three measurements were taken over a 15-year period and their study showed that the decrease in FEV_1 was comparable between smokers without asthma and non-smokers with asthma. The Busselton Health Study, which included 9317 patients, showed that asthma is associated with lower lung function in early adult life as well as increased rate of decline later in life.[30] These findings suggested the effect of asthma itself on lung function over time might be as potent as smoking.

Asthma is a longstanding chronic inflammatory condition, and evidence from several studies suggests that persistent inflammation may lead to irreversible airway remodeling over time.[31] Ulrik and Backer[32] conducted a 10-year follow-up study of life-long nonsmokers with asthma who had reversible airflow obstruction at the time of enrollment. Of the patients in this study, 23% developed irreversible airway obstruction over time. All of these patients were treated with high dose inhaled steroids and approximately two-thirds of these patients were on long-term corticosteroids, suggesting the presence of moderate to severe asthma. Tai and colleagues[33] also showed an association between childhood asthma and the development of COPD later in life. The odds ratio for developing COPD was 31.9 in patients with severe childhood asthma compared with 9.6 in all patients with childhood asthma.

Phenotype C in the Rhee study included patients who were long-term smokers with asthma who had features of both asthma and COPD, the "typical ACO patient".[34] Patients with phenotype D disease tend to lack a history of asthma or other allergic disease. The rationale to include these patients as ACO was the evidence that a significant number of patients with COPD tend to have bronchodilator reactivity and bronchial hyperresponsiveness, both of which have been associated with a decrease in lung function.[35,36] Joo and colleagues[9] applied the clinical phenotypes proposed by Rhee in their study of 103 patients with ACO. Putcha and colleagues[37] published data from the COPDGene and SPIROMICS in which they defined COPD subtypes by atopy and asthma overlap. More than one-half of the patients with COPD with asthma were nonatopic and most patients with atopy did not have asthma. Symptom burden was greatest and lung impairment was worst in the nonatopic group. The EUROSCOP study also published similar findings showing a subgroup of patients with atopic COPD who did not have asthma.[38] All these studies highlight that ACO is a heterogenous condition and has several different phenotypes.

PROPOSED CLINICAL PHENOTYPES

Based on evidence presented in this article, we propose that the following 4 ACO phenotypes could be used for future research purposes (**Fig. 1**).

1. *Phenotype A: Nonsmoking Asthmatics.* Age and severity of asthma has been described as the risk factors for decline in lung function. These patients have fixed airway obstruction and constitute phenotype A and B from the Rhee study.[6] Joo and colleagues[9] studied this subgroup and showed that these patients tend be younger females without a significant smoking history. These patients may or may not have evidence of eosinophilic inflammation.

2. *Phenotype B: Smoking Asthmatics.* These patients also have fixed obstruction and tend to be younger females with higher smoking history and more likely to have atopic features.[25,28] They tend to have higher use of short-acting beta2 agonists and inhaled and oral corticosteroids. Boulet and colleagues[28] showed that these

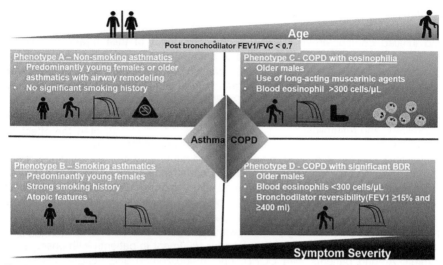

Fig. 1. Proposed classification and main characteristics of the 4 phenotypes of ACO. Phenotypes A and B are asthma predominant and phenotypes C and D are COPD predominant. The asthma-predominant phenotypes patients tend to be younger and have less severe disease as compared with COPD-predominant phenotypes. Fixed airway obstruction (postbronchodilator FEV_1/forced vital capacity of <0.7) is a feature of all phenotypes.

patients have higher residual volumes and a lower diffusion capacity corrected for alveolar volume, suggesting additional changes to asthma pathophysiology caused by smoking. Their use of health care services tends to be higher than patients with COPD with eosinophilia and COPD with high bronchodilator response.

3. *Phenotype C: COPD with Eosinophilia.* Patients in this group are more likely to be older males and tend to have higher eosinophil count (>300 cells/μL) and T helper cell type 2–related biomarkers compared with smoking asthmatics.[10] They are more likely to use long-acting muscarinic agents.[10] Their lung function tends to be similar to smoking asthmatics; however, they have lower health care use.

4. *Phenotype D: COPD with Significant Bronchodilator Response.* This is a group of patients with COPD who have marked positive results on bronchodilator testing (FEV_1 of $\geq$15% and $\geq$400 mL) as identified in Spanish guidelines[27,39] on ACO and the study by Toledo and associates.[10] These patients share several features with the COPD with eosinophilia phenotype in that these patients tend to be older males and their baseline lung function seems to be to be similar.[9,10] However, their blood eosinophil count tends to be less than 300 cells/μL.

ROLE OF PHENOTYPES IN THE MANAGEMENT OF ASTHMA–CHRONIC OBSTRUCTIVE PULMONARY DISEASE OVERLAP

One of the key components in the development of ACO is the risk factor that has contributed to the disease. As noted elsewhere in this article, smoking, age, and persistent airway inflammation have been identified as risk factors for greater declines in lung function and the development of irreversible airway obstruction later in life in patients with asthma. Similarly, patients with COPD can present with eosinophilia or high bronchodilator reactivity. There is a need for further studies to understand the natural history of the various phenotypes of ACO. Whether the phenotype is predominantly asthma or COPD may influence the choice of treatment.[6] Patients with asthma-predominant phenotypes are more likely to have eosinophilic inflammation and inhaled corticosteroids will be a key component of their treatment.[6] Long-acting beta agonists, leukotriene receptor antagonists, and long-acting muscarinic agents are the add-on medications when inhaled corticosteroids alone are not sufficient in controlling symptoms. In contrast, long-acting muscarinic agents will likely be the first-line agent in patients with COPD-predominant ACO with low eosinophil counts. Add-on therapies include long-acting beta agonists, inhaled corticosteroids, macrolides, and roflumilast.[6]

Data on the use of biologics in ACO is limited and inconsistent at times. In the Australian Xolair registry, omalizumab improved asthma control and quality of life.[40] Similarly, a post hoc analysis of PROSPERO noted that ACO treated with omalizumab had outcomes similar to asthmatics treated with this drug.[41] However, a more recent real-world study comparing response to biologics among asthmatics and patients with ACO showed that only 16% of the patients with ACO attained clinical control compared with 39.7% among patients with asthma.[42] Several anti–IL-5 and anti–IL-5Ra monoclonal antibodies are approved for treatment in patients with eosinophilic asthma. Among patients with COPD, only mepolizumab and benralizumab have been tested and have shown to decrease the rate of exacerbation in highly selected group of patients who have both COPD and high levels of eosinophils.[43] Dupilumab, which is an anti–IL-4Ra antibody, has been shown to improve lung function and severe exacerbation in severe asthma with even better response in patients with higher eosinophil counts.[44] However, its efficacy has not been established in patients with COPD or patients with ACO. Although biologic therapies are not the standard of care in patients with ACO at this time, it might be reasonable to choose a drug that has documented efficacy in asthma and eosinophilic COPD.

FUTURE DIRECTIONS

Despite the disagreements on the definition and identification of ACO as a distinct disease entity, most clinicians agree that there exists a subgroup of patients whose clinical presentation and course of illness does not correlate with the existing knowledge of either asthma or COPD. However, several questions remain unanswered, including the optimal treatment and the natural history of these ACO phentoypes.[2] Current studies on ACO phenotypes have not used all the available tools for the classification, and future studies should include a multitude of variables such as clinical, spirometry, FeNO, natural history of the disease, response to treatment, exacerbations, hospitalizations, development of comorbidities, survival, and blood and metabolic biomarkers to identify the composite determinants for a more precise phenotyping. Additional advanced omics studies could further improve the precision in phenotyping. The other critical area is to understand the stability of these phenotypes over long periods of time (decades), greater insights into their pathophysiology, and how these phenotypes can influence management decisions. Currently, there are only cross-sectional studies on ACO phenotypes and there is a need for longitudinal studies to understand these phenotypes better.

SUMMARY

The heterogeneity of patients with ACO led to development of several definitions that described key clinical, physiological, and biological features of this condition. It is obvious that ACO includes multiple phenotypes, which may influence the optimal choice of therapy and predict prognosis of the disease. Several ACO phenotypes have been proposed, based on host characteristics such as age and gender, symptom burden, spirometric features, smoking history, and underlying airway inflammation. Future longitudinal studies need to validate the stability of these phenotypes over time and determine their prognostic and predictive abilities to ensure a more precise approach to its management.

CLINICS CARE POINTS

- All ACO phenotypes have a postbronchodilator FEV_1/FVC ratio of less than 0.7 or below the lower limit of normal, where available.

- In addition to smoking, age and persistent airway inflammation have been identified as risk factors for increased decline in lung function and the development of irreversible airway obstruction later in life.

- There is no single biomarker for the diagnosis and differentiation of ACO phenotypes.

- Peripheral blood eosinophil counts and bronchodilator reversibility are helpful in phenotyping ACO.

- Total IgE, allergen-specific IgE, FeNO, periostin, YKL-40, chest imaging, and metabolic signatures may be useful in the clinical diagnosis, but their role in phenotyping ACO is yet to be determined.

- Based on available evidence, we propose 4 major phenotypes for ACO, namely, nonsmoking asthmatics, smoking asthmatics, COPD with eosinophilia, and COPD with HBR.

ACKNOWLEDGMENTS

The authors thank Ms Greeshma, MV, Research Scholar, JSS Medical College, JSSAHER, Mysore for help in designing the figure.

DISCLOSURE

The authors declare no relevant disclosures pertinent to this article. No funding was received for the manuscript.

REFERENCES

1. Garelli V, Petitpierre N, Nicod LP. Le syndrome de chevauchement asthme-BPCO [The asthma-COPD overlap syndrome]. Rev Med Suisse 2015;11(495):2145-50. French. PMID: 26742234.
2. Gibson PG, McDonald VM. Asthma-COPD overlap 2015: now we are six. Thorax 2015;70:683–91.
3. Ray A, Camiolo M, Fitzpatrick A, et al. Are we meeting the promise of endotypes and precision medicine in asthma? Physiol Rev 2020;100(3):983–1017.
4. Agache I, Akdis CA. Precision medicine and phenotypes, endotypes, genotypes, regiotypes, and theratypes of allergic diseases. J Clin Invest 2019;129(4): 1493–503.
5. Global Initiative for Asthma/Global Initiative for Chronic Obstructive Lung Disease. Diagnosis of diseases of chronic airflow limitation: asthma COPD and asthma-COPD overlap syndrome (ACOS) global initiative for chronic obstructive lung disease website. Available at: https://goldcopd.org/asthma-copd-asthma-copd-overlap-syndrome/. Accessed December 17, 2021.
6. Rhee CK. Phenotype of asthma-chronic obstructive pulmonary disease overlap syndrome. Korean J Intern Med 2015;30(4):443–9.

7. Fujino N, Sugiura H. ACO (asthma-COPD overlap) is independent from COPD, a case in favor: a systematic review. Diagnostics (Basel) 2021;11(5):859.

8. Lainez S, Court-Fortune I, Vercherin P, et al. Clinical ACO phenotypes: description of a heterogeneous entity. Respir Med Case Rep 2019;28:100929.

9. Joo H, Han D, Lee JH, et al. Heterogeneity of asthma-COPD overlap syndrome. Int J Chron Obstruct Pulmon Dis 2017;12:697–703.

10. Toledo-Pons N, van Boven JFM, Román-Rodríguez M, et al. ACO: time to move from the description of different phenotypes to the treatable traits. PLoS One 2019;14(1):e0210915.

11. LaPrad AS, Lutchen KR. Respiratory impedance measurements for assessment of lung mechanics: focus on asthma. Respir Physiol Neurobiol 2008;163(1–3):64–73.

12. Takeda T, Oga T, Niimi A, et al. Relationship between small airway function and health status, dyspnea and disease control in asthma. Respiration 2010;80(2):120–6.

13. Mikamo M, Shirai T, Mori K, et al. Predictors of expiratory flow limitation measured by forced oscillation technique in COPD. BMC Pulm Med 2014;14:23. https://doi.org/10.1186/1471-2466-14-23.

14. Shinke H, Yamamoto M, Hazeki N, et al. Visualized changes in respiratory resistance and reactance along a time axis in smokers: a cross-sectional study. Respir Investig 2013;51(3):166–74.

15. Gupta S, Siddiqui S, Haldar P, et al. Quantitative analysis of high-resolution computed tomography scans in severe asthma subphenotypes. Thorax 2010;65(9):775–81.

16. Karayama M, Inui N, Yasui H, et al. Physiological and morphological differences of airways between COPD and asthma-COPD overlap. Sci Rep 2019;9(1):7818.

17. Hardin M, Cho M, McDonald ML, et al. The clinical and genetic features of COPD-asthma overlap syndrome. Eur Respir J 2014;44(2):341–50.

18. Cai C, Bian X, Xue M, et al. Eicosanoids metabolized through LOX distinguish asthma-COPD overlap from COPD by metabolomics study. Int J Chron Obstruct Pulmon Dis 2019;14:1769–78.

19. Oh JY, Lee YS, Min KH, et al. Increased urinary I-histidine in patients with asthma-COPD overlap: a pilot study. Int J Chron Obstruct Pulmon Dis 2018;13:1809–18.

20. Ghosh N, Choudhury P, Kaushik SR, et al. Metabolomic fingerprinting and systemic inflammatory profiling of asthma COPD overlap (ACO). Respir Res 2020;21(1):126.

21. Sánchez Castillo S, Smith L, Díaz Suárez A, et al. Association between physical activity and comorbidities in Spanish people with asthma-COPD overlap. Sustainability 2021;13(14):7580.

22. Akmatov MK, Ermakova T, Holstiege J, et al. Comorbidity profile of patients with concurrent diagnoses of asthma and COPD in Germany. Sci Rep 2020;10(1):17945.

23. Yanagisawa S, Ichinose M. Definition and diagnosis of asthma-COPD overlap (ACO). Allergol Int 2018;67(2):172–8.

24. Sin DD, Miravitlles M, Mannino DM, et al. What is asthma-COPD overlap syndrome? Towards a consensus definition from a round table discussion. Eur Respir J 2016;48(3):664–73.

25. Pérez-de-Llano L, Cosio BG, CHACOS study group. Asthma-COPD overlap is not a homogeneous disorder: further supporting data. Respir Res 2017;18(1):183.

26. Cosío BG, Pérez de Llano L, Lopez Viña A, et al. on behalf of the CHACOS study group. Th-2 signature in chronic airway diseases: towards the extinction of asthma-COPD overlap syndrome? Eur Respir J 2017;49(5):1602397.

27. Miravitlles M, Alvarez-Gutierrez FJ, Calle M, et al. Algorithm for identification of asthma-COPD overlap: consensus between the Spanish COPD and asthma guidelines. Eur Respir J 2017;49(5):1700068.
28. Boulet LP, Boulay MÈ, Dérival JL, et al. Asthma-COPD overlap phenotypes and smoking: comparative features of asthma in smoking or non-smoking patients with an incomplete reversibility of airway obstruction. COPD 2018;15(2):130–8.
29. Lange P, Parner J, Vestbo J, et al. A 15-year follow-up study of ventilatory function in adults with asthma. N Engl J Med 1998;339(17):1194–200.
30. James AL, Palmer LJ, Kicic E, et al. Decline in lung function in the Busselton Health Study: the effects of asthma and cigarette smoking. Am J Respir Crit Care Med 2005;171(2):109–14.
31. Fabbri LM, Caramori G, Beghe B, et al. Physiologic consequences of long-term inflammation. Am J Respir Crit Care Med 1998;157:s195–8.
32. Ulrik CS, Backer V. Nonreversible airflow obstruction in life-long nonsmokers with moderate to severe asthma. Eur Respir J 1999;14(4):892–6.
33. Tai A, Tran H, Roberts M, et al. The association between childhood asthma and adult chronic obstructive pulmonary disease. Thorax 2014;69(9):805–10.
34. Perret JL, Dharmage SC, Matheson MC, et al. The interplay between the effects of lifetime asthma, smoking, and atopy on fixed airflow obstruction in middle age. Am J Respir Crit Care Med 2013;187(1):42–8.
35. Jamieson DB, Matsui EC, Belli A, et al. Effects of allergic phenotype on respiratory symptoms and exacerbations in patients with chronic obstructive pulmonary disease. Am J Respir Crit Care Med 2013;188(2):187–92.
36. Vestbo J, Edwards LD, Scanlon PD, et al. ECLIPSE Investigators. Changes in forced expiratory volume in 1 second over time in COPD. N Engl J Med 2011; 365(13):1184–92.
37. Putcha N, Fawzy A, Matsui EC, et al. Clinical phenotypes of atopy and asthma in COPD: a meta-analysis of SPIROMICS and COPDGene. Chest 2020;158(6): 2333–45.
38. Fattahi F, ten Hacken NH, Löfdahl CG, et al. Atopy is a risk factor for respiratory symptoms in COPD patients: results from the EUROSCOP study. Respir Res 2013;14(1):10.
39. Plaza V, Álvarez F, Calle M, et al. Consensus on the asthma-COPD overlap syndrome (ACOS) Between the Spanish COPD guidelines (GesEPOC) and the Spanish guidelines on the management of asthma (GEMA). Arch Bronconeumol 2017;53(8):443–9.
40. Nathan RA, Sorkness CA, Kosinski M, et al. Development of the asthma control test: a survey for assessing asthma control. J Allergy Clin Immunol 2004; 113(1):59–65.
41. Hanania NA, Chipps BE, Griffin NM, et al. Omalizumab effectiveness in asthma-COPD overlap: post hoc analysis of PROSPERO. J Allergy Clin Immunol 2019; 143(4):1629–33.e2.
42. Pérez de Llano L, Dacal Rivas D, Marina Malanda N, et al. The response to biologics is better in patients with severe asthma than in patients with asthma-COPD overlap syndrome. J Asthma Allergy 2022;15:363–9.
43. Donovan T, Milan SJ, Wang R, et al. Anti-IL-5 therapies for chronic obstructive pulmonary disease. Cochrane Database Syst Rev 2020;12(12):CD013432.
44. Castro M, Corren J, Pavord ID, et al. Dupilumab efficacy and safety in moderate-to-severe uncontrolled asthma. N Engl J Med 2018;378(26):2486–96.

Pharmacologic Management Strategies of Asthma-Chronic Obstructive Pulmonary Disease Overlap

Nicola A. Hanania, MD, MS[a],*, Marc Miravitlles, MD[b]

KEYWORDS

- Asthma • COPD • Treatment • Inhaled corticosteroids • Eosinophils
- Asthma COPD Overlap • Biologics • Pharmacologic therapies

KEY POINTS

- Asthma-chronic obstructive pulmonary disease (COPD) overlap (ACO) is a heterogenous entity applied to patients with clinical features of both asthma and COPD and has been associated with relative treatment refractoriness.
- Information is sparse about optimal treatment of ACO because of lack of randomized controlled trials in this population, and current treatment recommendations are based on consensus.
- Pharmacologic treatment of patients with ACO is based on treatment of underlying treatable traits and ideally should include an inhaled corticosteroid in addition to at least one long-acting bronchodilator.
- In patients with severe disease, biological therapies may be administered depending on the underlying phenotype, although use of such therapies in this population has not been well evaluated.
- A better understanding of the molecular mechanisms and drivers of airway inflammation in patients with ACO as well as the identification of novel biomarkers may lead to a more precise treatment approach for important unmet needs.

INTRODUCTION

Asthma-chronic obstructive pulmonary disease (COPD) overlap (ACO) is a term applied to patients with clinical features of both asthma and COPD. ACO has been associated with greater morbidity than asthma and COPD alone and with relative

[a] Section of Pulmonary and Critical Care Medicine, Baylor College of Medicine, 1504 Taub Loop, Houston, TX 77030, USA; [b] Pneumology Department, Hospital Universitari Vall d'Hebron/ Vall d'Hebron Research Institute (VHIR), Vall d'Hebron Barcelona Hospital Campus, P. Vall d'Hebron 119-129, Barcelona 08035, Spain
* Corresponding author.
E-mail address: Hanania@bcm.edu

Immunol Allergy Clin N Am 42 (2022) 657–669
https://doi.org/10.1016/j.iac.2022.05.002
0889-8561/22/© 2022 Elsevier Inc. All rights reserved.

immunology.theclinics.com

treatment refractoriness. However, accurate information is sparse about its optimal treatment, especially that it has several phenotypes, clinical presentation, and course. As discussed elsewhere in this series, much controversy exists about the exact definition and prevalence of ACO between studies, but most studies suggest that the prevalence of ACO ranges between 1.1% and 4.5% in the general population but is considerably higher in asthma and COPD populations, with a reported prevalence of 27% and 33%, respectively.[1–5]

Because of heterogeneity of ACO and lack of consensus on its definition, therapeutic approach to this disease is based on treating both the underlying asthma and COPD and has been based only on consensus statements and expert opinions[6–11]; this is compounded by the fact that patients with ACO have been excluded from clinical trials evaluating asthma and COPD therapies. Furthermore, patients with ACO have several phenotypes and clinical presentations, and thus having one therapeutic approach may be problematic. In this article, the authors provide an overview of the current recommendations for the pharmacologic approach to ACO based on existing knowledge and outline areas for future research.

DISCUSSION
Nonpharmacologic Approaches

Initial management of patients with ACO should adopt a similar approach to that used in patients with asthma or COPD. Identifying and limiting the patient's exposures as well a smoking cessation is particularly important in patients with ACO, because this irritant will affect the progression and symptoms. Furthermore, smoke exposure has been shown to decrease the response to inhaled corticosteroids (ICS).[12] Evaluation of other exposures such as biomass smoke, pollution, and other irritants needs to be considered. Delivering patient education and ensuring adequate inhaler technique are vital in this group of patients and should be encouraged at every visit.[13,14] Using an active management cycle in which patients are assessed, the response is reviewed, and the treatment is adjusted based on their symptoms and exacerbation history is also recommended. When selecting therapies, identifying underlying comorbidities is key, because increasing evidence shows that comorbid conditions may exert a considerable effect in patients with ACO, and considering diagnoses such as gastroesophageal reflux disease, osteoporosis, cardiovascular disease, and depression is essential.[15] Finally, encouraging exercise and, for those who have exercise limitation, referral to formal pulmonary rehabilitation is recommended.[16]

Inhaled Therapies

Therapy for mild-to-moderate disease in patients with ACO is centered on inhaled therapy. Treatment should follow a stepwise approach based on symptom control and history of exacerbations (**Fig. 1**). Patients with infrequent symptoms can be managed with as-needed short-acting bronchodilators. Nevertheless, as the symptoms progress, the introduction of ICS in patients with ACO is recommended to treat the asthma component and has been shown to reduce exacerbations and improve outcome especially in patients with high baseline blood eosinophil count.[14,17–23] Although the early use of ICS in this population has been recommended to target airway inflammation, because these patients often have concomitant airway obstruction, managing their symptoms should include adding one or more long-acting bronchodilators, often with the initial addition of a long-acting beta2-agonist (LABA).[24] The early use of ICS in combination with a LABA in treatment of patients with COPD who have a history of asthma is supported by a case-control study.[25] Gershon and

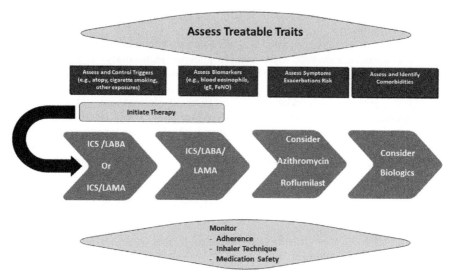

Fig. 1. Treatment algorithm for asthma-COPD overlap.

colleagues[25] obswerved that older adults with COPD and asthma treated with LABA/ICS had a significantly lower risk of the composite outcome of death or hospitalization compared with those treated with LABAs alone, was associated with a significantly lower risk of the composite outcome of death or COPD hospitalization.

Patients treated with ICS/LABA who continue to have symptoms are often treated with an additional long-acting bronchodilator, such as a long-acting muscarinic antagonists (LAMA).[26] Tiotropium bromide has been the most used LAMA in this situation because it is the only one currently approved for treatment of asthma. In a large, 12-week, randomized, double-blind, placebo controlled, parallel group, clinical trial, Magnussen and colleagues[27] demonstrated that patients with COPD who have concomitant asthma (ACO) achieve lung function improvements with tiotropium along with symptomatic benefit, as seen by reduced need for rescue medication. The use of tiotropium added to ICS in this population has also been shown to improve outcomes.[28] Triple inhaler therapy (ICS/LABA/LAMA) has been effective in both asthma and COPD and therefore should be considered if the patient's symptoms progress, especially if there is a history of frequent exacerbations.[18,29] If inhaler therapy is not sufficiently effective in these patients, advanced therapies based on phenotyping and identification of treatable traits may be considered. These therapies include the use of phosphodiesterase inhibitors, macrolides, and biologics.

Macrolides
Macrolides have been useful in various chronic pulmonary diseases, including in non-cystic bronchiectasis and cystic fibrosis. In asthma and COPD, various trials have been shown to provide benefits regarding exacerbations and other important outcomes. The mechanisms explaining these benefits are incompletely understood. The antimicrobial properties of these compounds may be beneficial in certain cases. Moreover, some evidence links toxins from *Mycoplasma pneumoniae* and infection with other atypical bacteria with T2 inflammatory responses and airway remodeling that may be mitigated with macrolides The potential antiinflammatory properties of macrolides also have been debated, but mounting evidence suggests that this class

of medications may affect the various inflammatory pathways and reduce airway reactivity and remodeling.

In relation to ACO, these potential benefits seem to extend to inflammation induced by smoke exposure. However, to the authors' knowledge, no study has evaluated prospectively the effects of macrolides in patients with ACO, and few data on the use of macrolides in ACO exist. Given the evidence from studies in both asthma and COPD populations, azithromycin can be considered as an adjunctive therapy in patients with ACO. However, this therapy should be reserved for patients whose condition remain uncontrolled despite ICS/LABA with or without LAMA, those whose condition has failed to respond to other therapies, or those considered at risk for future exacerbations. Long-term azithromycin use has been linked to increased antimicrobial resistance, and a careful risk/benefit evaluation should be done before initiating this therapy. Prescreening patients for the risk of cardiac arrhythmias and hearing problems and close postinitiation monitoring are recommended if the decision to start azithromycin is made.[30]

Phosphodiesterase inhibitors

Theophylline, a nonselective phosphodiesterase inhibitor, was one of the first medications used in treatment of patients with chronic airway diseases and in fact, is still used worldwide in milder forms of asthma and COPD. Doxofylline, another methylxanthine, has similar benefits in asthma compared with theophylline. To date, no studies have been conducted evaluating the efficacy of methylxanthines in an ACO population. In patients who have milder forms of ACO, this class of medications may be considered, but other safer and more effective therapies exist.

The oral phosphodiesterase-4 inhibitor, roflumilast, has been effective in improving lung function and decreased exacerbations rates in a subgroup of patients with COPD and those with a history of frequent exacerbations, a chronic bronchitis phenotype, and a FEV1 less than 50% predicted.[31-33] In asthma, roflumilast has shown consistent improvements of lung function in a meta-analysis of 14 trials.[34] No data exist on the effects of roflumilast in patients with ACO.[32,35] Interestingly, patients with COPD with higher counts of eosinophils had greater reduction in exacerbation rates.[36] Supporting these findings, a study of bronchial biopsies of patients with COPD indicated a decrease in tissue eosinophils after 16 weeks of therapy with roflumilast compared with placebo.[37] Other studies have shown antiinflammatory effects mediated by other cellular lines, such as neutrophils.[38] These findings on the studies on asthma and COPD, and the potential effects on eosinophils and other antiinflammatory properties, make roflumilast an attractive option to examine further in patients who have ACO who are at risk of frequent exacerbations.

Biologics and small molecule antagonists

Understanding the molecular mechanisms of airway inflammation in both asthma and COPD has led to the identification of novel targets for therapy that include cytokines and chemokines. Indeed, several monoclonal antibody biologics and small molecule inhibitors and antagonists have been developed and are either approved or currently being evaluated in clinical trials. The use of these therapies has been associated with significant reduction in exacerbations, emergency room visits, need for systemic corticosteroids, and improvements in quality of life, among other outcomes.[39] Because of the success of biologics in asthma, a similar strategy has been attempted in patients with COPD whose phenotypic characteristics may predict a favorable response, such as those with underlying T2 airway inflammation and eosinophilic features.[40]

Biomarkers, such as immunoglobulin E (IgE), peripheral blood eosinophils, and exhaled nitric oxide (FeNO), can identify patients who may benefit from these therapies.[41–43]

Therapies targeting interleukin (IL)-5 pathway (mepolizumab and benralizumab) have been examined in populations with COPD who have eosinophilia, and studies targeting IL-4 receptor (dupilumab) are ongoing. However, the results of the completed studies have shown mixed results.

Targeting pathways beyond IL-5, IL-4, and IL-13 are being considered for future therapies in both asthma and COPD and may have promising results in patients with ACO, for example, in asthma, targeting alarmins released by airway epithelial cells including thymic stromal lymphopoietin (TSLP), IL-25, and IL-33. Targeting these costimulatory cytokines can block T2 and non-T2 inflammatory response and may have important clinical implications. For example, tezepelumab, a monoclonal antibody targeting TSLP that was recently approved for treatment of severe asthma, was shown to decrease the rate of exacerbations in patients with uncontrolled moderate-to-severe asthma irrespective of blood eosinophil counts.[44]

Thus far, none of the aforementioned biologics have been systematically tested in large trials in the ACO population[45–47]; this is attributable to the varying definitions of ACO, wide range of disease severity, and exclusion and inclusion criteria for the different studies. Because many patients with ACO have allergic triggered symptoms, several studies and opinion pieces suggested a potential benefit for the use of omalizumab (anti-IgE) in this population.[45,48–51]

Omalizumab has been studied the most in patients with overlapping features. An analysis of 177 subjects from the Australian Xolair Registry indicated similar improvements in quality of life and asthma control in patients with severe allergic asthma compared with those with COPD overlapping features.[51] No improvements were observed in lung function. The PROSPERO study (Prospective Observational Study to Evaluate Predictors of Clinical Effectiveness in Response to Omalizumab) was an observational, real-life study that evaluated the effectiveness of omalizumab after 48 weeks of therapy. Current and prior smokers and patients with coexisting COPD were not excluded from this study. In a post hoc analysis of 737 patients from this cohort, patients with and without overlapping features had similar improvements in exacerbation rates and asthma control.[52] Nevertheless, because of the inherent limitations of a real-life study, these data should be interpreted with caution, because these types of studies have less rigor compared with the regulatory trials previously described.

The question remains as to whether one should use biologics on a routine basis in patients with ACO. Limited data are available to make a definitive recommendation regarding the use of these treatments in patients with overlapping features. In clinical practice, patients with uncontrolled asthma and coexisting COPD are encountered regularly. A real-life study showed that 22% to 30% of patients who receive biologicals for asthma have coexisting COPD,[53] which suggests that these patients are already receiving these therapies routinely. When all clinical management goals have been addressed, such as disease education, environmental measures, smoking cessation, and treatment of comorbid conditions, considering biological therapies in ACO is reasonable. Taking into consideration the robust evidence of improvements in multiple important asthma outcomes and understanding the limited ACO-specific studies, biologics should not be withheld in patients with ACO, particularly if patients' conditions remain uncontrolled with frequent exacerbations or chronic oral corticosteroids. Fortunately, biologics have been considered safe in the COPD population, but information of ongoing studies will provide additional safety information.

Targeting non-T2 airway inflammation including neutrophilic inflammation remains a great unmet need for treatment of severe asthma and COPD. Several agents, including biologics such those targeting IL-8, IL-17, and tumor necrosis factor alpha and small molecule antagonists such as CXCR2 and LTB4 antagonists, have failed to show benefits in clinical trials. Several other targets are being evaluated, but none of these has been evaluated in patients with ACO.

Guidelines' Recommendations for Treatment of Asthma-Chronic Obstructive Pulmonary Disease Overlap

As mentioned, the inclusion of ACO in the treatment guidelines for asthma or COPD has been controversial due to the lack of a universally accepted definition of the condition and the lack of evidence derived from randomized clinical trials in this population of patients. However, in 2014 the Global Initiative for Asthma (GINA) and the Global Initiative for Obstructive Lung Disease (GOLD) published a joint document on ACO. They included a list of characteristics that define either asthma or COPD and suggested that patents who shared characteristics of both diseases could be diagnosed with ACO.[54] Regarding treatment, they basically suggested that both components of the disease should be treated initially, the asthmatic component with ICS and the COPD components with inhaled long-acting bronchodilators. However, after the publication of the joint GINA-GOLD statement on ACO, the following updates of the GOLD document did not explicitly include the concept of ACO in their recommendations for management, instead the panel continued to classify the patients with the A–D classification according to the risk of exacerbations and intensity of symptoms. Moreover, in the 2020 update, the GOLD committee indicated that GOLD will no longer refer to ACO but recommended the use of blood eosinophil counts to direct the therapy with ICS and established some thresholds of blood eosinophilia to direct the use of ICS in COPD.[55] In summary, the GOLD document states that *"asthma and COPD may coexist in an individual patient,"* but do not use the concept of ACO for the recommendations of management.[55] Similarly, the GINA 2020 document referred to ACO or "asthma + COPD" as simple descriptors for patients who have features of both asthma and COPD and emphasized that these terms do not refer to a single disease entity. On the contrary, they included patients with several clinical phenotypes that are likely caused by a range of different underlying mechanisms.[56]

Despite the lack of interest for ACO in the global documents GOLD and GINA, some national guidelines for the management of COPD have included ACO in their recommendations of treatment. In 2007, the Canadian guidelines for COPD recognized that some patients with COPD may have an asthma component and may require different treatment, in particular an early introduction of ICS.[57] Three years later, in 2010, the Japanese guidelines on COPD included an article on "COPD complicated by asthma," which may be considered as what we now call ACO, but the name had not been proposed yet. The investigators also recommended the early introduction of ICS in these patients.[58] These 2 documents intuitively described the same type of patients, but they did not include a precise definition of the overlap between COPD and asthma; they only indicated that characteristics of both diseases may coexist in some patients and that this could have implications for treatment.

The term ACO appeared as such, for the first time, in the Spanish COPD guidelines in 2012.[59,60] This definition was adopted with minor modifications by other COPD guidelines such as the Czech,[61] the Finnish,[62] the Canadian,[63] the Middle East-North Africa Region,[64] and the Japanese.[65] The recent update of the Czech COPD guidelines recognized the 2 major phenotypes of ACO, the asthmatic smoker with nonfully reversible airflow limitation and the eosinophilic COPD, but still considered the requirements of major and minor criteria for its diagnosis[66] and required the presence of frequent exacerbations in addition to the ACO phenotype for prescription of ICS. However, other recent updates such as the 2019 update of the Canadian COPD guidelines did not include ACO as a phenotype of COPD directing the pharmacologic management; instead, the document recognized the role of blood eosinophil counts (one of the main criteria for ACO universally recognized) as the main factor to prescribe ICS.[67]

This Canadian approach followed the recommendations of the GOLD initiative that established the blood eosinophilia as the main biomarker to direct ICS treatment in COPD.[55] The 2017 update of the Spanish guidelines and the Portuguese guideline on COPD still included the ACO phenotype as composed by patients with COPD with coexistent asthma and eosinophilic COPD.[68,69] It was recognized that these 2 types of patients were different, but they were grouped together under the umbrella term of ACO because the therapeutic approach was the same.[68] However, in the last update in 2021 the Spanish guideline divided the 2 main phenotypes of ACO and considered the coexistence of asthma as a comorbidity in patients with COPD, that is, the real ACO, and included in the management recommendations the phenotype of the exacerbator with eosinophilia, irrespective of the characteristics of asthma.[70] It seems that the tendency for the future will be to differentiate a phenotype of eosinophilic COPD, based on blood eosinophil counts, and leave the concept of ACO for patients who fulfill the diagnostic criteria for both asthma and COPD simultaneously irrespective of blood eosinophil counts.[67,70,71]

Future Directions

Epidemiologic studies suggest that patients with ACO have worse outcomes and poorer response to treatment that those with asthma or COPD. It is therefore imperative to identify a more precise approach to its treatment. For this to happen, proper identification of its phenotypes and endotypes is needed. Existing therapies provide effective and safe approach to patients with mild or moderate disease. Although ICS are commonly used in treating patients with ACO, a great need remains to better understand the role of the long-term efficacy and safety of ICS in this population. Indeed, prospective clinical trials are required to validate (or refute) response to ICS and the cost-effectiveness of this approach. The efficacy and safety of biologics should also be explored in this population, which should include development of easy to use, reproducible biomarkers to help identify the different phenotypes. At the moment, identification of treatable traits is the recommended approach in patients with ACO.[7,10,72,73] These treatable traits should be clinically relevant, be easily identified and measured, and have therapeutic implications. Appropriate evaluation of these traits includes evaluation of respiratory symptoms, radiographic characteristics, comorbid conditions, history of exacerbations, or infections. Biological markers may also be helpful. Other than blood eosinophils and exhaled nitric oxide, use of experimental biomarkers such as serum periostin and chitinase-3-like protein 1 (YKL-40) has been shown to better characterize 3 populations of patients with chronic airway disease.[74] Patients with asthma and ACO had higher levels of periostin but not in COPD, whereas YKL-40 was high in COPD and ACO but not in asthma. Future studies need to explore ways to ensure more appropriate selection of patients, using these clinical traits and biomarkers to identify responders to certain therapies.

SUMMARY

ACO is a term applied to patients with clinical features of both asthma and COPD. There continues to be lots of controversies about the exact definition and phenotypes of ACO, and information is sparse about its course because most clinical studies evaluating patients with asthma and COPD have excluded patients with ACO. Current recommendations for therapy are based on expert opinion, roundtable discussions, and strategy documents. Such documents suggest that initial therapy for patients with ACO should include one or more long-acting bronchodilators, the cornerstone of COPD treatment, and an ICS, the cornerstone of asthma treatment. In severe disease, management should target treatable traits as well as should be driven by the phenotype/endotype of the patient. Several biological therapies are now available that target T2 airway inflammation in asthma but few of these have thus far been evaluated in ACO. Targeting non-T2 inflammation remains a major unmet need. Future studies need to determine best strategies for the treatment of these patients, focusing on a better and more in-depth understanding of the molecular mechanisms of ACO and its related phenotypes.

CLINICS CARE POINTS

- Limited evidence exists regarding the optimal initial therapy for patients with ACO.
- The use of inhaled corticosteroids early in the disease process is recommended to address airway inflammation.
- Inhaled long-acting bronchodilators need to be considered as add-on therapies to address the COPD component.
- In some phenotypes of ACO such as those with chronic bronchitis and recurrent exacerbations, the use of azithromycin and/or roflumilast may be considered.
- Biologics used in treatment of severe asthma may have a role in some patients with severe ACO; however, their use in this population requires further evaluation.

DISCLOSURE

Dr N. Hanania reports receiving consulting fees from GSK, Astra Zeneca, Sadslnofi, Regeneron, Teva, Amgen, Roche/Genentech, Boehringer Ingelheim, and Novartis; his institution has received research support from Boehringer Ingelheim, GlaxoSmithKline, and AstraZeneca, Sanofi, Teva, Genentech. M. Miravitlles has received speaker fees from AstraZeneca, Boehringer Ingelheim, Chiesi, Cipla, Menarini, Rovi, Bial, Sandoz, Zambon, CSL Behring, Grifols, and Novartis; consulting fees from Astra-Zeneca, Atriva Therapeutics, Boehringer Ingelheim, Chiesi, GlaxoSmithKline, Bial, Gebro Pharma, CSL Behring, Laboratorios Esteve, Ferrer, Mereo Biopharma, Verona Pharma, Spin Therapeutics, pH Pharma, Palobiofarma SL, Takeda, Novartis, Sanofi, and Grifols; and research grants from Grifols.

REFERENCES

1. Wurst KE, Kelly-Reif K, Bushnell GA, et al. Understanding asthma-chronic obstructive pulmonary disease overlap syndrome. Respir Med 2016;110:1–11.
2. Marco R de, Pesce G, Marcon A, et al. The coexistence of asthma and chronic obstructive pulmonary disease (COPD): prevalence and risk factors in young, middle-aged and elderly people from the general population. PLoS One 2013; 8(5):e62985.

3. Kumbhare S, Pleasants R, Ohar JA, et al. Characteristics and Prevalence of Asthma/Chronic Obstructive Pulmonary Disease Overlap in the United States. Ann Am Thorac Soc 2016;13(6):803–10.

4. Mendy A, Forno E, Niyonsenga T, et al. Prevalence and features of asthma-COPD overlap in the United States 2007-2012. Clin Respir J 2018;12(8):2369–77.

5. Boulet L-P, Hanania NA. The many faces of asthma-chronic obstructive pulmonary disease overlap. Curr Opin Pulm Med 2019;25(1):1–10.

6. Maselli DJ, Hardin M, Christenson SA, et al. Clinical approach to the therapy of asthma-COPD overlap. Chest 2019;155(1):168–77.

7. Maselli DJ, Hanania NA. Management of asthma COPD overlap. Ann Allergy Asthma Immunol 2019;123(4):335–44.

8. Miravitlles M. Diagnosis of asthma - COPD overlap: the five commandments. Eur Respir J 2017;49(5):170050.

9. Roman-Rodriguez M, Kaplan A. GOLD 2021 Strategy Report: Implications for Asthma-COPD Overlap. Int J Chron Obstruct Pulmon Dis 2021;16:1709–15.

10. Pérez de Llano L, Miravitlles M, Golpe R, et al. A Proposed Approach to Chronic Airway Disease (CAD) Using Therapeutic Goals and Treatable Traits: A Look to the Future. Int J Chron Obstruct Pulmon Dis 2020;15:2091–100.

11. Plaza V, Alvarez F, Calle M, et al. Consensus on the Asthma-COPD Overlap Syndrome (ACOS) Between the Spanish COPD Guidelines (GesEPOC) and the Spanish Guidelines on the Management of Asthma (GEMA). Arch Bronconeumol 2017;53(8):443–9. Available at: https://www.ncbi.nlm.nih.gov/pubmed/28495077.

12. Lazarus SC, Chinchilli VM, Rollings NJ, et al. Smoking affects response to inhaled corticosteroids or leukotriene receptor antagonists in asthma. Am J Respir Crit Care Med 2007;175(8):783–90.

13. Ding B, Small M, Scheffel G, et al. Maintenance inhaler preference, attribute importance, and satisfaction in prescribing physicians and patients with asthma, COPD, or asthma-COPD overlap syndrome consulting for routine care. Int J Chron Obs Pulmon Dis 2018;13:927–36. Available at: https://www.ncbi.nlm.nih.gov/pubmed/29588581.

14. Nili M, LeMasters TJ, Adelman M, et al. Initial maintenance therapy adherence among older adults with asthma-COPD overlap. Am J Manag Care 2021;27(11):463–70.

15. Maselli DJ, Hanania NA. Asthma COPD overlap: Impact of associated comorbidities. Pulm Pharmacol Ther 2018;52:27–31.

16. Mann DL, Reid MB. Exercise training and skeletal muscle inflammation in chronic heart failure: feeling better about fatigue. J Am Coll Cardiol 2003;42(5):869–72. Available at: https://www.ncbi.nlm.nih.gov/pubmed/12957434.

17. Bafadhel M, Peterson S, De Blas MA, et al. Predictors of exacerbation risk and response to budesonide in patients with chronic obstructive pulmonary disease: a post-hoc analysis of three randomised trials. Lancet Respir Med 2018;6(2):117–26.

18. Park S-Y, Kim S, Kim J-H, et al. A Randomized, Noninferiority Trial Comparing ICS + LABA with ICS + LABA + LAMA in Asthma-COPD Overlap (ACO) Treatment: The ACO Treatment with Optimal Medications (ATOMIC) Study. J Allergy Clin Immunol Pract 2021;9(3):1304–11.e2.

19. Song JH, Lee CH, Kim JW, et al. Clinical implications of blood eosinophil count in patients with non-asthma-COPD overlap syndrome COPD. Int J Chron Obs Pulmon Dis 2017;12:2455–64. Available from: https://www.ncbi.nlm.nih.gov/pubmed/28860740.

20. Takayama Y, Ohnishi H, Ogasawara F, et al. Clinical utility of fractional exhaled nitric oxide and blood eosinophils counts in the diagnosis of asthma-COPD overlap. Int J Chron Obstruct Pulmon Dis 2018;13:2525–32.

21. Jo YS, Hwang Y II, Yoo KH, et al. Effect of Inhaled Corticosteroids on Exacerbation of Asthma-COPD Overlap According to Different Diagnostic Criteria. J Allergy Clin Immunol Pract 2020;8(5):1625–33.e6.

22. Cheng W-C, Liao W-C, Wu B-R, et al. Clinical predictors of asthmatics in identifying subgroup requiring long-term tiotropium add-on therapy: a real-world study. J Thorac Dis 2019;11(9):3785–93.

23. Kendzerska T, Aaron SD, To T, et al. Effectiveness and Safety of Inhaled Corticosteroids in Older Individuals with Chronic Obstructive Pulmonary Disease and/or Asthma. A Population Study. Ann Am Thorac Soc 2019;16(10):1252–62.

24. Amegadzie JE, Gorgui J, Acheampong L, et al. Comparative safety and effectiveness of inhaled bronchodilators and corticosteroids for treating asthma-COPD overlap: a systematic review and meta-analysis. J Asthma 2021;58(3):344–59.

25. Gershon AS, Campitelli MA, Croxford R, et al. Combination long-acting β-agonists and inhaled corticosteroids compared with long-acting β-agonists alone in older adults with chronic obstructive pulmonary disease. JAMA 2014;312(11): 1114–21.

26. Qin J, Wang G, Han D. Benefits of LAMA in patients with asthma-COPD overlap: A systematic review and meta-analysis. Clin Immunol 2022;237:108986.

27. Magnussen H, Bugnas B, Noord J van, et al. Improvements with tiotropium in COPD patients with concomitant asthma. Respir Med 2008;102(1):50–6.

28. Xu H, Lu X. Inhaled Glucocorticoid with or without Tiotropium Bromide for Asthma-Chronic Obstructive Pulmonary Disease Overlap Syndrome. J Coll Physicians Surg Pak 2019;29(3):249–52.

29. Ishiura Y, Fujimura M, Ohkura N, et al. Triple Therapy with Budesonide/Glycopyrrolate/Formoterol Fumarate Improves Inspiratory Capacity in Patients with Asthma-Chronic Obstructive Pulmonary Disease Overlap. Int J Chron Obstruct Pulmon Dis 2020;15:269–77.

30. Albert RK, Connett J, Bailey WC, et al. Azithromycin for prevention of exacerbations of COPD. N Engl J Med 2011;365(8):689–98.

31. Chong J, Leung B, Poole P. Phosphodiesterase 4 inhibitors for chronic obstructive pulmonary disease. Cochrane Database Syst Rev 2017;9:CD002309.

32. Bodkhe S, Nikam M, Sherje AP, et al. Current insights on clinical efficacy of roflumilast for treatment of COPD, asthma and ACOS. Int Immunopharmacol 2020;88: 106906.

33. Martinez FJ, Calverley PMA, Goehring U-M, et al. Effect of roflumilast on exacerbations in patients with severe chronic obstructive pulmonary disease uncontrolled by combination therapy (REACT): a multicentre randomised controlled trial. Lancet 2015;385(9971):857–66.

34. Luo J, Yang L, Yang J, et al. Efficacy and safety of phosphodiesterase 4 inhibitors in patients with asthma: a systematic review and meta-analysis. Respirology 2018;23(5):467–77.

35. Zhang X, Chen Y, Fan L, et al. Pharmacological mechanism of roflumilast in the treatment of asthma-COPD overlap. Drug Des Devel Ther 2018;12:2371–9.

36. Martinez FJ, Rabe KF, Calverley PMA, et al. Determinants of Response to Roflumilast in Severe COPD: Pooled Analysis of Two Randomized Trials. Am J Respir Crit Care Med 2018;198(10):1268–78.

37. Rabe KF, Watz H, Baraldo S, et al. Anti-inflammatory effects of roflumilast in chronic obstructive pulmonary disease (ROBERT): a 16-week, randomised, placebo-controlled trial. Lancet Respir Med 2018;6(11):827–36.

38. Wells JM, Jackson PL, Viera L, et al. A randomized, placebo-controlled trial of roflumilast. effect on proline-glycine-proline and neutrophilic inflammation in chronic obstructive pulmonary disease. Am J Respir Crit Care Med 2015; 192(8):934–42.

39. Assaf SM, Hanania NA. Biological treatments for severe asthma. Curr Opin Allergy Clin Immunol 2019;19(4):379–86.

40. Saha S, Brightling CE. Eosinophilic airway inflammation in COPD. Int J Chron Obstruct Pulmon Dis 2006;1(1):39–47.

41. Cosio BG, Perez de Llano L, Lopez Vina A, et al. Th-2 signature in chronic airway diseases: towards the extinction of asthma-COPD overlap syndrome? Eur Respir J 2017;49(5). Available at: https://www.ncbi.nlm.nih.gov/pubmed/28461299.

42. Narendra D, Blixt J, Hanania NA. Immunological biomarkers in severe asthma. Semin Immunol 2019;46:101332.

43. Kobayashi S, Hanagama M, Yamanda S, et al. Inflammatory biomarkers in asthma-COPD overlap syndrome. Int J Chron Obs Pulmon Dis 2016;11: 2117–23. Available at: https://www.ncbi.nlm.nih.gov/pubmed/27660429.

44. Menzies-Gow A, Corren J, Bourdin A, et al. Tezepelumab in Adults and Adolescents with Severe, Uncontrolled Asthma. N Engl J Med 2021;384(19):1800–9.

45. Ricciardi L, Papia F, Liotta M, et al. Omalizumab in middle-aged or older patients with severe allergic asthma-COPD overlap. Postep dermatologii i Alergol 2022; 39(1):88–93.

46. Pérez de Llano L, Dacal Rivas D, Marina Malanda N, et al. The Response to Biologics is Better in Patients with Severe Asthma Than in Patients with Asthma-COPD Overlap Syndrome. J Asthma Allergy 2022;15:363–9.

47. Isoyama S, Ishikawa N, Hamai K, et al. Efficacy of mepolizumab in elderly patients with severe asthma and overlapping COPD in real-world settings: A retrospective observational study. Respir Investig 2021;59(4):478–86.

48. Sposato B, Scalese M, Milanese M, et al. Should omalizumab be used in severe asthma/COPD overlap? J Biol Regul Homeost Agents 2018;32(4):755–61.

49. Tat TS, Cilli A. Omalizumab treatment in asthma-COPD overlap syndrome. J Asthma 2016;53(10):1048–50.

50. Yalcin AD, Celik B, Yalcin AN. Omalizumab (anti-IgE) therapy in the asthma-COPD overlap syndrome (ACOS) and its effects on circulating cytokine levels. Immunopharmacol Immunotoxicol 2016;38(3):253–6.

51. Maltby S, Gibson PG, Powell H, et al. Omalizumab Treatment Response in a Population With Severe Allergic Asthma and Overlapping COPD. Chest 2017;151(1): 78–89. Available at: https://www.ncbi.nlm.nih.gov/pubmed/27742181.

52. Hanania NA, Chipps BE, Griffin NM, et al. Omalizumab effectiveness in asthma-COPD overlap: Post hoc analysis of PROSPERO. J Allergy Clin Immunol 2019; 143(4):1629–33.e2.

53. Llanos J-P, Bell CF, Packnett E, et al. Real-world characteristics and disease burden of patients with asthma prior to treatment initiation with mepolizumab or omalizumab: a retrospective cohort database study. J Asthma Allergy 2019;12: 43–58.

54. GINA-GOLD Diagnosis of disease of chronic airflow limitation: Asthma, COPD and asthma-COPD overlap syndrome (ACOS). Available at: https://ginasthma. org/wp-content/uploads/2019/11/GINA_GOLD_ACOS_2014-wms.pdf. Accessed 25 April 2022.

55. Global Initiative for Chronic Obstructive Lung Disease (GOLD). Global strategy for the diagnosis, management, and prevention of COPD 2020. Available at: https://goldcopd.org/wp-content/uploads/2019/12/GOLD-2020-FINAL-ver1.2-03Dec19_WMV.pdf. Accessed 25 April 2022.

56. Global Initiative for Asthma (GINA). 2020. Available at: https://ginasthma.org/wp-content/uploads/2020/06/GINA-2020-report_20_06_04-1-wms.pdf. Accessed 23 March 2022.

57. O'Donnell DE, Aaron S, Bourbeau J, et al. Canadian Thoracic Society recommendations for management of chronic obstructive pulmonary disease 2007 update. Can Respir J 2007;14(Suppl B):5B–32B.

58. Nagai A. [Guidelines for the diagnosis and management of chronic obstructive pulmonary disease: 3rd edition]. Nihon Rinsho 2010;69(10):1729–34.

59. Miravitlles M, Soler-Cataluña JJ, Calle M, et al. Spanish COPD guidelines (GesEPOC). Pharmacological treatment of stable COPD. Arch Bronconeumol 2012;48: 247–57.

60. Soler-Cataluña JJ, Cosío B, Izquierdo JL, et al. Consensus document on the overlap phenotype COPD-asthma in COPD. Arch Bronconeumol 2012;48:331–7.

61. Koblizek V, Chlumsky J, Zindr V, et al. Chronic Obstructive Pulmonary Disease: Official diagnosis and treatment guidelines Biomed of the Czech Pneumological and Phthisiological society: a novel phenotypic approach to COPD with patient-oriented care- Pap. Med Fac Univ Palacky Olomouc Czech Repub 2013;157: 189–201.

62. Kankaanranta H, Harju T, Kilpeläinen M, et al. Diagnosis and pharmacotherapy of Stable Chronic Obstructive Pulmonary Disease: The Finish Guidelines Basic. Clin Pharmacol Toxicol 2015;116:291–307.

63. Bourbeau J, Bhutani M, Hernandez P, et al. CTS position statement: pharmacotherapy in patients with COPD—an update. Can J Respir Crit Care Sleep Med 2017;1(4):222–41.

64. Mahboud BH, Vats MG, Al Zaabi A, et al. Joint Statament for the diagnosis, management, and prevention of chronic obstructive pulmonary disease for Gulf Cooperation Council countries and Middle East-North Africa region, 2017. Int J Chron Obstruct Pulmon Dis 2017;12:2869–90.

65. Yanagisawa S, Ichinose M. definition and diagnosis of asthma-COPD overlap (ACO). Allergol Int 2018;67:172–8.

66. Zatloukal J, Brat K, Neumannova K, et al. Chronic obstructive pulmonary disease - diagnosis and management of stable disease; a personalized approach to care, using the treatable traits concept based on clinical phenotypes. Position paper of the Czech Pneumological and Phthisiological Society. Biomed Pap Med Fac Univ Palacky Olomouc Czech Repub 2020;164(4):325–56.

67. Bourbeau J, Bhutani M, Hernandez P, et al. Canadian Thoracic Society Clinical Practice Guideline on pharmacotherapy in patients with COPD – 2019 update of evidence. Can J Respir Crit Care Sleep Med 2019;3(4):210–32.

68. Miravitlles M, Alvarez-Gutierrez F, Calle M, et al. Algorithm for identification of ACO: Consensus between the Spanish COPD and asthma guidelines. Eur Respir J 2017;49:1700068.

69. Araújo D, Padrão E, Morais-Almeida M, et al. Asthma-chronic obstructive pulmonary disease overlap syndrome - Literature review and contributions towards a Portuguese consensus. Rev Port Pneumol (2006) 2017;23(2):90–9.

70. Miravitlles M, Calle M, Molina J, et al. Update of the Spanish guideline for COPD (GesEPOC) 2021: Pharmacological treatment of stable COPD. Arch Bronconeumol 2022;58:69–81.

71. Montes de Oca M, López Varela MV, Acuña A, et al. Incorporating New Evidence on Inhaled Medications in COPD. The Latin American Chest Association (ALAT) 2019. Arch Bronconeumol 2020;56(2):106–13.
72. Milne S, Mannino D, Sin DD. Asthma-COPD Overlap and Chronic Airflow Obstruction: Definitions, Management, and Unanswered Questions. J Allergy Clin Immunol Pract 2020;8(2):483–95.
73. Gaspar Marques J, Lobato M, Leiria Pinto P, et al. Asthma and COPD "overlap": a treatable trait or common several treatable-traits? Eur Ann Allergy Clin Immunol 2020;52(4):148–59.
74. Shirai T, Hirai K, Gon Y, et al. Combined Assessment of Serum Periostin and YKL-40 May Identify Asthma-COPD Overlap. J Allergy Clin Immunol Pract 2019;7(1):134–45.e1.

Novel Therapeutic Strategies in Asthma-Chronic Obstructive Pulmonary Disease Overlap

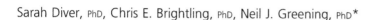

Sarah Diver, PhD, Chris E. Brightling, PhD, Neil J. Greening, PhD*

KEYWORDS

- Asthma • ACO • COPD • Dysbiosis • Inflammation • Mucus • Therapies
- Remodeling

KEY POINTS

- Precision medicine can be achieved by targeting specific phenotypes where asthma and COPD overlap.
- Many agents show promise in ameliorating type 2 eosinophilic inflammation and are progressing through clinical trials; however, novel therapies targeting neutrophilic inflammation have been less successful.
- Specific biomarkers are required to identify those likely to benefit from antimicrobial interventions in airways disease.
- Therapeutic agents targeting inflammation may have a positive impact on airway remodeling or mucous hypersecretion; however, further studies in larger numbers are required to evaluate both specific agents in current development and novel approaches.

INTRODUCTION

Heterogeneity is well recognized in airways diseases like asthma and chronic obstructive pulmonary disease (COPD), and characterization of distinct phenotypes has highlighted where pathologic processes overlap. Asthma-COPD overlap (ACO) has been used to describe individuals with clinical features of both diseases. More specificity, however, is required because treatments are increasingly targeted to specific disease traits and established biomarkers rather than traditional disease labels. The underpinning mechanisms for many of the novel therapies within are common and likely to be effective in the correctly identified individual, irrespective of a disease label such as asthma, COPD, or ACO.

Department of Respiratory Sciences, Leicester NIHR BRC, Institute for Lung Health, University of Leicester, Leicester, UK
* Corresponding author.
E-mail address: neil.greening@leicester.ac.uk

Immunol Allergy Clin N Am 42 (2022) 671–690
https://doi.org/10.1016/j.iac.2022.04.005
0889-8561/22/© 2022 Elsevier Inc. All rights reserved.
immunology.theclinics.com

In this article, the authors discuss novel therapeutic agents according to several phenotypes recognized in both asthma and COPD, including the more widely established T2 eosinophilic inflammation, particularly noted in asthma, as well as other pathways such as neutrophilic inflammation and dysbiosis more commonly reported in COPD. Specifically, the following treatment topics are reviewed (**Fig. 1**):

- T2-mediated, eosinophilic inflammation
- Non-T2 (neutrophilic) inflammation
- Dysbiosis
- Mucous hypersecretion
- Airways remodeling

T2 Eosinophilic Inflammation

T2-mediated eosinophilic inflammation is the most common inflammatory endotype in asthma and may be underestimated due to the suppressive effects of treatment, with only 5% of patients persistently "T2-low" following T2 biomarker-based corticosteroid optimization.[1] Inflammation in COPD is more commonly Th1 mediated and neutrophilic; however, sputum eosinophilia is recorded in 10% to 40% of patients.[2]

Eosinophilic inflammation has been the recent focus of pharmacotherapy in asthma, with multiple agents now licensed or in development; however, there are currently no licensed T2 biologics available for use in COPD.

ANTI-IMMUNOGLOBULIN E

Omalizumab is approved for use in children and adults with moderate-to-severe asthma and proven aeroallergen sensitization. Omalizumab reduces circulating immunoglobulin E (IgE) in the blood and interstitial space and inhibits IgE binding to high- and low-affinity receptors on mast cells, basophils, and dendritic cells. Clinically, omalizumab reduces asthma exacerbations and oral corticosteroid dependence.[3]

Data suggest that atopy is present in roughly one-third of patients with COPD[4]; however, it is associated with a lower risk of acute exacerbation. Independent of allergic status, upregulation of the high-affinity FcεRI receptors on plasma dendritic cells implicated in the asthmatic response to omalizumab has also been demonstrated in severe COPD[5] indicating that selected patients with COPD could benefit from anti-IgE treatment.

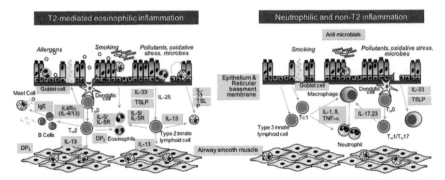

Fig. 1. Inflammatory pathways and therapeutic targets in airways disease. RBM, Reticular basement membrane.

Although omalizumab use in COPD has not been studied, small studies in allergic asthma with comorbid COPD, consistent with ACO, suggest a positive impact. A post-hoc analysis of Prospective Observational Study to Evaluate Predictors of Clinical Effectiveness in Response to Omalizumab (PROSPERO) evaluated ~50 patients with ACO, based on 2 different definitions: indicating similar improvements in exacerbations and asthma control compared with those observed in asthmatic subjects without ACO.[6] Similarly, data from the Australian Xolair Registry reported that 17 patients with ACO demonstrated improvements in asthma control and quality of life compared with those with no COPD, although associated improvements in forced expiratory volume in 1 second (FEV_1) were not observed in this subgroup.[7] A further analysis examined the response to omalizumab in subgroups of asthma with and without fixed airflow obstruction (FAO), demonstrating a positive impact on exacerbations in those with high but not low bronchodilator reversibility (BDR) in both of these groups, whereas improvements in FEV_1 were observed only in those with high BDR and absent FAO.[8]

ANTI-INTERLEUKIN-5/5R

Interleukin (IL)-5 is produced by T-helper type 2 lymphocytes, innate lymphoid type 2 cells, and eosinophils and is a key cytokine involved in recruitment, maturation, activation, and survival of eosinophils. Biological agents are available targeting both IL-5 and the IL-5 receptor. In severe eosinophilic asthma, these agents have consistently reduced acute exacerbation rates and successfully allowed reduction of oral corticosteroid burden.[9-15] Sputum IL-5 levels are elevated in eosinophilic COPD[16] suggesting that targeting this pathway could be of clinical benefit.

Benralizumab in COPD: In an initial phase 2a trial in eosinophilic COPD, treatment did not meet the primary end point of reducing exacerbation rates. However, reduction in sputum eosinophils was associated with a significant improvement in FEV_1 and there was a trend toward reduced exacerbations in those with higher blood eosinophils, suggesting treatment could be beneficial in some.[17] The subsequent phase 3 trial found no significant reduction in exacerbation rate despite substantial depletion of sputum and blood eosinophils.[18] Further analysis was performed, aiming to identify the population of subjects with COPD most likely to benefit from treatment, with the greatest treatment effect in those with blood eosinophils greater than or equal to 220 cells/μL, particularly in the presence of increased exacerbation frequency and severe airflow obstruction (FEV_1 <40%).[19] Another trial of benralizumab for acute exacerbations of eosinophilic airways disease, including both subjects with asthma and COPD, is ongoing.[20]

Mepolizumab in COPD: Two phase 3 trials (Mepolizumab vs. Placebo as Add-on Treatment for Frequently Exacerbating COPD Patients (METREX) and Mepolizumab vs. Placebo as Add-on Treatment for Frequently Exacerbating COPD Patients Characterized by Eosinophil Level (METREO)) evaluated the impact of anti-IL-5 on COPD exacerbation rates in subjects who were uncontrolled despite triple therapy.[21] Outcomes were assessed across a range of baseline blood eosinophil counts. In eosinophilic COPD, moderate and severe exacerbation rates were reduced by 18% and 20%, respectively, whereas no benefit was observed in those who were noneosinophilic. The phase 3 Mepolizumab as Add-on Treatment IN Participants With COPD Characterized by Frequent Exacerbations and Eosinophil Level (MATINEE)[22] trial is recruiting subjects with eosinophilic COPD who are persistent exacerbators with an elevated blood eosinophil count at baseline (≥300 cells/μL) and will assess the effect on annualized exacerbation rates. The Mepolizumab for COPD Hospital Eosinophilic

Admissions Pragmatic Trial (COPD-HELP) trial is also evaluating the effect of mepolizumab on acute exacerbations of COPD.[23]

TARGETING INTERLEUKIN-4/13

Despite being an integral T2 cytokine, therapies targeting IL-13 alone in asthma have failed to meet the primary end point of reducing asthma exacerbations, and development has ceased.[24,25] The efficacy of lebrikizumab was examined in patients with moderate-to-severe COPD and a history of exacerbations but did not reduce exacerbations,[26] and development has ceased.

The monoclonal antibody dupilumab targets IL-4Rα, blocking downstream activity in both IL-13 and IL-4 pathways. In asthma, this has led to significant clinical improvements both with regard to exacerbation rates and physiology.[27] Consequently, this agent is being evaluated in moderate-to-severe COPD with evidence of T2 inflammation.[28]

Targeting Epithelial Cytokines

The epithelial cytokines IL-25, IL-33, and Thymic stromal lymphopoietin perpetuate T2 inflammation via downstream effects on various cells including Th2 cells, innate lymphoid cells, and dendritic cells. Therapies targeting these upstream mediators are more advanced in asthma but are now in trials for appropriate subgroups of patients with COPD.

Interleukin-33: IL-33 is a member of the IL-1 family and signals via the ST2 pathway to promote Th2 immunity and inflammation. IL-33 levels are increased in asthma with bronchial epithelial cells as an important source. A role in asthma pathophysiology is supported by genome association studies.[29,30] A phase 2a clinical trial of anti-IL-33 in asthma was positive for a reduction in loss of control events.[31]

IL-33 levels and levels of the soluble ST2 receptor are also known to be increased in COPD, with IL-33 levels correlating positively with blood eosinophil count[32] and associated with an increased risk of exacerbation. Rabe and colleagues[33] demonstrated that the genetic risk of COPD is reduced by loss-of-function mutation in the IL-33 gene. The investigators subsequently randomized 343 patients with COPD to itepekimab or placebo. Although the study was negative overall, subgroup analysis revealed that exacerbations were reduced and FEV_1 improved in former smokers, whereas therapy had no impact on clinical outcomes in those who continued to smoke.[33] Phase 3 trials will aid understanding of whether this represents a therapeutic option in certain patients.

Targeting the ST2 receptor has also shown promise. In a phase 2 trial in asthma, the ST2 receptor antagonist, astegolimab, significantly reduced acute exacerbations, including in those with blood eosinophils less than 300 cells/μL.[34] A similar phase 2a trial has recently been published in COPD, although it did not meet statistical significance.[35] Subgroup analysis indicated that effects were greatest in those with blood eosinophil counts less than 170 cells/μL and exploring the effects of treatment on other exacerbation drivers, such as respiratory viral infection, may help to clarify these effects in future.

TSLP: TSLP is another epithelial cytokine that is elevated in asthma. A mechanistic trial in severe asthma showed that the anti-TSLP agent tezepelumab successfully attenuates eosinophilic inflammation in the airway submucosa,[36] whereas concurrent phase 3 clinical trials reported a significant reduction in acute exacerbations and improvement in other clinical outcomes.[37]

Targeting TSLP in COPD is being studied in the Tezepelumab COPD Exacerbation Study (COURSE) trial, a phase 2a multicenter randomized controlled trial to assess the effect of tezepelumab on moderate or severe exacerbation rate ratios.[38]

OTHERS

DP$_2$: Selective DP$_2$ inhibitors were an attractive prospect for targeting eosinophilic inflammation in airways disease due to expression of the receptor on key inflammatory cells, and involvement in regulating both allergic and non-allergic pathways.[39] However, phase 2 data demonstrating significant reductions in airway eosinophilia in asthma[40] were not reflected in 4 further phase 3 trials.[41,42] Earlier studies of another DP$_2$ antagonist, AZD1981, in COPD had been negative, with no significant impact on FEV$_1$ or Clinical COPD Questionnaire scores.[43]

SB010 (GATA3 inhibitor): GATA3 is an integral transcription factor directly involved in Th2 differentiation and initial expression of T2 cytokines.[44] The inhaled DNA enzyme SB010 cleaves GATA3 mRNA and has been shown to attenuate Th2 inflammatory responses in both asthma[45] and eosinophilic COPD.[46] Drug development remains ongoing. It has also been suggested that sirtuin 6 activators could decrease the T2 immune response through decreased acetylation of GATA3.[47,48]

Dexpramipexole: Dexpramipexole is an oral, synthetic aminobenzothiazole initially developed as treatment of amyotrophic lateral sclerosis. Despite failing to meet phase 3 outcomes in this area, a significant and targeted depletion of blood eosinophils in subjects receiving the drug was observed during the development program, related to inhibition of eosinophil maturation. Subsequent positive studies in hypereosinophilic syndrome[49] and chronic rhinosinusitis with nasal polyps[50] have led to extension of clinical trials into asthma. A phase 2 trial in moderate-to-severe eosinophilic ($\geq$0.3 $\times$ 10^9/L) asthma reported that 300 mg dexpramipexole led to an 80% decrease in blood eosinophils with an associated trend toward improvement in FEV$_1$,[51] indicating a potential benefit in other eosinophilic airways diseases such as eosinophilic COPD.

Non-T2 Inflammation, T1/17, and Neutrophilic Inflammation

Neutrophilic inflammation is well recognized as the predominant inflammatory characteristic of COPD but is also a recognized phenotype of asthma, so it is of relevance to those with ACO. However, to date interventions to target neutrophilic inflammation have been disappointing and none are currently or imminently licensed. A summary of trialed therapies, both past and ongoing, are described in **Table 1**.

Airways Dysbiosis

The development of culture-independent techniques for in-depth characterization of airway ecology means this is an evolving field. It is known that some clinical outcomes, such as exacerbations, in airways disease relate to bacterial, viral, or fungal airway infection, and that these may or may not be associated with a chronically altered airway ecology. Understanding the relationship between airway organisms and inflammation is likely to indicate several novel therapeutic targets in future, irrespective of disease label.

Macrolide therapy

Long-term macrolide therapy is a well-established therapy in COPD[52] and should be considered in moderate-to-severe asthma[53,54] wherein the benefits are thought to outweigh the risks. Although many patients currently benefit from this therapy, appropriate patient selection will help to reduce the wider public health risks from antibiotic

Table 1
Key trials of therapies targeting mediators of non-T2 inflammation in airways disease

Target	Evidence in Asthma	Evidence in COPD	Current Perspective for ACO
TNF-α	Increased rates of malignancy in the treatment group[97] (golimumab)	No impact on health status, lung function, or physical activity including in subgroups selected by elevated baseline TNF or CRP Concern for increased rates of malignancy[98] (infliximab)	Despite use in other conditions, the unacceptable adverse event profile has prevented use of anti-TNF agents in airways disease
IL-1	Improved late-phase allergen response[99] (canakinumab) Agents targeting the NLRP3 inflammasome have reduced airway inflammation and airway hyperresponsiveness in animal models[104]	Reduced blood neutrophils and CRP but no effect on exacerbation rates or quality of life (MEDI8968)[100] No impact on lung function (canakinumab)[101]	Further trials of canakinumab in asthma have been halted due to the SARS-CoV-2 pandemic[102] Many NLRP3 inhibiting agents are in early-phase development; however, RRx-001 (an oncological treatment) potently inhibits NLRP3 without significant safety concerns and is in phase 3 clinical trials[103]; this could potentially be of benefit in airways disease
IL-6	No effect on late-phase allergen response in mild asthma, although participants were unselected and predominantly T2 high (tocilizumab)[105]	No clinical trial data	Although no studies are currently in progress, specific asthma and COPD phenotypes have been linked to IL-6 trans-signalling, so there may be a basis for targeting IL-6 in selected groups in future

	Asthma	COPD	Comment
IL-17	No impact on asthma control, asthma symptoms, or lung function (brodalumab).[106] Follow-up trials refuted any benefit in subjects with high bronchodilator reversibility[107]	No impact on lung function, symptom scores, and rescue medication use. No measurement made of biological mediators limiting ability to examine effects in specific endotypes (CNTO 6785)[109]	Considerable interest remains in the Th17 pathway as a key mediator of neutrophilic inflammation in airways disease, and early studies in animal models suggest that this pathway could also be targeted, for example, through the Th17 transcription factor RORγt[110] Further characterization of this pathway and the relationships with other inflammatory pathways may indicate whether IL-17-targeted therapies could improve outcomes in selected patients with airways disease
IL-23	No improvement in lung function or asthma control in T2-low, uncontrolled moderate-to-severe asthma (CJM112)[108] Despite evidence for a biological effect, median time to asthma worsening increased in the treatment group (risankizumab)[111]	No reported clinical trials of anti-IL23 in COPD	
CXCR2	No effect on severe exacerbations, lung function, symptoms, or quality of life in subjects with low blood eosinophils and IgE (AZD5069)[112]	Improved FEV_1, particularly in smokers, but high rates of treatment discontinuation due to neutropenia and increased infections on continued monitoring (navarixin)[113] Improved patient-reported dyspnoea outcomes in a small study (anti-IL8)[114]	The role of CXCR2 in regulation of neutrophil extracellular trap formation[115] presents the opportunity to refine the use of anti-CXCR2 in specific disease phenotypes of severe asthma and COPD
Kinase inhibitors: PI3K	Reduced sputum proinflammatory cytokines but no impact on clinical outcomes (nemiralisib)[116]	Evidence of reduced inflammation and improved time to recovery when given at time of acute exacerbation; however, no improvement in FEV_1 and no effect on future exacerbations (nemiralisib)[117–119]	Multiple kinases drive inflammation and remodeling in the lung and therefore represent potential therapeutic strategies in both asthma and COPD; however, off-target effects and lack of specificity have been some of the issues stalling development. Agents targeting JAK1 and spleen tyrosine kinases remain in early-phase development[120–122]
P38 MAPK	No reported trials in asthma	Well tolerated but no effect on exercise tolerance or lung function including in subgroups without eosinophilia (losmapimod)[123–125]	

(continued on next page)

Table 1
(continued)

Target	Evidence in Asthma	Evidence in COPD	Current Perspective for ACO
PDE3/4	Improvement in lung function in asthma but not progressed in clinical trials (roflumilast)[126]	Roflumilast a currently licensed therapy recognized to have some positive impact on FEV$_1$ and exacerbations; however, poorly tolerated due to gastrointestinal and psychiatric adverse effects associated with treatment[127]	Although roflumilast is already licensed in COPD, the side effect profile has limited use. Development of agents delivered directly to the respiratory tract may minimize the systemic effects. Attenuation of Th1 cytokines indicates there may be specific populations within airways disease more likely to benefit[128]
	Inhaled PDE4 reduces the late-phase allergen response (CHF6001)[129]	Inhaled PDE3/4 inhibitors reduce inflammation and improve FEV$_1$ (ensifentrine)[130,131]	

Abbreviations: CRP, C-reactive protein; CXCR2, C-X-C motif chemokine receptor 2; JAK1, Janus kinase 1; MAPK, mitogen-activated protein kinase; NLRP3, NLR family pyrin domain containing 3; PDE, phosphodiesterase; PI3K, phosphoinositide 3 kinase; RORγt, RAR-related orphan receptor gamma; SARS-CoV-2, severe acute respiratory syndrome coronavirus 2; T2, type 2 inflammation; TNF, tumor necrosis factor.

resistance[55]; therefore identifying the target population most likely to respond remains an unmet clinical need.

In asthma, Brusselle and colleagues[56] indicated that the benefits of macrolide therapy were observed in noneosinophilic subgroups only; however, this was refuted by the Effect of azithromycin on asthma exacerbations and quality of life in adults with persistent uncontrolled asthma (AMAZES) trial, which reported benefits independent of inflammatory status,[57] although subgroup analysis demonstrated maximal effects in those with positive bacterial cultures. Posthoc analysis of the AMAZES trial has, however, suggested that airway abundance of *Haemophilus influenzae* predicts response to azithromycin therapy.[58] At present, widely accessible biomarkers of dysbiosis are not available; however, in future it is likely that these will be useful to indicate those most likely to benefit. In COPD, the Gammaproteobacteria to Firmicutes ratio (γP:F) has shown promise in identifying those likely to benefit from antimicrobials in the context of acute exacerbation.[59]

Probiotics and prebiotics

Probiotics are live microorganisms that confer health benefits on their recipient host and include the genera *Lactobacillus* and *Bifidobacteria*. Prebiotics are indigestible carbohydrates metabolized by gut bacteria but not host cells, thereby stimulating growth and/or activity of beneficial organisms. These strategies have been used in asthma with the aim of modulating the gut microbiome to achieve an antiinflammatory effect.[60] Probiotics have demonstrated mixed success in terms of improving clinical outcomes in asthma but remain in clinical trials. A current trial in COPD is seeking to ascertain whether modulating the lower respiratory microbiome will reduce exacerbations in moderate-to-very severe COPD, comparing an oral probiotic intervention with inhalation of amikacin, combined administration of the influenza and pneumococcal vaccine, and current standard of care.[61]

Phage therapy

Bacteriophages are natural biological entities that kill bacteria with species-specific precision, indicating a promising strategy to target pathogens known to be implicated in chronic lung diseases. Although bacteriophages were discovered over a century ago, there has been renewed interest recently in view of increasing antibiotic resistance and slowed development of new antibiotic agents.[62] In COPD, bacteriophage abundance decreased during viral infection, suggesting a possible mechanism for increased susceptibility to bacterial infection in this context.[63] Virome study in asthma also indicates that bacteriophage abundance was severely reduced compared with healthy controls, and correlated with ACT and FEV_1.[64] Clinical trials in obstructive airways disease are awaited; however, in preclinical studies of chronic lung infection, phage therapy was shown to be efficacious against *Pseudomonas aeruginosa*.[65]

Antifungal and antiviral interventions

Viral infection, particularly rhinovirus, is a well-recognized etiological factor in exacerbations and is associated with suboptimal interferon responses. Although a trial of inhaled interferon-β did not improve asthma control questionnaire-6 scores in those with asthma with acquired viral infection, analysis of the subgroup with moderate-to-severe disease demonstrated a significant improvement compared with placebo.[66] In vitro bronchial epithelial cells pretreated with azithromycin had an augmented interferon response when infected with rhinovirus,[67] suggesting that the positive effects observed in clinical trials in asthma and COPD may relate to the effect on viral immunity; however, whereas studies of azithromycin in acute exacerbations of COPD trended toward reducing treatment failure,[68] studies in acute exacerbations of asthma were negative, albeit potentially underpowered.[69]

The clinical significance of fungal infection in COPD is incompletely understood, and likely to be underestimated; however, *Aspergillus* spp are isolated in ~15% at exacerbation and follow-up, with hypersensitivity to *Aspergillus* reported in 8% to 15%, associated with reduced lung function.[70] It is unknown whether antifungal therapies may improve lung function in COPD, and treatment is only recommended where there is a concurrent diagnosis of fungal lung disease. Fungal sensitization is more common in severe asthma, reported in up to 50%[71]; however, to date antifungal treatment in severe asthma not meeting criteria for allergic bronchopulmonary aspergillosis has not been efficacious in reducing severe exacerbations or improving quality of life.[72]

Mucous Hypersecretion

Mucus is an aqueous solution of lipids, proteins, and mucins. Mucins are encoded by MUC genes and synthesized in goblet cells and submucosal glands.[73]

In asthma, mucous hypersecretion is linked to overexpression of the cytokine IL-13, which increases the number of goblet cells in the airway. Studies in COPD have linked goblet cell hyperplasia and mucin production to activation of the epidermal growth factor receptor (EGFR) cascade.

Several mucolytic agents are licensed for use in airways disease; however, development of novel agents to inhibit mucin synthesis has been limited by lack of both efficacy and selectivity resulting in poor tolerance (eg, targeting EGFR[74] and MAPK13[75]). Bio-11006, an agent aiming to reduce mucin secretion via inhibition of myristoylated alanine-rich C-kinase substrate (MARCKS), remains in development for COPD having demonstrated an improvement in mucous hypersecretion with associated increase in lung function in an initial phase 2 trial[76]; however, there are no active trials in asthma at present.

Several bronchoscopic techniques have been proposed for the treatment of chronic bronchitis, characterized by increased mucous production and goblet cell hyperplasia. The RejuvenAir System (CSA Medical, Inc. Lexington, MA) metered cryospray aims to destroy hyperplastic goblet cells and excessive airway mucous glands with topical liquid nitrogen spray. Small studies have demonstrated the technique to be safe,[77] and further trials assessing the effects of treatment on acute exacerbations (NCT03893370) and goblet cell density (NCT03892694) are ongoing. In bronchial rheoplasty, the RheOx catheter delivers bursts of high-frequency electrical energy to the airway using a monopolar electrode, targeting abnormal goblet cells and glands. Despite some early serious adverse events (SAEs), this technique reduced goblet cell hyperplasia score and improved patient-reported outcomes at 12 months.[78] These bronchoscopic techniques have not yet been trialed in patients with asthma, or evaluated subgroups with features of ACO.

Targeting mucin synthesis or secretion in airways disease will require development of agents with greater selectivity. Other novel approaches have been proposed further, such as lysis of occlusive mucous plugs in the context of acute clinical deterioration.[79]

Airways Remodeling

Airway remodeling occurs in both asthma and COPD, affecting both small and large airways in asthma and predominantly small airways in COPD. Common remodeling features include loss of epithelial integrity, mucous hypersecretion, increased airway smooth muscle (ASM) mass, and alterations to levels of extracellular matrix proteins and airway microvasculature. Inflammation is closely linked to remodeling, and one approach is to target the inflammatory pathways responsible for structural changes in the airway. Physiologic changes including airflow limitation and airway hyperresponsiveness occur in both conditions to differing degrees.[80]

Targeting airway smooth muscle

Therapies targeting ASM have been more extensively studied in asthma because ASM area in COPD airways is similar to that in healthy smokers and nonsmokers, although with increased localization of neutrophils.[81] The anti-DP_2 agent, fevipiprant, reduced ASM mass compared with placebo[82] with computational modeling indicating that both attenuation of eosinophilic inflammation and decreased myofibroblast recruitment were responsible; however, as discussed earlier, this agent is no longer in development for asthma or COPD. Other biologic agents in asthma have not reported reductions in ASM compared with placebo,[36,82,83] and indeed a recent cluster analysis based on fluctuations in lung function in asthma and COPD suggests that remodeling is not directly related to T2 inflammation.[84]

Bronchial thermoplasty (BT) in severe asthma involves pulsed application of radiofrequency energy to the airway wall via a bronchoscopically inserted catheter and led to improvements in exacerbations and hospitalizations in clinical trials.[85,86] The positive impacts reported following BT are thought to relate to reduction in ASM as a direct response to heat; however, biopsy studies have shown an improvement in epithelial integrity post-BT, and mathematical modeling suggests that other mechanisms may contribute to ASM reduction.[87] Small retrospective studies of BT in subjects with ACO and severe asthma with smoking history suggest that a benefit is still observed in these groups; however, further data are required.[88–91] In COPD, targeted lung denervation aims to disrupt parasympathetic nerve transmission to and from the lung through the application of radiofrequency energy via a dual cooled catheter, reducing ASM contraction and mucous production and increasing acetylcholine production. The Targeted Lung Denervation for Patients With Moderate to Severe COPD-2 (AIRFLOW-2) trial indicated that those receiving treatment experienced fewer events, and were less likely to be hospitalized for COPD exacerbation, than those in the sham procedure group.[92] The AIRFLOW-3 trial will study the technique in a larger number of subjects.[93–95]

Novel remodeling targets

Several novel bronchodilator targets are in preclinical development and may demonstrate efficacy in asthma, COPD, and ACO in future; these include the selective phosphodiesterase inhibitors discussed in see **Table 1**, bitter taste receptor agonists, E-prostanoid receptor 4 agonists, Rho kinase inhibitors, calcilytics, agonists of peroxisome proliferator-activated receptor-γ, agonists of relaxin receptor 1, soluble guanylyl cyclase activators, and pepducins.[96]

With increasing recognition of heterogeneity in asthma and COPD, characterization of underlying disease mechanisms has highlighted numerous potential therapeutic targets. Agents directed toward these may have benefit only in specific subgroups, although pathways may be common across asthma and COPD, and future clinical trials will need to carefully select both appropriate subjects for inclusion and clinical outcome measures to ensure that the effects of new treatments can be interpreted with confidence. The lack of a clear definition for ACO increases the complexity of performing prospective clinical trials in this group; however, where evidence is consistent across phenotype-specific populations in asthma and COPD, extrapolation may be possible.

As there is increasing success in outcomes such as reducing exacerbations across airways disease, focus should shift to other treatment goals where current agents have demonstrated less success, although the contribution of extrathoracic factors such as obesity, deconditioning, and comorbidities may play a significant role here. Expectations will then need to be raised further to include cure and disease prevention.

SUMMARY

Novel therapeutic options in asthma, COPD, and ACO have started to come into clinical practice over the last decade, initially targeting anti-IL-5 pathways, but will continue to expand and indications widen. The specificity of treatment group, alongside relatively expensive cost, means they are likely to remain specialist interventions requiring phenotypic workup; this makes their application in ACO more challenging but does mean careful patient characterization and workup is needed to ensure the right patient receives the right therapy.

To date, most therapies have targeted T2 inflammation and eosinophil-driven disease, with limited success in antineutrophilic interventions. Other pathways, such as dysbiosis, mucous hypersecretion, and airways remodeling provide considerable opportunities for increased therapeutic targets over the next 15 years.

CLINICS CARE POINTS

- Targeted therapies are unlikely to be licensed in ACO due to the lack of formal diagnostic criteria; this could potentially limit access where there is a potential benefit for patients.

- Standalone trials, or posthoc analyses of interventions in subgroups with specific treatable traits like fixed airflow obstruction, but without disease labels, could provide evidence to support the use of targeted therapies in certain groups.

- We suggest that when assessing a patient for specific therapeutic strategies, clinicians could clearly identify and document the mechanism or treatable trait that a therapy will target rather than utilizing broad disease labels, such as ACO, for example, "eosinophilic airway inflammation with recurrent exacerbations" or "recurrent lower respiratory tract infections with growth of *Haemophilus influenzae* in sputum."

- Although patients with ACO may have wider-ranging disease features, it is important to acknowledge that they may still demonstrate features consistent with the inclusion criteria of clinical trials of targeted therapies in either asthma or COPD that justify the use of these agents.

DISCLOSURE

S. Diver has no relevant disclosures. C. E. Brightling has received grants from Astra-Zeneca, GSK, Roche/Genentech, BI, Novartis, Chiesi, MSD, Sanofi, Regeneron, 4DPharma, Mologic and consulting fee (paid to institution) from Astra Zeneca, GSK, Roche/Genentech, BI, Novartis, Chiesi, MSD, Sanofi, Regeneron, and 4DPharma. N. J. Greening has received grants from GSK and Roche/Genentech and consulting fee from AstraZeneca, BI, Chiesi, GSK, and Genentech.

REFERENCES

1. Heaney LG, Busby J, Hanratty CE, et al. Composite type-2 biomarker strategy versus a symptom-risk-based algorithm to adjust corticosteroid dose in patients with severe asthma: a multicentre, single-blind, parallel group, randomised controlled trial. Lancet Respir Med 2021;9(1):57–68.

2. George L, Brightling CE. Eosinophilic airway inflammation: role in asthma and chronic obstructive pulmonary disease. Ther Adv Chronic Dis 2016;7(1):34–51.

3. Normansell R, Walker S, Milan SJ, et al. Omalizumab for asthma in adults and children. Cochrane Database Syst Rev 2014;1:CD003559.

4. Putcha N, Fawzy A, Matsui EC, et al. Clinical Phenotypes of Atopy and Asthma in COPD: A Meta-analysis of SPIROMICS and COPDGene. Chest 2020;158(6): 2333–45.

5. Stoll P, Bähker A, Ulrich M, et al. The dendritic cell high-affinity IgE receptor is overexpressed in both asthma and severe COPD. Clin Exp Allergy 2016; 46(4):575–83.

6. Hanania NA, Chipps BE, Griffin NM, et al. Omalizumab effectiveness in asthma-COPD overlap: Post hoc analysis of PROSPERO. J Allergy Clin Immunol 2019; 143(4):1629–33.e2.

7. Maltby S, Gibson PG, Powell H, et al. Omalizumab Treatment Response in a Population With Severe Allergic Asthma and Overlapping COPD. Chest 2017; 151(1):78–89.

8. Hanania NA, Fortis S, Haselkorn T, et al. Omalizumab in Asthma with Fixed Airway Obstruction: Post Hoc Analysis of EXTRA. J Allergy Clin Immunol Pract 2022;10(1):222–8.

9. Pavord ID, Korn S, Howarth P, et al. Mepolizumab for severe eosinophilic asthma (DREAM): a multicentre, double-blind, placebo-controlled trial. Lancet 2012;380(9842):651–9.

10. Bel EH, Wenzel SE, Thompson PJ, et al. Oral glucocorticoid-sparing effect of mepolizumab in eosinophilic asthma. N Engl J Med 2014;371(13):1189–97.

11. Ortega HG, Liu MC, Pavord ID, et al. Mepolizumab treatment in patients with severe eosinophilic asthma. N Engl J Med 2014;371(13):1198–207.

12. Castro M, Zangrilli J, Wechsler ME, et al. Reslizumab for inadequately controlled asthma with elevated blood eosinophil counts: results from two multicentre, parallel, double-blind, randomised, placebo-controlled, phase 3 trials. Lancet Respir Med 2015;3(5):355–66.

13. Bleecker ER, FitzGerald JM, Chanez P, et al. Efficacy and safety of benralizumab for patients with severe asthma uncontrolled with high-dosage inhaled corticosteroids and long-acting beta2-agonists (SIROCCO): a randomised, multicentre, placebo-controlled phase 3 trial. Lancet 2016;388(10056):2115–27.

14. FitzGerald JM, Bleecker ER, Nair P, et al. Benralizumab, an anti-interleukin-5 receptor alpha monoclonal antibody, as add-on treatment for patients with severe, uncontrolled, eosinophilic asthma (CALIMA): a randomised, double-blind, placebo-controlled phase 3 trial. Lancet 2016;388(10056):2128–41.

15. Nair P, Wenzel S, Rabe KF, et al. Oral Glucocorticoid-Sparing Effect of Benralizumab in Severe Asthma. N Engl J Med 2017;376(25):2448–58.

16. Bafadhel M, McCormick M, Saha S, et al. Profiling of sputum inflammatory mediators in asthma and chronic obstructive pulmonary disease. Respiration 2012; 83(1):36–44.

17. Brightling CE, Bleecker ER, Panettieri RA Jr, et al. Benralizumab for chronic obstructive pulmonary disease and sputum eosinophilia: a randomised, double-blind, placebo-controlled, phase 2a study. Lancet Respir Med 2014; 2(11):891–901.

18. Criner GJ, Celli BR, Brightling CE, et al. Benralizumab for the Prevention of COPD Exacerbations. N Engl J Med 2019;381(11):1023–34.

19. Criner GJ, Celli BR, Singh D, et al. Predicting response to benralizumab in chronic obstructive pulmonary disease: analyses of GALATHEA and TERR-ANOVA studies. Lancet Respir Med 2020;8(2):158–70.

20. ClinicalTrials.gov. Acute Exacerbations Treated With BenRAlizumab (The ABRA Study) (ABRA). 2021. Available at: https://clinicaltrials.gov/ct2/show/NCT04098718. Accessed 17 Sept 2021.

21. Pavord ID, Chanez P, Criner GJ, et al. Mepolizumab for Eosinophilic Chronic Obstructive Pulmonary Disease. N Engl J Med 2017;377(17):1613–29.

22. ClinicalTrials.gov. Mepolizumab as Add-on Treatment IN Participants With COPD Characterized by Frequent Exacerbations and Eosinophil Level (MATI-NEE). 2021. Available at: https://clinicaltrials.gov/ct2/show/NCT04133909. Accessed 3 Dec 2021.

23. ClinicalTrials.gov. Mepolizumab for COPD Hospital Eosinophilic Admissions Pragmatic Trial (COPD-HELP). 2021. Available at: https://clinicaltrials.gov/ct2/show/NCT04075331. Accessed December 3 2021.

24. Hanania NA, Korenblat P, Chapman KR, et al. Efficacy and safety of lebrikizumab in patients with uncontrolled asthma (LAVOLTA I and LAVOLTA II): replicate, phase 3, randomised, double-blind, placebo-controlled trials. Lancet Respir Med 2016;4(10):781–96.

25. Panettieri RA Jr, Sjöbring U, Péterffy A, et al. Tralokinumab for severe, uncontrolled asthma (STRATOS 1 and STRATOS 2): two randomised, double-blind, placebo-controlled, phase 3 clinical trials. Lancet Respir Med 2018;6(7):511–25.

26. Yousuf A, Ibrahim W, Greening NJ, et al. T2 Biologics for Chronic Obstructive Pulmonary Disease. J Allergy Clin Immunol Pract 2019;7(5):1405–16.

27. Castro M, Corren J, Pavord ID, et al. Dupilumab Efficacy and Safety in Moderate-to-Severe Uncontrolled Asthma. N Engl J Med 2018;378(26):2486–96.

28. ClinicalTrials.gov. Pivotal Study to Assess the Efficacy, Safety and Tolerability of Dupilumab in Patients With Moderate-to-severe COPD With Type 2 Inflammation (BOREAS). 2021. Available at: https://clinicaltrials.gov/ct2/show/NCT03930732. Accessed 3 Dec 2021.

29. Aneas I, Decker DC, Howard CL, et al. Asthma-associated genetic variants induce IL33 differential expression through an enhancer-blocking regulatory region. Nat Commun 2021;12(1):6115.

30. Ketelaar ME, Portelli MA, Dijk FN, et al. Phenotypic and functional translation of IL33 genetics in asthma. J Allergy Clin Immunol 2021;147(1):144–57.

31. Wechsler ME, Ruddy MK, Pavord ID, et al. Efficacy and Safety of Itepekimab in Patients with Moderate-to-Severe Asthma. N Engl J Med 2021;385(18):1656–68.

32. Kim SW, Rhee CK, Kim KU, et al. Factors associated with plasma IL-33 levels in patients with chronic obstructive pulmonary disease. Int J Chron Obstruct Pulmon Dis 2017;12:395–402.

33. Rabe KF, Celli BR, Wechsler ME, et al. Safety and efficacy of itepekimab in patients with moderate-to-severe COPD: a genetic association study and randomised, double-blind, phase 2a trial. Lancet Respir Med 2021;9(11):1288–98.

34. Kelsen SG, Agache IO, Soong W, et al. Astegolimab (anti-ST2) efficacy and safety in adults with severe asthma: A randomized clinical trial. J Allergy Clin Immunol 2021;148(3):790–8.

35. Yousuf AJ, Mohammed S, Carr L, et al. Late Breaking Abstract - Astegolimab, an anti-ST2, in chronic obstructive pulmonary disease - COPD-ST2OP: a phase IIa, placebo-controlled trial. Eur Respir J 2021;58(suppl 65):RCT206.

36. Diver S, Khalfaoui L, Emson C, et al. Effect of tezepelumab on airway inflammatory cells, remodelling, and hyperresponsiveness in patients with moderate-to-severe uncontrolled asthma (CASCADE): a double-blind, randomised, placebo-controlled, phase 2 trial. Lancet Respir Med 2021;9(11):1299–312.

37. Menzies-Gow A, Colice G, Griffiths JM, et al. NAVIGATOR: a phase 3 multicentre, randomized, double-blind, placebo-controlled, parallel-group trial to evaluate the efficacy and safety of tezepelumab in adults and adolescents with severe, uncontrolled asthma. Respir Res 2020;21(1):266.

38. ClinicalTrials.gov. Tezepelumab COPD Exacerbation Study (COURSE). 2021. Available at: https://clinicaltrials.gov/ct2/show/NCT04039113. Accessed 3 Dec 2021.

39. Brightling CE, Brusselle G, Altman P. The impact of the prostaglandin D(2) receptor 2 and its downstream effects on the pathophysiology of asthma. Allergy 2020;75(4):761–8.

40. Gonem S, Berair R, Singapuri A, et al. Fevipiprant, a prostaglandin D2 receptor 2 antagonist, in patients with persistent eosinophilic asthma: a single-centre, randomised, double-blind, parallel-group, placebo-controlled trial. Lancet Respir Med 2016;4(9):699–707.

41. Castro M, Kerwin E, Miller D, et al. Efficacy and safety of fevipiprant in patients with uncontrolled asthma: Two replicate, phase 3, randomised, double-blind, placebo-controlled trials (ZEAL-1 and ZEAL-2). EClinicalMedicine 2021;35: 100847.

42. Brightling CE, Gaga M, Inoue H, et al. Effectiveness of fevipiprant in reducing exacerbations in patients with severe asthma (LUSTER-1 and LUSTER-2): two phase 3 randomised controlled trials. Lancet Respir Med 2021;9(1):43–56.

43. Snell N, Foster M, Vestbo J. Efficacy and safety of AZD1981, a CRTH2 receptor antagonist, in patients with moderate to severe COPD. Respir Med 2013; 107(11):1722–30.

44. Bowen H, Kelly A, Lee T, et al. Control of cytokine gene transcription in Th1 and Th2 cells. Clin Exp Allergy 2008;38(9):1422–31.

45. Krug N, Hohlfeld JM, Kirsten AM, et al. Allergen-induced asthmatic responses modified by a GATA3-specific DNAzyme. N Engl J Med 2015;372(21):1987–95.

46. Greulich T, Hohlfeld JM, Neuser P, et al. A GATA3-specific DNAzyme attenuates sputum eosinophilia in eosinophilic COPD patients: a feasibility randomized clinical trial. Respir Res 2018;19(1):55.

47. Jang HY, Gu S, Lee SM, et al. Overexpression of sirtuin 6 suppresses allergic airway inflammation through deacetylation of GATA3. J Allergy Clin Immunol 2016;138(5):1452–5.e13.

48. Ma K, Lu N, Zou F, et al. Sirtuins as novel targets in the pathogenesis of airway inflammation in bronchial asthma. Eur J Pharmacol 2019;865:172670.

49. Panch SR, Bozik ME, Brown T, et al. Dexpramipexole as an oral steroid-sparing agent in hypereosinophilic syndromes. Blood 2018;132(5):501–9.

50. Laidlaw TM, Prussin C, Panettieri RA, et al. Dexpramipexole depletes blood and tissue eosinophils in nasal polyps with no change in polyp size. Laryngoscope 2019;129(2):E61–6.

51. ClinicalTrials.gov. Dexpramipexole Dose-Ranging Biomarker Study in Subjects With Eosinophilic Asthma (AS201). 2021. Available at: https://clinicaltrials.gov/ct2/show/NCT04046939. Accessed 17 Sept 2021.

52. Herath SC, Normansell R, Maisey S, et al. Prophylactic antibiotic therapy for chronic obstructive pulmonary disease (COPD). Cochrane Database Syst Rev 2018;10(10):Cd009764.

53. Global Initiative for Asthma. Global Strategy for Asthma Management and Prevention. Scientific Report 2021. Available at: https://ginasthma.org/gina-reports/.

54. Holguin F, Cardet JC, Chung KF, et al. Management of severe asthma: a European Respiratory Society/American Thoracic Society guideline. Eur Respir J 2020;55(1):1900588.

55. Taylor SL, Leong LEX, Mobegi FM, et al. Long-Term Azithromycin Reduces Haemophilus influenzae and Increases Antibiotic Resistance in Severe Asthma. Am J Respir Crit Care Med 2019;200(3):309–17.

56. Brusselle GG, Vanderstichele C, Jordens P, et al. Azithromycin for prevention of exacerbations in severe asthma (AZISAST): a multicentre randomised double-blind placebo-controlled trial. Thorax 2013;68(4):322–9.

57. Gibson PG, Yang IA, Upham JW, et al. Effect of azithromycin on asthma exacerbations and quality of life in adults with persistent uncontrolled asthma (AMAZES): a randomised, double-blind, placebo-controlled trial. Lancet 2017; 390(10095):659–68.

58. Taylor SL, Ivey KL, Gibson PG, et al. Airway abundance of Haemophilus influenzae predicts response to azithromycin in adults with persistent uncontrolled asthma. Eur Respir J 2020;56(4):2000194.

59. Haldar K, Bafadhel M, Lau K, et al. Microbiome balance in sputum determined by PCR stratifies COPD exacerbations and shows potential for selective use of antibiotics. PLoS One 2017;12(8):e0182833.

60. Chung KF. Airway microbial dysbiosis in asthmatic patients: A target for prevention and treatment? J Allergy Clin Immunol 2017;139(4):1071–81.

61. Hua JL, Hu WP, Zuo YH, et al. Prevention of Acute Exacerbation in Subjects with Moderate-to-very Severe COPD by Modulating Lower Respiratory Microbiome: Protocol of a Prospective, Multicenter, Randomized Controlled Trial. Int J Chron Obstruct Pulmon Dis 2020;15:2985–90.

62. Nale JY, Clokie MR. Preclinical data and safety assessment of phage therapy in humans. Curr Opin Biotechnol 2021;68:310–7.

63. van Rijn AL, van Boheemen S, Sidorov I, et al. The respiratory virome and exacerbations in patients with chronic obstructive pulmonary disease. PLoS One 2019;14(10):e0223952.

64. Choi S, Sohn KH, Jung JW, et al. Lung virome: New potential biomarkers for asthma severity and exacerbation. J Allergy Clin Immunol 2021;148(4):1007–15.e9.

65. Waters EM, Neill DR, Kaman B, et al. Phage therapy is highly effective against chronic lung infections with Pseudomonas aeruginosa. Thorax 2017;72(7):666–7.

66. Djukanovic R, Harrison T, Johnston SL, et al. The effect of inhaled IFN-beta on worsening of asthma symptoms caused by viral infections. A randomized trial. Am J Respir Crit Care Med 2014;190(2):145–54.

67. Gielen V, Johnston SL, Edwards MR. Azithromycin induces anti-viral responses in bronchial epithelial cells. Eur Respir J 2010;36(3):646–54.

68. Vermeersch K, Gabrovska M, Aumann J, et al. Azithromycin during Acute Chronic Obstructive Pulmonary Disease Exacerbations Requiring Hospitalization (BACE). A Multicenter, Randomized, Double-Blind, Placebo-controlled Trial. Am J Respir Crit Care Med 2019;200(7):857–68.

69. Johnston SL, Szigeti M, Cross M, et al. Azithromycin for Acute Exacerbations of Asthma : The AZALEA Randomized Clinical Trial. JAMA Intern Med 2016; 176(11):1630–7.

70. Leung JM, Tiew PY, Mac Aogáin M, et al. The role of acute and chronic respiratory colonization and infections in the pathogenesis of COPD. Respirology 2017; 22(4):634–50.
71. O'Driscoll BR, Powell G, Chew F, et al. Comparison of skin prick tests with specific serum immunoglobulin E in the diagnosis of fungal sensitization in patients with severe asthma. Clin Exp Allergy 2009;39(11):1677–83.
72. Agbetile J, Bourne M, Fairs A, et al. Effectiveness of voriconazole in the treatment of Aspergillus fumigatus-associated asthma (EVITA3 study). J Allergy Clin Immunol 2014;134(1):33–9.
73. Ha EV, Rogers DF. Novel Therapies to Inhibit Mucus Synthesis and Secretion in Airway Hypersecretory Diseases. Pharmacology 2016;97(1–2):84–100.
74. Woodruff PG, Wolff M, Hohlfeld JM, et al. Safety and efficacy of an inhaled epidermal growth factor receptor inhibitor (BIBW 2948 BS) in chronic obstructive pulmonary disease. Am J Respir Crit Care Med 2010;181(5):438–45.
75. Alevy YG, Patel AC, Romero AG, et al. IL-13-induced airway mucus production is attenuated by MAPK13 inhibition. J Clin Invest 2012;122(12):4555–68.
76. Van As A, Kraft M, Hanania NA, et al. Inhibition of airway mucus hypersecretion and inflammation with bio-11006, A novel dual action drug, results in improvement of indices of bronchitis and lung function in chronic obstructive pulmonary disease (COPD), 2011. American Thoracic Society Congress; 2011. Colorado Convention Center: American Journal of Respiratory and Critical Care Medicine; 2011.
77. Garner JL, Shaipanich T, Hartman JE, et al. A prospective safety and feasibility study of metered cryospray for patients with chronic bronchitis in COPD. Eur Respir J 2020;56(6):2000556.
78. Valipour A, Fernandez-Bussy S, Ing AJ, et al. Bronchial Rheoplasty for Treatment of Chronic Bronchitis. Twelve-Month Results from a Multicenter Clinical Trial. Am J Respir Crit Care Med 2020;202(5):681–9.
79. Dunican EM, Watchorn DC, Fahy JV. Autopsy and Imaging Studies of Mucus in Asthma. Lessons Learned about Disease Mechanisms and the Role of Mucus in Airflow Obstruction. Ann Am Thorac Soc 2018;15(Suppl 3):S184–91.
80. Liu G, Philp AM, Corte T, et al. Therapeutic targets in lung tissue remodelling and fibrosis. Pharmacol Ther 2021;225:107839.
81. Baraldo S, Turato G, Badin C, et al. Neutrophilic infiltration within the airway smooth muscle in patients with COPD. Thorax 2004;59(4):308–12.
82. Saunders R, Kaul H, Berair R, et al. Fevipiprant reduces airway smooth muscle mass in asthmatics via PGD2 receptor antagonism. Eur Respir J 2017;50(suppl 61):OA283.
83. Chachi L, Diver S, Kaul H, et al. Computational modelling prediction and clinical validation of impact of benralizumab on airway smooth muscle mass in asthma. Eur Respir J 2019;54(5):1900930.
84. Delgado-Eckert E, James A, Meier-Girard D, et al. Lung function fluctuation patterns unveil asthma and COPD phenotypes unrelated to type 2 inflammation. J Allergy Clin Immunol 2021;148(2):407–19.
85. Castro M, Rubin AS, Laviolette M, et al. Effectiveness and safety of bronchial thermoplasty in the treatment of severe asthma: a multicenter, randomized, double-blind, sham-controlled clinical trial. Am J Respir Crit Care Med 2010; 181(2):116–24.
86. Wechsler ME, Laviolette M, Rubin AS, et al. Bronchial thermoplasty: Long-term safety and effectiveness in patients with severe persistent asthma. J Allergy Clin Immunol 2013;132(6):1295–302.

87. Chernyavsky IL, Russell RJ, Saunders RM, et al. In vitro, in silico and in vivo study challenges the impact of bronchial thermoplasty on acute airway smooth muscle mass loss. Eur Respir J 2018;51(5):1701680.

88. Hu SY, Long F, Long L, et al. [Analysis of the clinical efficacy and safety of bronchial thermoplasty in the treatment of patients with severe asthma and asthma-chronic obstructive pulmonary disease overlap]. Zhonghua Yi Xue Za Zhi 2021; 101(15):1071–6.

89. Otoshi R, Baba T, Aiko N, et al. Effectiveness and Safety of Bronchial Thermoplasty in the Treatment of Severe Asthma with Smoking History: A Single-Center Experience. Int Arch Allergy Immunol 2020;181(7):522–8.

90. Slebos DJ, Klooster K, Koegelenberg CF, et al. Targeted lung denervation for moderate to severe COPD: a pilot study. Thorax 2015;70(5):411–9.

91. Valipour A, Asadi S, Pison C, et al. Long-term safety of bilateral targeted lung denervation in patients with COPD. Int J Chron Obstruct Pulmon Dis 2018;13: 2163–72.

92. Slebos DJ, Shah PL, Herth FJF, et al. Safety and Adverse Events after Targeted Lung Denervation for Symptomatic Moderate to Severe Chronic Obstructive Pulmonary Disease (AIRFLOW). A Multicenter Randomized Controlled Clinical Trial. Am J Respir Crit Care Med 2019;200(12):1477–86.

93. Slebos DJ, Degano B, Valipour A, et al. Design for a multicenter, randomized, sham-controlled study to evaluate safety and efficacy after treatment with the Nuvaira® lung denervation system in subjects with chronic obstructive pulmonary disease (AIRFLOW-3). BMC Pulm Med 2020;20(1):41.

94. Zakarya R, Chan YL, Rutting S, et al. BET proteins are associated with the induction of small airway fibrosis in COPD. Thorax 2021;76(7):647–55.

95. Tian B, Hosoki K, Liu Z, et al. Mucosal bromodomain-containing protein 4 mediates aeroallergen-induced inflammation and remodeling. J Allergy Clin Immunol 2019;143(4):1380–94.e9.

96. Cazzola M, Rogliani P, Matera MG. The future of bronchodilation: looking for new classes of bronchodilators. Eur Respir Rev 2019;28(154).

97. Wenzel SE, Barnes PJ, Bleecker ER, et al. A randomized, double-blind, placebo-controlled study of tumor necrosis factor-alpha blockade in severe persistent asthma. Am J Respir Crit Care Med 2009;179(7):549–58.

98. Rennard SI, Fogarty C, Kelsen S, et al. The safety and efficacy of infliximab in moderate to severe chronic obstructive pulmonary disease. Am J Respir Crit Care Med 2007;175(9):926–34.

99. Pascoe S, Kanniess F, Bonner J, et al. A monoclonal antibody to IL-1B attenuates the late asthmatic response to antigen challenge in patients with mild asthma. Suppl. 5028. Eur Respir J; 2006. p. 752. European Respiratory Journal.

100. Calverley PMA, Sethi S, Dawson M, et al. A randomised, placebo-controlled trial of anti-interleukin-1 receptor 1 monoclonal antibody MEDI8968 in chronic obstructive pulmonary disease. Respir Res 2017;18(1):153.

101. Rogliani P, Calzetta L, Ora J, et al. Canakinumab for the treatment of chronic obstructive pulmonary disease. Pulm Pharmacol Ther 2015;31:15–27.

102. Osei ET, Brandsma CA, Timens W, et al. Current perspectives on the role of interleukin-1 signalling in the pathogenesis of asthma and COPD. Eur Respir J 2020;55(2).

103. Oronsky B, Reid TR, Larson C, et al. REPLATINUM Phase III randomized study: RRx-001 + platinum doublet versus platinum doublet in third-line small cell lung cancer. Future Oncol 2019;15(30):3427–33.

104. Williams EJ, Negewo NA, Baines KJ. Role of the NLRP3 inflammasome in asthma: Relationship with neutrophilic inflammation, obesity, and therapeutic options. J Allergy Clin Immunol 2021;147(6):2060–2.

105. Revez JA, Bain LM, Watson RM, et al. Effects of interleukin-6 receptor blockade on allergen-induced airway responses in mild asthmatics. Clin Transl Immunol 2019;8(6):e1044.

106. Busse WW, Holgate S, Kerwin E, et al. Randomized, double-blind, placebo-controlled study of brodalumab, a human anti-IL-17 receptor monoclonal antibody, in moderate to severe asthma. Am J Respir Crit Care Med 2013; 188(11):1294–302.

107. ClinicalTrials.gov. Study of Efficacy and Safety of Brodalumab Compared With Placebo in Inadequately Controlled Asthma Subjects With High Bronchodilator Reversibility. 2016. Available at: https://clinicaltrials.gov/ct2/show/ NCT01902290. Accessed 3 Dec 2021.

108. ClinicalTrials.gov. Study to Assess the Efficacy and Safety of CJM112 in Patients With Inadequately Controlled Severe Asthma. 2021. Available at: https:// clinicaltrials.gov/ct2/show/study/NCT03299686. Accessed 3 Dec 2021.

109. Eich A, Urban V, Jutel M, et al. A Randomized, Placebo-Controlled Phase 2 Trial of CNTO 6785 in Chronic Obstructive Pulmonary Disease. COPD 2017;14(5): 476–83.

110. Whitehead GS, Kang HS, Thomas SY, et al. Therapeutic suppression of pulmonary neutrophilia and allergic airway hyperresponsiveness by a RORγt inverse agonist. JCI Insight 2019;5(14):e125528.

111. Brightling CE, Nair P, Cousins DJ, et al. Risankizumab in Severe Asthma - A Phase 2a, Placebo-Controlled Trial. N Engl J Med 2021;385(18):1669–79.

112. O'Byrne PM, Metev H, Puu M, et al. Efficacy and safety of a CXCR2 antagonist, AZD5069, in patients with uncontrolled persistent asthma: a randomised, double-blind, placebo-controlled trial. Lancet Respir Med 2016;4(10):797–806.

113. Rennard SI, Dale DC, Donohue JF, et al. CXCR2 Antagonist MK-7123. A Phase 2 Proof-of-Concept Trial for Chronic Obstructive Pulmonary Disease. Am J Respir Crit Care Med 2015;191(9):1001–11.

114. Mahler DA, Huang S, Tabrizi M, et al. Efficacy and safety of a monoclonal antibody recognizing interleukin-8 in COPD: a pilot study. Chest 2004;126(3): 926–34.

115. Uddin M, Watz H, Malmgren A, et al. NETopathic Inflammation in Chronic Obstructive Pulmonary Disease and Severe Asthma. Front Immunol 2019;10:47.

116. Khindri S, Cahn A, Begg M, et al. A Multicentre, Randomized, Double-Blind, Placebo-Controlled, Crossover Study To Investigate the Efficacy, Safety, Tolerability, and Pharmacokinetics of Repeat Doses of Inhaled Nemiralisib in Adults with Persistent, Uncontrolled Asthma. J Pharmacol Exp Ther 2018;367(3):405–13.

117. Cahn A, Hamblin JN, Begg M, et al. Safety, pharmacokinetics and dose-response characteristics of GSK2269557, an inhaled PI3Kδ inhibitor under development for the treatment of COPD. Pulm Pharmacol Ther 2017;46:69–77.

118. Cahn A, Hamblin JN, Robertson J, et al. An Inhaled PI3Kδ Inhibitor Improves Recovery in Acutely Exacerbating COPD Patients: A Randomized Trial. Int J Chron Obstruct Pulmon Dis 2021;16:1607–19.

119. Fahy WA, Homayoun-Valiani F, Cahn A, et al. Nemiralisib in Patients with an Acute Exacerbation of COPD: Placebo-Controlled, Dose-Ranging Study. Int J Chron Obstruct Pulmon Dis 2021;16:1637–46.

120. Braithwaite IE, Cai F, Tom JA, et al. Inhaled JAK inhibitor GDC-0214 reduces exhaled nitric oxide in patients with mild asthma: A randomized, controlled, proof-of-activity trial. J Allergy Clin Immunol 2021;148(3):783–9.

121. Li S, Hui Y, Yuan J, et al. Syk-Targeted, a New 3-Arylbenzofuran Derivative EAPP-2 Blocks Airway Inflammation of Asthma-COPD Overlap in vivo and in vitro. J Inflamm Res 2021;14:2173–85.

122. Ramis I, Otal R, Carreño C, et al. A novel inhaled Syk inhibitor blocks mast cell degranulation and early asthmatic response. Pharmacol Res 2015;99:116–24.

123. Watz H, Barnacle H, Hartley BF, et al. Efficacy and safety of the p38 MAPK inhibitor losmapimod for patients with chronic obstructive pulmonary disease: a randomised, double-blind, placebo-controlled trial. Lancet Respir Med 2014; 2(1):63–72.

124. Marks-Konczalik J, Costa M, Robertson J, et al. A post-hoc subgroup analysis of data from a six month clinical trial comparing the efficacy and safety of losmapimod in moderate-severe COPD patients with ≤2% and >2% blood eosinophils. Respir Med 2015;109(7):860–9.

125. Pascoe S, Costa M, Marks-Konczalik J, et al. Biological effects of p38 MAPK inhibitor losmapimod does not translate to clinical benefits in COPD. Respir Med 2017;130:20–6.

126. Luo J, Yang L, Yang J, et al. Efficacy and safety of phosphodiesterase 4 inhibitors in patients with asthma: A systematic review and meta-analysis. Respirology 2018;23(5):467–77.

127. Janjua S, Fortescue R, Poole P. Phosphodiesterase-4 inhibitors for chronic obstructive pulmonary disease. Cochrane Database Syst Rev 2020;5(5): Cd002309.

128. Southworth T, Kaur M, Hodgson L, et al. Anti-inflammatory effects of the phosphodiesterase type 4 inhibitor CHF6001 on bronchoalveolar lavage lymphocytes from asthma patients. Cytokine 2019;113:68–73.

129. Singh D, Leaker B, Boyce M, et al. A novel inhaled phosphodiesterase 4 inhibitor (CHF6001) reduces the allergen challenge response in asthmatic patients. Pulm Pharmacol Ther 2016;40:1–6.

130. Singh D, Beeh KM, Colgan B, et al. Effect of the inhaled PDE4 inhibitor CHF6001 on biomarkers of inflammation in COPD. Respir Res 2019;20(1):180.

131. Singh D, Lea S, Mathioudakis AG. Inhaled Phosphodiesterase Inhibitors for the Treatment of Chronic Obstructive Pulmonary Disease. Drugs 2021;81(16): 1821–30.

Unmet Needs and the Future of Asthma-Chronic Pulmonary Obstructive Disease Overlap

Mario Cazzola, MD[a,*], Paola Rogliani, MD[a],
Maria Gabriella Matera, MD, PhD[b]

KEYWORDS

- Asthma • COPD • ACO • Overlap • Airway inflammation • Biomarkers
- Omics signatures • Personalized medicine

KEY POINTS

- There are aspects related to definition, approach to diagnosis, and management of asthma-chronic obstructive pulmonary disease (ACO) that are still debated because they are not clearly defined. They must be regarded as unmet needs, and their understanding is an absolute necessity.
- It is challenging to give a univocal definition of ACO, which is not a single entity but a group of phenotypes or, better, endo-phenotypes, and any definition used would not fully describe the molecular and clinical heterogeneity of these endophenotypes.
- The need to identify new biomarkers specific to ACO that can differentiate it from asthma and COPD is urgent. "Multi-omics" platforms (genomics, transcriptomics, proteomics, metabolomics, lipidomics, glycomics, epigenomics) can help with this.
- A treatment choice not supported by evidence of efficacy in the specific endo-phenotypes of the patient with ACO is another unmet need with many questions for which the answers remain pending.
- There is an urgent need to determine how, when, and in whom to use targeted therapies, including biological antibodies targeting cytokines and inflammatory precursors.

INTRODUCTION

Disagreement regarding the definition, approach to diagnosis, and management of asthma-chronic obstructive pulmonary disease (COPD) overlap (ACO) is quite

[a] Department of Experimental Medicine, Unit of Respiratory Medicine, University of Rome "Tor Vergata", Via Montpellier 1, 00133 Rome, Italy; [b] Department of Experimental Medicine, Unit of Pharmacology, University of Campania "Luigi Vanvitelli", Via Santa Maria di Costantinopoli, 16 80138 Naples, Italy
* Corresponding author.
E-mail address: mario.cazzola@uniroma2.it

Immunol Allergy Clin N Am 42 (2022) 691–700
https://doi.org/10.1016/j.iac.2022.04.006
0889-8561/22/© 2022 Elsevier Inc. All rights reserved.
immunology.theclinics.com

common among clinicians and researchers. There are, in fact, aspects that are still debated, and their clarification becomes an absolute necessity. These are unmet needs that must be addressed to understand ACO better. Here, we present a brief overview of the current landscape of the ACO and what we believe are the major current unmet needs, which, if addressed, will allow for progressive optimization of care for these patients (**Box 1**).

The Definition

It has been authoritatively pointed out that although ACO is a particularly challenging concept for clinicians and researchers, its relevance as a separate disease entity is still extremely controversial.[1] The presence of many and sometimes conflicting definitions of ACO[2,3] has not yet allowed the formulation of a clear, simple, and unambiguous definition of this pathologic condition that is globally accepted. Unfortunately, this lack makes it impossible to understand whether ACO really exists and, if it does, what its prevalence and characteristics are and what the most appropriate treatment is.

Therefore, an unambiguous definition of ACO, the lack of which is certainly a fundamental unmet need, is urgently needed.

However, the Global Initiative for Chronic Obstructive Lung Disease (GOLD) no longer wants to refer to ACO, although it recognizes that some traits and clinical aspects common to asthma and COPD may be present at the same time in a single patient.[4] Even the Global Initiative for Asthma (GINA) now affirms that the term ACO does not refer to a single disease entity but includes patients with different clinical phenotypes that are probably caused by several different underlying mechanisms.[5]

Provided that ACO is not a single entity but a group of phenotypes or, better, endophenotypes,[6] it is likely that a definition of ACO that can be globally accepted will remain an unmet need also in the future. To be globally acceptable, the definition of

---

Box 1
Unmet needs that must be addressed to better understand ACO

- Identification of potentially distinct molecular mechanisms (endotypes) associated with specific clinical manifestations (phenotypes).

- Longitudinal studies to prospectively determine the stability of these endo-phenotypes and their subsequent outcomes.

- Determining which diagnostic tests, biomarkers, and imaging techniques should be used to diagnose ACO accurately.

- Identifying new biomarkers specific to ACO that can differentiate it from asthma and COPD.

- Validation of clinical relevance of omics signatures by specifically designed RCTs.

- Need to deconstruct obstructive airway disease, including ACO, into its component parts to identify accuraterly and then target/treat relevant features in an individual.

- Broadening knowledge of the mechanisms underlying treatable traits to guide targeted treatment properly.

- Need to determine how, when, and in whom to use targeted therapies, including biological antibodies targeting cytokines and inflammatory precursors.

- Development of biological therapies that can simultaneously interfere with both neutrophilic and eosinophilic components of inflammation.

ACO should be specific enough to be clinically useful but also include a huge number of criteria to ensure the inclusion of all ACO endo-phenotypes.[7] However, it is impossible to provide an unambiguous definition capable of describing the molecular and clinical heterogeneity of these endo-phenotypes.

Abandoning attempts to standardize the definition of ACO implies the need to deepen the phenotyping approach down to the genome level.[1] The identification of potentially distinct molecular mechanisms (endotypes) associated with specific clinical manifestations (phenotypes) may help to better understand heterogeneous diseases and to effectively manage therapy. Clearly, longitudinal data are needed to prospectively determine the stability of these endo-phenotypes and their subsequent outcomes. Unfortunately, there is currently a paucity of prospective studies to better understand these fundamental issues and to formulate treatment guidelines.

The Approach to Diagnosis

The need to escape a rigid definition of ACO has led to the formulation of straightforward diagnostic approaches based on either direct[8] or indirect[9] recognition of the simultaneous presence of asthma and COPD. However, ensuring that both asthma and COPD are present is not easy because differentiating the 2 conditions can be difficult.[10] The diagnosis of asthma or COPD is generally neither objective nor quantitative. It is made by considering subjective symptoms that are easily influenced by background characteristics, such as age, sex, lifestyle habits, and predisposition of the patient.[11] Moreover, it is never accurate because it is based only on pulmonary function tests, chest radiographs, and peripheral blood eosinophil counts.

A more sophisticated diagnostic approach is, therefore, needed. However, the presence of many different endo-phenotypes raises the pressing question of which diagnostic tests, biomarkers, and imaging techniques should be used to diagnose ACO accurately.[12] The answer to this question indeed represents a primary and urgent need for everyone who wants to face ACO, but it is currently difficult and, in any case, unsatisfying.

Identification of valid biomarkers is likely to be the highest priority. They reflect the activation of different inflammatory pathways underlying COPD and asthma and are activated to varying extents in patients with ACO. A panel of biomarkers could likely help to identify these different inflammatory pathways and overcome the low sensitivity and specificity of individual biomarkers.[13] The most straightforward approach would be to combine validated biomarkers of COPD and asthma and measure their levels. However, fibrinogen is the only circulating biomarker of COPD approved by the US Food and Drug Administration and European Medicines Agency.[14] On the other side of the spectrum, fractional exhaled nitric oxide (FeNO) and blood eosinophils are the only biomarkers of asthma in clinical use in which elevated levels reflect ongoing type-2 inflammation. In contrast, other biomarkers, such as immunoglobulin E (IgE), periostin, and serpin β2, do not help identify type-2 high endotype.[15]

There is uncertainty about which combination of biomarkers to use (**Table 1**). For example, the combination of FeNO and blood eosinophil counts helps to establish that the patient does not have COPD, but not to state that the patient has ACO and is not suffering from asthma.[16] Looking at the other side of the spectrum, it was documented that serum interleukin (IL)-5 was lower and IL-8 was higher in patients with COPD than in patients with asthma. Still, there was no difference in these levels between patients with COPD and ACO.[17] These are just 2 examples, but the literature is so full of documentation of the currently limited utility of the use of biomarkers alone or in combination in ACO that it is impossible to report individual references because there are just too many of them. The combination of biomarkers may be of utility in

Table 1 Potential asthma-chronic obstructive pulmonary disease overlap biomarkers					
	Serum Periostin	Serum YKL-40	Blood IgE	Blood Eosinophils	FeNO
Asthma	High	Low	High	High	High
COPD	Low	High	Low	Low	Low
ACO	High	High	High	High	High

identifying ACO as in the case of serum periostin and YKL-40.[18] However, it is easy to indicate their limitations immediately. In fact, it is now established that serum periostin and YKL-40 are biomarkers of subtypes of asthma or COPD and not of ACO.[19] Therefore, it can be correctly stated that there are currently no biomarkers that can help accurately distinguish ACO from asthma or COPD.

The lack of effective biomarkers is certainly an important unmet need. Unfortunately, for both asthma and COPD, and thus also for their overlap, the observed lack of association between unmet clinical needs and putative biomarkers may depend on the considerable heterogeneity in airway inflammation between different patients and on the unclear correlation between biomarkers in the systemic and pulmonary compartments.[14,20]

Therefore, it is urgent to identify new biomarkers specific to ACO that can differentiate it from asthma and COPD. The development of "multi-omic" (genomics, transcriptomics, proteomics, metabolomics, lipidomics, glyconomics, epigenomics) platforms that measure even millions of analytes, typically of a specific type, on a single sample will hopefully enable the identification of potential robust biomarkers.[21] It can be expected that the use of multiple combined biomarkers, identified by different omics technologies, may enhance our ability to differentiate ACO from pure asthma and pure COPD and place the patient who exhibits features of both disorders at a precise point in the intersection of these 2 extremes.

However, none of the omics signatures have been translated into clinical practice, which is one of its most important limitations. It will be essential to understand the optimal analysis techniques for analyzing omics and whether there will be a real need for all omics/biomarkers to implement this approach in new biomarker discovery.[22] Once biomarkers are identified, it will be necessary to understand how strong they will be in enabling better clinical classification of patients with ACO, rather than remaining mere information for further research; this means that the clinical relevance of omics must be validated by specifically designed randomized controlled trials (RCTs).

The Management

Even a diligent specialist often has difficulty predicting whether the patient with shared COPD and asthmatic features will respond to the treatment he/she is prescribing. Understanding which pharmacologic therapies can improve clinical outcomes in patients with ACO is undoubtedly a challenging task considering that ACO is a blend of conditions as opposed to a single entity. However, there is always a continuous inflammation of the airways at its root.

The difficulty in distinguishing the components of asthma and COPD that predominate in the individual patient with ACO is the cause of the possible undertreatment the patient receives.[12] Underutilization of medications such as inhaled corticosteroids (ICSs) and biological therapies that could potentially modify the disease[23] may cause worse lung function, more respiratory symptoms, and more emergency visits than individuals with asthma or COPD alone.[24] Quite frequently, the clinician, in the absence of reliable tools that might guide him/her in clinical therapeutic decision-making, proceeds based on his/her own feeling that the disease is more like asthma or more like COPD.[25] Unfortunately, asthma and COPD are extremely heterogeneous conditions, and there remains a significant unmet need for both asthma and COPD treatments.[26] This heterogeneity is therefore also inherent in ACO. It is evident that having difficulty addressing this heterogeneity is an unmet need in ACO management.

Empiricism in treatment choice is surely also a consequence of the fact that patients with overlapping asthma and COPD were excluded in large RCTs in asthma or COPD. Current treatment of ACO is based on recommendations made by expert opinion, roundtable conclusions, and extrapolating concepts from strategy documents (ie, GINA and GOLD) because of a lack of evidence-based information.[27] This means that the best therapeutic regimen and response to therapy of ACO remains undefined, although there have been attempts to codify the therapeutic approach to ACO.

Thus, the Japanese Respiratory Society simplified things by recommending that the ACO patient be treated with ICSs in the presence of characteristics of asthma in addition to bronchodilators.[28] The 2015 Spanish GEMA guideline did not differ from the Japanese guidelines by recommending the combination of an ICS with a long-acting β-agonist (LABA) as the first treatment choice and suggesting the possibility of adding a long-acting muscarinic antagonist (LAMA) if patients remain uncontrolled.[29] However, the recommendation to use triple therapy is present in both the GOLD[4] and GINA[5] strategies, although with a substantial difference between the 2 strategies. GOLD recommends adding an LAMA to an ICS/LABA combination or an ICS to an LABA/LAMA combination considering the presence of dyspnea or exacerbations and referring to the blood eosinophil count.[4] In contrast, GINA plans to add an LAMA to ICS/LABA when the disease is not well controlled and before escalating to treatment with biologics or oral corticosteroids.[5] Triple therapy is therefore recommended in patients with a severe clinical picture of chronic obstructive airway disorder, regardless of whether the pathology they suffer from is called COPD, asthma, or ACO.

There is no doubt that a treatment choice not supported by evidence of efficacy in the specific endo-phenotypes of the patient with ACO is another unmet need with many questions for which the answers remain pending.[1] It is not yet clear whether it will be sufficient to produce a standardized, globally accepted definition of ACO or, exploiting the advantages offered by omics technology, get up to genome level to endo-phenotyping the patient. A deep endo-phenotyping could identify new biomarkers, and it is widely accepted that the identification of more selective biomarkers (or panels of biomarkers) is essential not only for an adequate diagnosis of ACO but also to be able to identify the right patient to be administered the right drug at the right time.[15] However, identifying of new biomarkers is not enough because we must always establish how it is possible to translate them into clinical practice.

Another approach may involve dropping the asthma, COPD, and ACO labels and focusing on the possible next trend in the treatment of patients with chronic obstructive airway disorders, namely treating treatable traits.[30] However, there is a lack of RCTs supporting a treatable traits approach. Consequently, we still do not know which outcome measures are most appropriate and clinically meaningful to evaluate when following this approach in patients with ACO.[1] One evaluative possibility might be to incorporate the clinical impact of treatment on treatable traits while maintaining the indispensable elements of the current system, namely spirometry,[7] but this remains an option without clinical validation.

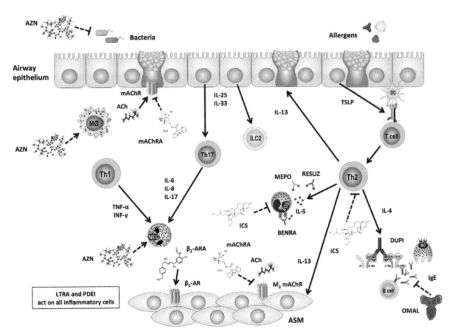

Fig. 1. Mechanisms in the airway inflammatory processes that may be the target of current and future pharmacologic therapies for asthma, COPD, and ACO.Abbreviations: ACh, acetylcholine; ASM, airway smooth muscle; AZN, azithromycin; BC, B cell; BENRA, benralizumab; DC, dendritic cell; DUPI, dupilumab; EOS, eosinophil; ICS, inhaled corticosteroid; IFN-γ, interferon-γ; IL, interleukin; ILC2, immune lymphocyte cell 2; LTRA, leukotriene receptor antagonist; mAChR, muscarinic receptor; mAChRA, mAChR antagonist; MC, mast cell; MEPO, mepolizumab; MØ, macrophage; NEU, neutrophil; OMAL, omalizumab; PDEI, phosphodiesterase inhibitor; RESLIZ, reslizumab; Th1, Th1 lymphocyte; Th17, Th17 lymphocyte; Th2, Th2 lymphocyte; TNF-α, tumor necrosis factor α; TSLP, thymic stromal lymphopoietin; β2-AR, β2-adrenoceptor; β2-ARA, β2-AR agonist. *Modified from* Leung C, Sin DD. Asthma-COPD Overlap: What Are the Important Questions? Chest. 2022 Feb;161(2):330-344.

However, the great heterogeneity of ACO and its broad spectrum of overlapping features suggest that there is a need for treatment that is more precise than the current treatable traits approach, which consists of deconstructing obstructive airway disease, including ACO, into its parts to identify accurately and then target/treat relevant traits in an individual.[15] Additional knowledge about the mechanisms underlying these treatable traits is needed to guide targeted treatment correctly.

Given the growing, but still limited, understanding of the inflammatory pathways involved in ACO and the possibility of interfacing with an inflammation that is sometimes neutrophilic and other times eosinophilic predominant and that is considered by many to be a treatable trait,[31] more knowledge is needed regarding pharmacologically targeting the inflammatory pathways within ACO (**Fig. 1**). There is an absolute need to determine as soon as possible how, when, and in whom to use targeted therapies, including biological antibodies targeting cytokines and inflammatory precursors[28]; this will facilitate the development of personalized medicine also for ACO.

Regrettably, waiting for novel ACO specific biomarkers, the physician treating the patient with ACO is forced to use biomarkers used in asthma studies. Elevated levels of FeNO and blood eosinophils reflect ongoing type-2 inflammation and suggest that an effective biological treatment in asthma will also be effective in this form of ACO.

However, the few available data[32–34] show that we are still far from understanding what the specific target for biological therapies is in the individual patient with ACO, considering that the targets of the type-2 pathway include, for what is known so far, IgE, IL-5, IL-4 receptor α (receptor for both IL-4 and IL-13), IL-13, and thymic stromal lymphopoietin[35]; this is the same problem as in allergic asthma, and only understanding the underlying mechanisms, with the development of specific biomarkers, can help guide effective treatment.

Even more problematic is the use of biological therapies when the goal is to target the neutrophilic component of inflammation that is predominant in COPD and can also be found in a subgroup of patients with asthma. So far, little is known on potential predictive and prognostic biomarkers for neutrophilic airway inflammation, which remains as a diagnosis of exclusion if type-2 inflammation is low or absent,[36] and attempts to target neutrophilic inflammation with biological therapies directly have led to disappointing results to date.[37] The lack of biomarkers for neutrophilic airway inflammation is a further unmet need. It will be necessary to broaden the understanding of what drives neutrophilic inflammation, mainly when it occurs in an asthmatic individual, to use appropriate preventive measures and treatments.[36]

We need to understand if influencing eosinophilic inflammation with currently available targeted therapies could increase neutrophilic inflammation. If so, it becomes critical to understand if it will be possible to develop biological therapies that can simultaneously interfere with both types of inflammation.

SUMMARY

There is a clear need to change the taxonomy of chronic obstructive airway disorder as soon as possible, abandoning the terms asthma, COPD, and ACO and using the terms by which new phenotypes and underlying endotypes will be progressively identified.[38]

It is foreseeable that soon, through the clever and accurate application of the "-omic" sciences, there will be a substantial broadening of our knowledge of inflammatory patterns that will help us to classify patients with chronic obstructive airway disorder. Translating this into routine practice will allow the implementation of personalized medicine for obstructive airway disorder that will enable us to offer our patients the best treatment option in each defined endo-phenotype and identify new traits/targets and therefore new treatments.

CLINICS CARE POINTS

- There is an urgent need to ensure that the identified endo-phenotypes remain stable over time and that their outcomes do not change.

- A panel of specific biomarkers, identified as knowledge improves, will be key to a personalized management approach to different endo-phenotypes.

- A truly personalized drug treatment will only be possible when we can focus exclusively on the traits that need to be treated in the patient we are dealing with.

- An alternative to the approach focused on treatable traits may be to develop biological therapies that can interfere with inflammation in a decisive way regardless of its type.

DISCLOSURE

Mario Cazzola participated as a faculty member and advisor in scientific meetings and courses under the sponsorship of Abdi Ibrahim, Almirall, AstraZeneca, Boehringer

Ingelheim, Chiesi Farmaceutici, Cipla, Edmond Pharma, GlaxoSmithKline, Glenmark, Lallemand, Menarini Group, Mundipharma, Novartis, Pfizer, Teva, Verona Pharma, and Zambon and is or was a consultant to ABC Farmaceutici, AstraZeneca, Chiesi Farmaceutici, Edmond Pharma, Lallemand, Novartis, Ockham Biotech, Verona-Pharma, and Zambon. Paola Rogliani reported grants and personal fees from Almirall, AstraZeneca, Biofutura, Boehringer Ingelheim, Chiesi Farmaceutici, GlaxoSmithKline, Menarini Group, Mundipharma, and Novartis and participated as a lecturer and advisor in scientific meetings and courses under the sponsorship of Almirall, AstraZeneca, Biofutura, Boehringer Ingelheim, Chiesi Farmaceutici, Edmond Pharma, GlaxoSmithKline, Menarini Group, Mundipharma, and Novartis. Her department was funded by Almirall, Boehringer Ingelheim, Chiesi Farmaceutici, Novartis, and Zambon. Maria Gabriella Matera participated as a faculty member and advisor in scientific meetings and courses under the sponsorship of ABC Farmaceutici, Almirall, AstraZeneca, Chiesi Farmaceutici, GlaxoSmithKline, and Novartis and was a consultant to Chiesi Farmaceutici and GlaxoSmithKline. Her department was funded by GlaxoSmithKline and Novartis. The authors have no other relevant affiliations or financial involvement with any organization or entity with a financial interest in or financial conflict with the subject matter or materials discussed in the manuscript apart from those disclosed.

REFERENCES

1. Milne S, Mannino D, Sin DD. Asthma-COPD overlap and chronic airflow obstruction: definitions, management, and unanswered questions. J Allergy Clin Immunol Pract 2020;8(2):483–95.
2. Cazzola M, Rogliani P. Do we really need asthma-chronic obstructive pulmonary disease overlap syndrome? J Allergy Clin Immunol 2016;138(4):977–83.
3. Halpin DMG. What is asthma chronic obstructive pulmonary disease overlap? Clin Chest Med 2020;41(3):395–403.
4. Global Initiative for Chronic Obstructive Lung Disease. Global strategy for diagnosis, management and prevention of chronic obstructive pulmonary disease. 2022. Available at. https://goldcopd.org/wp-content/uploads/2021/11/GOLD-REPORT-2022-v1.1-22Nov2021_WMV.pdf. Accessed Dec 4th, 2021.
5. Global Inititative for Asthma. Global strategy for asthma management and prevention. 2021. Available at. https://ginasthma.org/wp-content/uploads/2021/05/GINA-Main-Report-2021-V2-WMS.pdf. Accessed Dec 4th, 2021.
6. Boulet LP, Hanania NA. The many faces of asthma-chronic obstructive pulmonary disease overlap. Curr Opin Pulm Med 2019;25(1):1–10.
7. Tu X, Donovan C, Kim RY, et al. Asthma-COPD overlap: current understanding and the utility of experimental models. Eur Respir Rev 2021;30(159):190185.
8. Mekov E, Nuñez A, Sin DD, et al. Update on asthma-COPD overlap (ACO): a narrative review. Int J Chron Obstruct Pulmon Dis 2021;16:1783–99.
9. Sam A, Kraft M. Asthma-COPD overlap. Curr Pulmonol Rep 2022. https://doi.org/10.1007/s13665-021-00284-0. Epub ahead of print.
10. Rogliani P, Ora J, Puxeddu E, et al. Airflow obstruction: is it asthma or is it COPD? Int J Chron Obstruct Pulmon Dis 2016;11:3007–13.
11. Yanagisawa S, Ichinose M. Definition and diagnosis of asthma-COPD overlap (ACO). Allergol Int 2018;67(2):172–8.
12. Leung C, Sin DD. Asthma-COPD overlap: what are the important questions? Chest 2022;161(2):330–44.

13. Kobayashi S, Hanagama M, Yamanda S, et al. Inflammatory biomarkers in asthma-COPD overlap syndrome. Int J Chron Obstruct Pulmon Dis 2016;11: 2117–23.
14. Cazzola M, Puxeddu E, Ora J, et al. Evolving concepts in chronic obstructive pulmonary disease blood-based biomarkers. Mol Diagn Ther 2019;23(5):603–14.
15. Cazzola M, Ora J, Cavalli F, et al. Treatable mechanisms in asthma. Mol Diagn Ther 2021;25(2):111–21.
16. Shi B, Li W, Hao Y, et al. Characteristics of inflammatory phenotypes among patients with asthma: relationships of blood count parameters with sputum cellular phenotypes. Allergy Asthma Clin Immunol 2021;17(1):47.
17. de Llano LP, Cosío BG, Iglesias A, et al. Mixed Th2 and non-Th2 inflammatory pattern in the asthma-COPD overlap: a network approach. Int J Chron Obstruct Pulmon Dis 2018;13:591–601.
18. Shirai T, Hirai K, Gon Y, et al. Combined assessment of serum periostin and YKL-40 may identify asthma-COPD overlap. J Allergy Clin Immunol Pract 2019;7(1): 134–45.
19. Izuhara K, Barnes PJ. Can we define asthma-COPD overlap (ACO) by biomarkers? J Allergy Clin Immunol Pract 2019;7(1):146–7.
20. Pérez de Llano L, Martínez-Moragón E, Plaza Moral V, et al. Unmet therapeutic goals and potential treatable traits in a population of patients with severe uncontrolled asthma in Spain. ENEAS Study Respir Med 2019;151:49–54.
21. Ray A, Camiolo M, Fitzpatrick A, et al. Are we meeting the promise of endotypes and precision medicine in asthma? Physiol Rev 2020;100(3):983–1017.
22. Abdel-Aziz MI, Neerincx AH, Vijverberg SJ, et al. Omics for the future in asthma. Semin Immunopathol 2020;42(1):111–26.
23. Reddel HK, Vestbo J, Agustí A, et al. Heterogeneity within and between physician-diagnosed asthma and/or COPD: NOVELTY cohort. Eur Respir J 2021; 58(3):2003927.
24. Ekerljung L, Mincheva R, Hagstad S, et al. Prevalence, clinical characteristics and morbidity of the Asthma-COPD overlap in a general population sample. J Asthma 2018;55(5):461–9.
25. Desai M, Oppenheimer J, Tashkin DP. Asthma-chronic obstructive pulmonary disease overlap syndrome: What we know and what we need to find out. Ann Allergy Asthma Immunol 2017;118(3):241–5.
26. Heaney LG, McGarvey LP. Personalised medicine for asthma and chronic obstructive pulmonary disease. Respiration 2017;93(3):153–61.
27. Maselli DJ, Hanania NA. Management of asthma COPD overlap. Ann Allergy Asthma Immunol 2019;123(4):335–44.
28. Japanese Respiratory Society. The JRS guidelines for the management of ACO 2018. (In Japanese). Tokyo: Medical Review; 2018.
29. GEMA4.0. [Guidelines for asthma management. (In Spanish)]. Arch Bronconeumol 2015;51(Suppl. 1):2–54.
30. Gaspar Marques J, Lobato M, Leiria Pinto P, et al. Asthma and COPD "overlap": a treatable trait or common several treatable-traits? Eur Ann Allergy Clin Immunol 2020;52(4):148–59.
31. Morissette M, Godbout K, Côté A, et al. Asthma COPD overlap: Insights into cellular and molecular mechanisms. Mol Aspects Med 2022;85:101021.
32. Brightling CE, Bleecker ER, Panettieri RA Jr, et al. Benralizumab for chronic obstructive pulmonary disease and sputum eosinophilia: a randomised, double-blind, placebo-controlled, phase 2a study. Lancet Respir Med 2014;2(11): 891–901.

33. Pavord ID, Chanez P, Criner GJ, et al. Mepolizumab for eosinophilic chronic obstructive pulmonary disease. N Engl J Med 2017;377(17):1613–29.

34. Hanania NA, Chipps BE, Griffin NM, et al. Omalizumab effectiveness in asthma-COPD overlap: post hoc analysis of PROSPERO. J Allergy Clin Immunol 2019; 143(4):1629–33.

35. Akar-Ghibril N, Casale T, Custovic A, et al. Allergic endotypes and phenotypes of asthma. J Allergy Clin Immunol Pract 2020;8(2):429–40.

36. Assaf SM, Hanania NA. Eosinophilic vs. neutrophilic asthma. Curr Pulmonol Rep 2020;9:28–35.

37. Cazzola M, Ora J, Cavalli F, et al. An overview of the safety and efficacy of monoclonal antibodies for the chronic obstructive pulmonary disease. Biologics 2021; 15:363–74.

38. Bateman ED, Reddel HK, van Zyl-Smit RN, et al. The asthma-COPD overlap syndrome: towards a revised taxonomy of chronic airways diseases? Lancet Respir Med 2015;3(9):719–28.

Printed and bound by CPI Group (UK) Ltd, Croydon, CR0 4YY

03/10/2024

01040476-0002